Rare Genitourinary Tumors

Lance Pagliaro
Editor

Rare Genitourinary Tumors

Springer

Editor
Lance Pagliaro
Division of Medical Oncology
Department of Oncology
Mayo Clinic
Rochester, MN
USA

ISBN 978-3-319-30044-3 ISBN 978-3-319-30046-7 (eBook)
DOI 10.1007/978-3-319-30046-7

Library of Congress Control Number: 2016940903

Printed on acid-free paper

This Springer imprint is published by Springer Nature
The registered company is Springer International Publishing AG Switzerland

Contents

Editor Biography

Dr. Lance Pagliaro earned his medical degree at Albany Medical College and received postgraduate training at The George Washington University Hospital and The University of Texas MD Anderson Cancer Center. In the course of his career spanning 20 years at MD Anderson, Dr. Pagliaro specialized in the treatment of adults with genitourinary cancers. He became recognized as an expert in the curative treatment of penile cancer, advanced metastatic testicular cancer, and mediastinal germ cell tumors. He led numerous prospective clinical trials and important retrospective studies in these and the more common cancers of the prostate, bladder, and kidneys. His many contributions to the literature have included studies of chemotherapy and targeted therapy for penile cancer, a rare tumor, leading to a new standard of care for that disease. Dr. Pagliaro is currently a professor of oncology at the Mayo Clinic College of Medicine. He practices medical oncology at Mayo Clinic, where he frequently lectures and is active in clinical research and medical education.

Contributors

E. Jason Abel Department of Urology, University of Wisconsin School of Medicine and Public Health, Madison, WI, USA

Mehrad Adibi Department of Urology, The University of Texas MD Anderson Cancer Center, Houston, TX, USA

Neeraj Agarwal Division of Medical Oncology, Huntsman Cancer Institute, University of Utah, Salt Lake City, UT, USA

Dan Albertson Department of Pathology, Huntsman Cancer Institute, University of Utah, Salt Lake City, UT, USA

Marc Barry Department of Pathology, University of New Mexico School of Medicine, Albuquerque, NM, USA

Axel Bex Division of Surgical Oncology, Department of Urology, The Netherlands Cancer Institute, Amsterdam, The Netherlands

Leonardo D. Borregales Department of Urology, The University of Texas MD Anderson Cancer Center, Houston, TX, USA

Jad Chahoud Department of Internal Medicine, The University of Texas Health Science Center, University of Texas Medical School at Houston, Houston, TX, USA

Marcela G. del Carmen Division of Gynecologic Oncology, Vincent Obstetrics and Gynecology, Massachusetts General Hospital, Harvard Medical School, Boston, MA, USA

Tracy M. Downs Department of Urology, University of Wisconsin School of Medicine and Public Health, Madison, WI, USA

Patricia J. Eifel Department of Radiation Oncology, The University of Texas MD Anderson Cancer Center, Houston, TX, USA

John Paul Flores Division of Hematology-Oncology, Tufts Medical Center, Boston, MA, USA

Paul K. Hegarty Department of Andrology, Urological and Reconstructive Surgery, Mater Misericordiae University Hospital, Dublin 7, Republic of Ireland

Winston W. Huh Department of Pediatrics, The University of Texas MD Anderson Cancer Center, Houston, TX, USA

Wen-Jen Hwu Department of Melanoma Medical Oncology, The University of Texas MD Anderson Cancer Center, Houston, TX, USA

David F. Jarrard Department of Urology, University of Wisconsin School of Medicine and Public Health, Madison, WI, USA

Ashish M. Kamat Department of Urology, The University of Texas MD Anderson Cancer Center, Houston, TX, USA

Jose A. Karam Department of Urology, The University of Texas MD Anderson Cancer Center, Houston, TX, USA

Richard Lauer Division of Hematology/Oncology, Department of Internal Medicine, University of New Mexico School of Medicine, Albuquerque, NM, USA

Dara Lundon Department of Andrology, Urological and Reconstructive Surgery, Mater Misericordiae University Hospital, Dublin 7, Republic of Ireland

Kimberly A. Maciolek Department of Urology, University of Wisconsin School of Medicine and Public Health, Madison, WI, USA

Ankit Madan Department of Medicine, Section of Hematology-Oncology, University of Alabama at Birmingham (UAB), Birmingham, AL, USA

Midhun Malla Internal Medicine, St. Joseph's Hospital and Medical Center, Phoenix, AZ, USA

Gabriel G. Malouf Department of Medical Oncology, Groupe Hospitalier Pitié-Salpêtrière, Hopitaux de Paris, Faculty of Medicine Pierre et Marie Curie, Institut Universitaire de Cancérologie GRC5, Paris, France

Paul Mathew Division of Hematology-Oncology, Department of Medicine, Tufts University School of Medicine, Boston, MA, USA

Marc R. Matrana Hematology/Oncology Section, The Gayle and Tom Benson Cancer Center, Ochsner Medical Center, New Orleans, LA, USA

Ochsner Clinical School, The University of Queensland School of Medicine, New Orleans, LA, USA

Richard Meijer Department of Urology, University Medical Center Utrecht, Utrecht, The Netherlands

Adam R. Metwalli Urologic Oncology Branch, Center for Cancer Research, National Cancer Institute, Bethesda, MD, USA

Priyadharsini Nagarajan Department of Pathology, The University of Texas MD Anderson Cancer Center, Houston, TX, USA

Fardod O'Kelly Department of Andrology, Urological and Reconstructive Surgery, Mater Misericordiae University Hospital, Dublin 7, Republic of Ireland

Lance Pagliaro Division of Medical Oncology, Department of Oncology, Mayo Clinic, Rochester, MN, USA

Sachin Pai Ochsner Medical Oncology Fellowship Program, Ochsner Clinic Foundation, New Orleans, LA, USA

Sumanta K. Pal Department of Medical Oncology and Experimental Therapeutics, City of Hope, Comprehensive Cancer Center, Duarte, CA, USA

Curtis A. Pettaway Department of Urology, The University of Texas MD Anderson Cancer Center, Houston, TX, USA

Louis L. Pisters Department of Urology, The University of Texas MD Anderson Cancer Center, Houston, TX, USA

Victor G. Prieto Department of Pathology, The University of Texas MD Anderson Cancer Center, Houston, TX, USA

Arpit Rao Division of Hematology/Oncology, Department of Internal Medicine, University of New Mexico School of Medicine, Albuquerque, NM, USA

Mila Pontremoli Salcedo The Department of Obstetrics and Gynecology, Federal University of Health Sciences Porto Alegre (UFCSPA) / Irmandade Santa Casa de Misericordia de Porto Alegre, Porto Alegre, Brazil

Kathleen M. Schmeler Department of Gynecologic Oncology and Reproductive Medicine, The University of Texas MD Anderson Cancer Center, Houston, TX, USA

Arlene O. Siefker-Radtke Department of Genitourinary Medical Oncology, The University of Texas MD Anderson Cancer Center, Houston, TX, USA

Parminder Singh Division of Hematology and Medical Oncology, University of Arizona Cancer Center, Banner University Medical Center, Tucson, AZ, USA

Guru Sonpavde Department of Medicine, Section of Hematology-Oncology, University of Alabama at Birmingham (UAB), Birmingham, AL, USA

Pranav Sharma Department of Urology, Moffitt Cancer Center, Tampa, FL, USA

Austen Slade Department of Urology, The University of Texas MD Anderson Cancer Center, Houston, TX, USA

Philippe E. Spiess Department of Urology, Moffitt Cancer Center, Tampa, FL, USA

Ramaprasad Srinivasan Urologic Oncology Branch, Center for Cancer Research, National Cancer Institute, Bethesda, MD, USA

Daniel Su Urologic Oncology Branch, Center for Cancer Research, National Cancer Institute, Bethesda, MD, USA

Nizar M. Tannir Department of Genitourinary Medical Oncology, The University of Texas MD Anderson Cancer Center, Houston, TX, USA

Michael Tetzlaff Department of Pathology, The University of Texas MD Anderson Cancer Center, Houston, TX, USA

Arun Z. Thomas Department of Urology, The University of Texas MD Anderson Cancer Center, Houston, TX, USA

Van Anh Trinh Department of Melanoma Medical Oncology, The University of Texas MD Anderson Cancer Center, Houston, TX, USA

Jeffrey Wang Baylor University, College of Arts and Sciences, Waco, TX, USA

Jue Wang Genitourinary Oncology Division, University of Arizona Cancer Center at St. Joseph's Hospital and Medical Center, Phoenix, AZ, USA

Stephen B. Williams Department of Urology, The University of Texas MD Anderson Cancer Center, Houston, TX, USA

Christopher G. Wood Department of Urology, The University of Texas MD Anderson Cancer Center, Houston, TX, USA

Kamran Zargar-Shoshtari Department of Urology, Moffitt Cancer Center, Tampa, FL, USA

Papillary Renal Carcinoma

1

Daniel Su, Adam R. Metwalli, and Ramaprasad Srinivasan

Introduction

Renal cell carcinoma (RCC) arising from the renal parenchyma accounts for more than 90 % of adult kidney cancers [1]. RCC is composed of multiple genetically, histologically, pathologically, and metabolically distinct disease entities [2]. Over the past two decades, our ability to distinguish between various RCC subtypes has improved significantly; as we begin to better characterize these subtypes, it is becoming increasingly clear that a successful approach to the treatment of RCC should take into account the prevailing heterogeneity. Papillary RCC (pRCC) is the second most common histologic subtype of RCC after clear cell renal cell carcinoma (ccRCC) and accounts for 10–15 % of all RCC [1]. Both sporadic and familial forms of pRCC have been described. A higher incidence of sporadic pRCC is thought to occur in patients with end-stage renal disease (ESRD) and acquired renal cystic disease (ARCD) when compared to the general population [3, 4]. However, the risk association of ESRD with pRCC was not seen in a more recent study [5]. Familial forms of pRCC are associated with hereditary papillary renal carcinoma (HPRC) and hereditary leiomyomatosis and renal cell carcinoma (HLRCC); papillary RCC has also been described as a component of Birt-Hogg-Dubé (BHD), although this histology is only infrequently encountered in BHD patients [6, 7].

pRCC is a heterogeneous group of malignancies that are characterized by the presence of a papillary architecture on histopathologic examination. Based on histologic features, two subtypes of papillary RCC are recognized: type I and type II. pRCC can be divided clinically into organ-confined and metastatic disease states, with some studies showing better survival compared to ccRCC in localized states and worse prognosis in the metastatic state [8–10]. pRCC localized to the kidneys

D. Su, MD • A.R. Metwalli, MD • R. Srinivasan, MD, PhD (✉)
Urologic Oncology Branch, Center for Cancer Research, National Cancer Institute, Building 10 – Hatfield CRC, Room 1-5940, Bethesda, MD 20892, USA
e-mail: metwallia@mail.nih.gov; ramasrin@mail.nih.gov

L. Pagliaro (ed.), *Rare Genitourinary Tumors*,
DOI 10.1007/978-3-319-30046-7_1

is generally managed surgically with overall good outcomes; the approach to advanced disease is less satisfactory and the standard of care continues to evolve. Although agents targeting the VEGF and mTOR pathways have led to improved outcomes in patients with advanced ccRCC [11], patients with metastatic pRCC are generally unresponsive to these agents [12]. However, recent insights into the mechanisms underlying some variants of pRCC have led to the development of promising clinical strategies that are currently under evaluation [13].

Epidemiology and Risk Stratification

It is estimated that 61,560 new cases of renal cell carcinoma will be diagnosed in the United States in 2015, resulting in 14,080 deaths [14]. Worldwide, RCC is the 13th most common malignancy, with 271,000 new cases diagnosed in 2008 [15]. The incidence of RCC experienced an upward trend in the past decade but has stabilized and started to show a decline partly due to the success of smoking cessation programs and improvements in occupation protection [1].

While extensive epidemiologic data pertaining to kidney cancer are available, these do not address specific subtypes. Since ccRCC accounts for 85–90 % of all RCC, this subtype heavily influences the published epidemiologic data and trends. In general, RCC occurs about twice as often in males as in females, and the average age of diagnosis of sporadic forms of RCC is in the early sixth decade [1, 16].

Several studies have suggested racial disparities in the incidence of pRCC. In the United States, papillary RCC appears to be more common in blacks than in other races. In a review of 204 patients who underwent partial or radical nephrectomy, including 97 (47.5 %) patients with ccRCC, 65 (31.9 %) patients with pRCC, and 13 (6.4 %) patients with chromophobe RCC (chRCC), Sankin et al. found that 47.9 % of renal tumors in black patients were pRCC, compared to only 10.3 % of the tumors in non-black patients ($p<0.001$) [17]. Chow et al. drew similar conclusions from an analysis of 39,350 RCC patients in the SEER database from 1992 to 2007 [18]. In this analysis, black patients were more frequently diagnosed with pRCC subtypes when compared to white patients (12.5 % vs. 4.5 %). Additionally, 5-year relative survival rates in black patients with pRCC was inferior to that of white patients (80.5 % [95 % CI 74.8–85)] vs. 87.5 % [95 % CI 84.3–90.1]). Interestingly, ccRCC was found to be associated with a worse prognosis than pRCC, but the survival advantage for white patients spanned both histologic subtypes. Another analysis based on the Surveillance, Epidemiology, and End Results (SEER) program dataset evaluated 52,924 RCC patients and similarly observed a racial disparity in the incidence of pRCC [19]. The authors of this study concluded that black patients are more likely to have pRCC than white patients (23 % vs. 9 %, respectively); furthermore, pRCC incidence (cases per 100,000 men and women) increased more rapidly for black patients than white patients during the study period of 2001–2009 (increasing from 1.6 to 4.0 for black patients vs. 0.7 to 1.3 for white patients; $p<0.01$).

The natural history of papillary RCC and the prognosis of affected patients vary considerably depending on the subtype of papillary RCC. Several analyses have attempted to compare the prognosis and clinical course of this entity with those of clear cell RCC. A large series from the Mayo Clinic (3,062 patients with all subtypes of RCC, 33 years of follow-up) sought to determine if RCC histology/subtype influenced outcome [10]. This study included 2,466 (80.5 %) patients with ccRCC, 438 (14.3 %) patients with pRCC, and 158 (5.2 %) patients with chRCC and concluded that ccRCC histology was a significant predictor for metastasis (hazard ratio [HR] 2.76, 95 % CI 2.05–3.72 $p<0.001$) and cancer-specific death (HR 1.77, 95 % CI 1.38–2.26 $p<0.001$). However, these analyses did not account for disparities in clinical and pathological stage comparison between histologic subtypes.

A more recent study employed the SEER database to evaluate impact of RCC histologic subtypes on overall survival and cancer-specific survival [20]. The authors identified 17,605 patients from 2000 to 2005 who were treated for RCC with radical or partial nephrectomy; 78.6 % had ccRCC, 12.9 % pRCC, 5.4 % chRCC, 2.5 % sarcomatoid differentiation, and 0.6 % collecting duct subtype. In this study, patients with pRCC were less likely to present with T3 or greater disease (17.6 % for pRCC vs. 28 % for ccRCC, 82.8 % for sarcomatoid, and 55.7 % for collecting duct, $p<0.001$). The impact of this finding on prognosis was unclear, as pRCC histology only showed a trend toward better cancer-specific survival (HR 0.85, 95 % CI 0.70–1.02) in a multivariate analysis. There was no significant difference in overall survival between ccRCC and pRCC.

Another retrospective study evaluated 4,063 patients with RCC; the authors evaluated histology, age, TNM stage, Fuhrman grade, and performance status for prognostic significance [21]. 87.7 % of the patients had ccRCC histology, 9.7 % pRCC, and 2.5 % chRCC. A trend toward better survival in patients with pRCC and chRCC was identified on univariate analysis ($p=0.0007$) when compared to ccRCC patients. However histologic subtype was not found to be predictive of outcome in multivariate analysis ($p<0.001$).

It is generally believed that type II pRCC tends have a more aggressive course whereas type I pRCC exhibits a relatively indolent course [22]. Antonelli et al. used their prospectively collected institutional database of 1,150 patients who were treated surgically for RCC; of these, 132 (11.5 %) had a papillary histology confirmed by a single genito-urologic pathology (including 57 [43 %] patients with type I and 75 [57 %] patients with type II). With an average follow-up of 50 months, nine patients (14 %) developed metastatic disease in the type II pRCC group, with no metastatic disease identified in the type I group. While type I histology was associated with better 36-month disease-free survival when compared to type II on univariate analysis ($p<0.004$), this difference was not statistically significant on multivariate analysis ($p=0.937$).

A second study of 130 patients with pRCC suggested that type II pRCC is associated with worse cancer-specific survival and overall survival [23]. Type II tumors were associated with higher stage, grade, and microvascular invasion at the time of surgery ($p<0.001$). During a median follow-up of 48 months, 5 (7 %) type I pRCC patients and 62 (47.7 %) type II pRCC patients died from cancer-specific causes ($p=0.002$). On univariate analysis, type II histology was associated with worse overall survival (HR 4.34, 95 % CI 1.60–11.82, $p=0.002$)

and worse disease-free survival (HR 7.69, 95 % CI 2.96–20.00, $p<0.001$). On multivariate analysis histologic subtype (HR 3.22, 95 % CI 1.09–9.49, $p=0.034$) and TNM stage of III–IV (HR 12.27, 95 % CI 4.95–30.40, $p<0.001$) remained statistically significant as factors affecting cancer-specific survival. A meta-analysis of three studies including 2,455 nccRCC patients demonstrated similar results, with type II pRCC associated with worse outcome than type I pRCC [24].

Clinical Findings

Physical Exam Findings

RCC is an insidious disease with manifestations that often remain occult until late in the clinical course. The classic triad of hematuria, flank pain, and flank mass is uncommon and when present is often associated with advance disease. Most RCC, especially small renal masses, are now incidentally discovered on imaging studies performed for other indications [25, 26].

Symptoms associated with paraneoplastic syndrome are found in approximately 20 % of RCC patients and include hypertension, polycythemia, and hypercalcemia [27]. Physical examination, while important, has a limited role in the diagnostic evaluation of RCC; familial pRCC is an exception, and a thorough physical exam is often a crucial aid in diagnosis. In advanced disease, physical exam findings such as palpable flank or abdominal mass, lymphadenopathy, unilateral varicocele, and lower extremity edema can be found.

With a few exceptions, the clinical presentation of papillary RCC is indistinguishable from that of other kidney cancer variants. Patients usually present from the third to eighth decade of life, with a male to female ratio that ranges from 2:1 to 3.9:1, although pediatric cases of pRCC have been described in HLRCC [14, 28]. While the majority of pRCC cases present with unilateral and unifocal disease, pRCC is the most common multifocal or bilateral RCC variant [29]. In patients with papillary RCC associated with the hereditary kidney cancer syndromes HLRCC or HPRC, a family history of papillary RCC may provide clues to the diagnosis. Additionally, patients with HLRCC may present with cutaneous or early-onset uterine leiomyomas or provide a family history of these disease sequelae [28]. Patients with pRCC are also much more likely to develop malignant ascites than are those with ccRCC [30].

It was believed that in hemodialysis patients developing RCC, a disproportionately large percentage presented with pRCC when compared to the general population. In a study evaluating 43 RCC patients with ESRD on hemodialysis (HD) 21 (48.8 %), patients had pRCC, which was significantly higher than the incidence in the general population ($p<0.001$) [3]. However, this predilection for developing pRCC was not seen in a larger, more recent study of 401 patients with ESRD on HD who underwent radical nephrectomy for RCC [5]. In this study, the incidence of ccRCC (308/401, 76.8 %) and pRCC, (84/401, 20.9 %) was consistent with that expected in the general population.

Imaging Findings

High-resolution computed tomography (CT) before and after administration of intravenous contrast is the gold standard for evaluation of solid renal masses, but magnetic resonance imaging (MRI) is an acceptable alternative [31]. MRI is often performed when optimal CT imaging cannot be performed, such as in case of severe iodinated contrast allergy, pregnancy, or renal dysfunction. However, with its multiplanar capability, MRI is particularly useful in some circumstances, such as delineation of a tumor thrombus [32, 33].

While radiologic features alone should not form the basis for differentiation between individual RCC subtypes, a few characteristics are noteworthy. Sporadic pRCC is often characterized by less intratumoral vascularity when compared to ccRCC. Clinically, this is reflected in the observation that pRCC tumors demonstrate less post-contrast enhancement than ccRCC on CT imaging [34, 35].

Larger (>3 cm) pRCC tumors can appear heterogeneous on CT; they often have areas of necrosis and hemorrhage [36]. This is a useful characteristic to differentiate pRCC from chRCC, as large chRCC tend to appear homogenous [37]. The opposite is true with small (<3 cm) pRCC when compared to ccRCC, where pRCC appears more homogenous [36].

There is no large study that compares differences in imaging characteristics between type I and type II pRCC. However, in a small series of 19 patient, the authors reported that type II pRCC tend be more heterogeneous with necrotic areas and have indistinct borders when compared to type I pRCC [38] (Fig. 1.1a).

The low degree of enhancement seen with pRCC can cause diagnostic difficulties when either a simple renal cyst or a hyperdense renal cyst is in the differential. In most cases, a simple cyst does not enhance more than 10–20 HU from non-contrast to post-contrast imaging. Any enhancement of greater than 10 HU should alert the clinician to investigate further. In the scenario where a cyst possess pseudoenhancement, additional imaging modalities such as ultrasound or MRI can provide useful information [39].

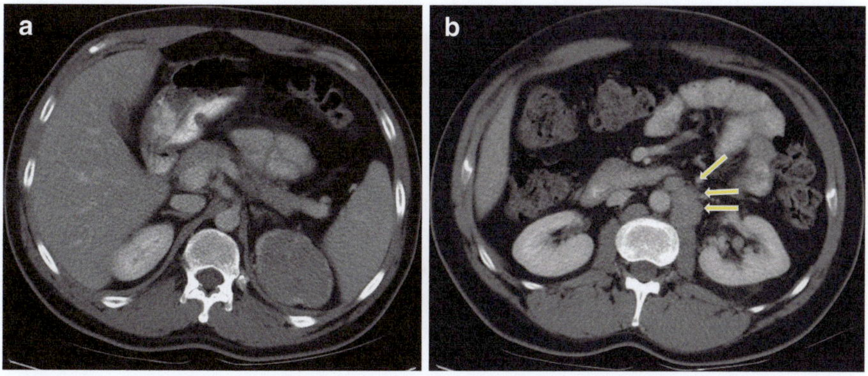

Fig. 1.1 (**a**) Large infiltrating left kidney lesion with irregular borders. CT scan of the abdomen and pelvis in a 55-year-old male with HLRCC; this scan demonstrates a left-side kidney lesion with irregular border. (**b**) Left-side para-aortic lymphatic metastatic disease. CT scan of the abdomen and pelvis in a 55-year-old male with HLRCC, demonstrating para-aortic lymphadenopathy

In a study that evaluated the characteristics of small pRCC (<3 cm) on contrast-enhanced MRI, the authors found several features that may help differentiate pRCC and ccRCC [40]. As is the case with CT imaging, pRCC display less enhancement due to its relative hypovascularity when compared to ccRCC when studied on MRI. pRCC frequently have low signal intensity on both T1- and T2-weighted images and often display a pseudocapsule. In contrast, ccRCC often demonstrate a higher intensity signal on T2-weighted MRI images. Lastly, pRCC often exhibited a homogenous pattern on T2-weighted images whereas ccRCC displayed a hyperintense heterogeneous pattern.

Sporadic Papillary RCC

Pathology

Papillary renal cell carcinoma appears grossly as a well-circumscribed white or beige mass often with a thick fibrous capsule or pseudocapsule; the cut surface is usually yellow or brown in color [41]. There is considerable variation in the size of pRCC primaries at resection, ranging from 1.2 to 26 cm [42]. While smaller pRCC tend to be solid masses, larger pRCC frequently show cystic changes, necrosis, and hemorrhage [43]. pRCC can present in a multifocal fashion, with both multiple tumors on the same kidney and also bilateral tumors [29, 43].

A pathological hallmark of pRCC is the presence of true papillae with fibrovascular cores lined with neoplastic cells [43]. Morphologically, at least two types of pRCC have been described [42]. Type I pRCC have small basophilic cells with scant pale cytoplasm arranged in a single layer on the papillary basement membrane; these tumors tend to have low nuclear grade and often demonstrate the presence of macrophages. Type II pRCC comprises a heterogeneous group of malignancies and are classically described as having high-grade eosinophilic cells with pseudostratified nuclei on papillary cores, often with voluminous cytoplasm. The immunohistochemical profile of the two subtypes is different as well; type I pRCC tend to show expression of CK7, vimentin, and MUC1, whereas CK20 and E-cadherin expression is more frequently seen with type 2 pRCC [42, 44, 45].

It is important to note that there is considerable variation in classification of pRCC by pathologists; this is further made difficult by pRCC mimics such as clear cell tubulopapillary RCC, mucinous tubular and spindle carcinoma, and oncocytic pRCC [46, 47]. During a preconference survey at the International Society of Urological Pathology (ISUP) in 2013, only 59 % of conference participants answered they classified pRCC into type I and type II, only 10 % of the participating pathologists incorporated oncocytic pRCC into their practice. Of the remaining 31 %, 16 % used Fuhrman grading only and 10 % used other criteria. This highlights an important point that papillary RCC is a heterogeneous disease group, likely consisting of several distinct entities that are not well characterized or consistently described currently.

Genetics

Multiple chromosomal abnormalities are associated with papillary RCC, including trisomy of chromosome 3q, 7, 8, 12, 16, 17, and 20 and loss of the Y chromosome in male patients [29, 48]. There is some evidence that type I and type II pRCC have different genetic profiles; type I pRCC seem to exhibit chromosome 7p and 17p gains, whereas type II pRCC seems to have a higher frequency of allelic imbalance on 9p than type I [22, 49]. Somatic mutations of the MET gene are seen in approximately 15 % of pRCC tumors [50–52] and are believed to play a role in the pathogenesis of these tumors. The Cancer Genome Atlas (TCGA) project recently undertook a comprehensive genomic and molecular analysis of 161 papillary renal tumors. Preliminary data from this analysis suggests that alterations of the *MET* gene are seen primarily in type 1 papillary RCC [51]. In addition to activating mutations in *MET* (seen in 11.2 % of patients), other alterations including splice variants (seen in 5 % of patients) and gain of chromosome 7 are commonly seen in type 1 pRCC. Type 2 pRCC is comprised of a heterogeneous group of tumors, sharing some histologic similarities but nonetheless demonstrating considerable histologic and genetic variations. The genetic alterations underlying sporadic type 2 pRCC tumors are yet to be fully elucidated. Recent reports suggest that mutations in genes regulating the nuclear factor (erythroid-derived 2)-like 2 (NRF2) oxidative stress response pathway are seen in some tumors with type 2 papillary histology [53].

Molecular Pathways Important in Papillary RCC

Our understanding of the molecular pathways driving different forms of pRCC is based largely on studies of hereditary forms of pRCC and continues to evolve as newer technologies become available. Comprehensive approaches to molecular and genetic analyses that combine genomic, proteomic, and other platforms to interrogate aberrant or oncogenic pathways are currently being used to better understand the critical drivers of pRCC and are likely to elucidate at least some mechanisms at play. Although the key molecular and biochemical pathways driving the majority of pRCC are still not fully understood, there are at least two well-defined pathways that appear to operate in distinct subtypes of pRCC. Both pathways are summarized briefly here and discussed in more detail in the section on hereditary papillary cancers. The hepatocyte growth factor (HGF)/MET pathway mediates a number of important cellular functions including cell growth, tissue repair, and regeneration and is believed to be important in a subset of patients with type 1 papillary RCC [54] (Fig. 1.2). Patients with HPRC, who carry a germline-activating mutation of *MET*, provide the most compelling evidence that this pathway is activated in pRCC. Additionally, somatic *MET* mutations are seen in a small proportion of patients with sporadic pRCC [50, 51]. Trisomy of chromosome 7 is a relatively common event in pRCC, and since the genes for both *MET* and its ligand *HGF* are located on chromosome 7, it has been suggested that increased copy number of chromosome 7 may lead to activation of the HGF/MET pathway [55].

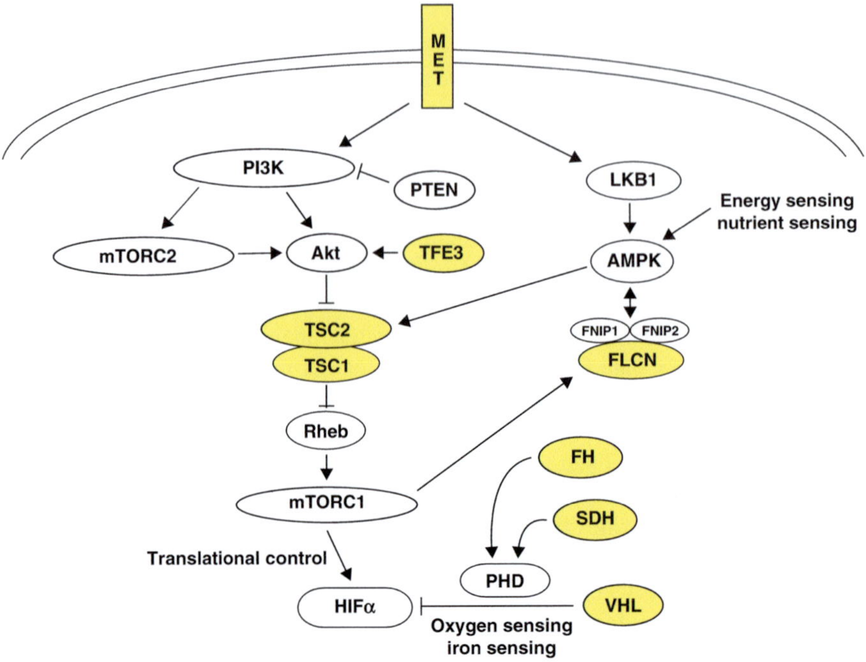

Fig. 1.2 Consequences MET inactivation. The HGF/Met signaling pathway regulates a large number of downstream signaling pathways, some of them critical in carcinogenesis. The RAS/mitogen-activated protein kinase (MAPK) pathway mediates cell scattering and proliferation signals. The PI3K pathway has been implicated in cell motility and remodeling of the extracellular matrix. PI3K also triggers activation of the AKT pathway, which is related to cell survival (Reproduced with permission from Linehan et al. [120])

NRF2, Kelch-like erythroid-derived cap-n-collar homology-associated protein 1 (KEAP1), and cullin 3 (CUL3) are part of a cellular process that regulates response to oxidative stress [56]. Activation of the NRF2 pathway has been demonstrated in both papillary RCC associated with HLRCC and in some forms of sporadic type 2 papillary RCC. Fumarate, a metabolic intermediate generated in the tricarboxylic acid (TCA) cycle, is a substrate for the enzyme fumarate hydratase (FH) and plays an important role in the regulation of this cascade. When fumarate hydratase is inactivated, as in HLRCC-associated tumors, fumarate accumulates intracellularly, leading to a specific posttranslational modification of KEAP1 (succination) [57]. This modification leads to impaired binding of KEAP1 with NRF2, preventing ubiquitin-mediated degradation and nuclear accumulation of the latter. Although somatic mutation of FH does not appear to be common in sporadic pRCC, mutations in KEAP1, NRF2, CUL3, and the sirtuin family of protein may be responsible for NRF2 activation in sporadic pRCC [53, 58] (Fig. 1.3).

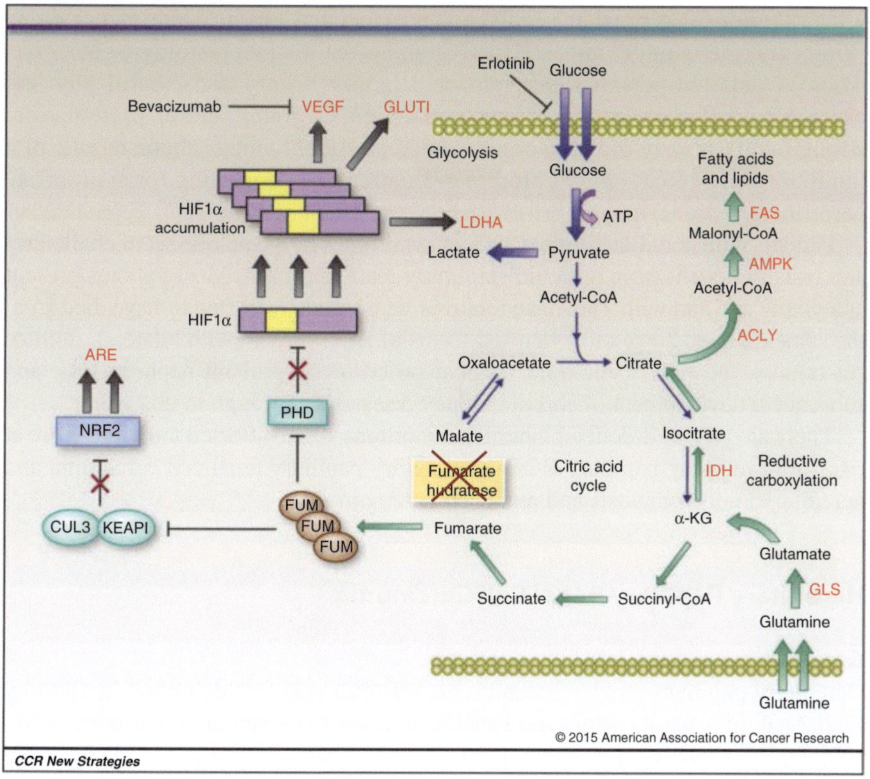

Fig. 1.3 Consequences of fumarate hydratase inactivation. When fumarate hydratase (FH) is inactivated, intracellular accumulation of fumarate occurs. Fumarate accumulation leads to succination of KEAP1, which in turn lead to nuclear accumulation of NRF2. High levels of fumarate also lead to competitive inhibition of PHD, which in turn leads to downstream translation activation of VEGF and GLUT1. Loss of FH also leads to changes in cellular metabolism, with an increased reliance on glucose and glutamine for macromolecular generation (Reproduced with permission from Srinivasan et al. [82])

Hereditary Papillary RCC

Although most cases of RCC are sporadic in nature, it is estimated that 1–4 % are the result of hereditary cancer syndromes [59, 60]. However, this is likely an underestimate and the true prevalence is not known; with the identification and recognition of new familial forms of RCC and heightened awareness of these entities among practitioners, it is estimated that a higher proportion of kidney cancers may have a heritable component [61].

Familial forms of kidney cancer are characterized by early age of onset and often present with bilateral and multifocal renal tumors [60]. Patients with hereditary renal cancer syndromes may present with a family history of RCC, bilateral/multifocal renal masses, known associated physical findings such as skin or uterine leiomyomas in HLRCC, and often distinct histologic characteristics. A detailed personal, surgical, and family history and careful physical exam are invaluable in this patient population. A young age of presentation, strong family history of RCC, or associated physical findings characteristic of a familial form of RCC should prompt evaluation and counseling for appropriate germline genetic testing.

Patients with hereditary kidney cancer syndromes face a unique set of challenges and usually benefit from a multidisciplinary team approach. Most patients present at a young age and will often have relatives who are also affected or have died from the same disease. Since most familial forms of RCC present with bilateral, mulifocal tumors, the risk of multiple surgical procedures, resultant nephron loss, and subsequent development of chronic kidney disease is very high in this group.

There are two well-defined inherited conditions where affected individuals are at risk for developing papillary RCC – hereditary papillary renal cell carcinoma and hereditary leiomyomatosis and renal cell carcinoma.

Hereditary Papillary Renal Cell Carcinoma

Genetics

Hereditary papillary renal cell carcinoma (HPRC) was first described in 1994 by Zbar et al. in a family with type I pRCC in members spanning three generations [62]. HPRC shows an autosomal dominant inheritance pattern and is highly penetrant with an average age of onset of renal manifestations in the sixth decade. The only known phenotype is the development of bilateral multifocal papillary type I RCC. Although renal manifestations of HPRC are identified relatively late, Schmidt et al. identified an early-onset form, where the median age of presentation was 46, compared to the sixth decade described earlier [63] (Fig. 1.4a, b).

Individuals who are affected with HPRC have a germline gain of function or activating mutation in the tyrosine kinase (TK) domain of the *MET* proto-oncogene, located on chromosome 7q [64]. Mutations in the TK domain of *MET* lead to constitutive activation of the MET pathway, believed to play a key role in tumorigenesis in this group of patients. Additionally, tumors from HPRC patients demonstrate gain of chromosome 7, resulting from nonrandom duplication of the chromosome bearing the mutant *MEt* allele.

Pathology

Kidneys of patients with HPRC often harbor multiple macroscopic and microscopic (incipient) lesions, ranging from tumors that are less than the size of a single tubule, to papillary adenoma (<0.5 cm), to pRCC (>0.5 cm) [65]. It is estimated that 1,100–3,400 papillary tumors are present in a single kidney in patients with HPRC [66]. Renal tumors associated with HPRC are morphologically consistent with type I pRCC and usually exhibit low nuclear grade. Focal areas of clear cells with intracytoplasmic lipid and glycogen were also present in up to 94 % of tumors from HPRC patients; however these areas can be distinguished from conventional ccRCC tumors by the presence of small basophilic nuclei and the lack of a fine vascular network (Fig. 1.5). Tumors from all but two patients contained foamy macrophages in fibrovascular cores [65].

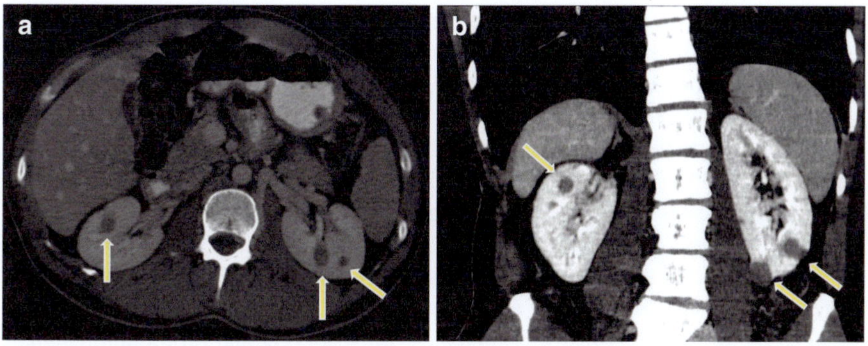

Fig. 1.4 (**a**) Bilateral multifocal hypointense renal lesions, axial view. CT scan of the abdomen and pelvis in a 40-year-old male with HPRC demonstrating multiple, bilateral, hypointense renal lesions. Same patient as (**b**), in axial view. (**b**) Bilateral multifocal hypointense renal lesions, coronal view. CT scan of the abdomen and pelvis in a 40-year-old male with HPRC demonstrating multiple, bilateral, hypointense renal lesions. Same patient as (**a**), in coronal view

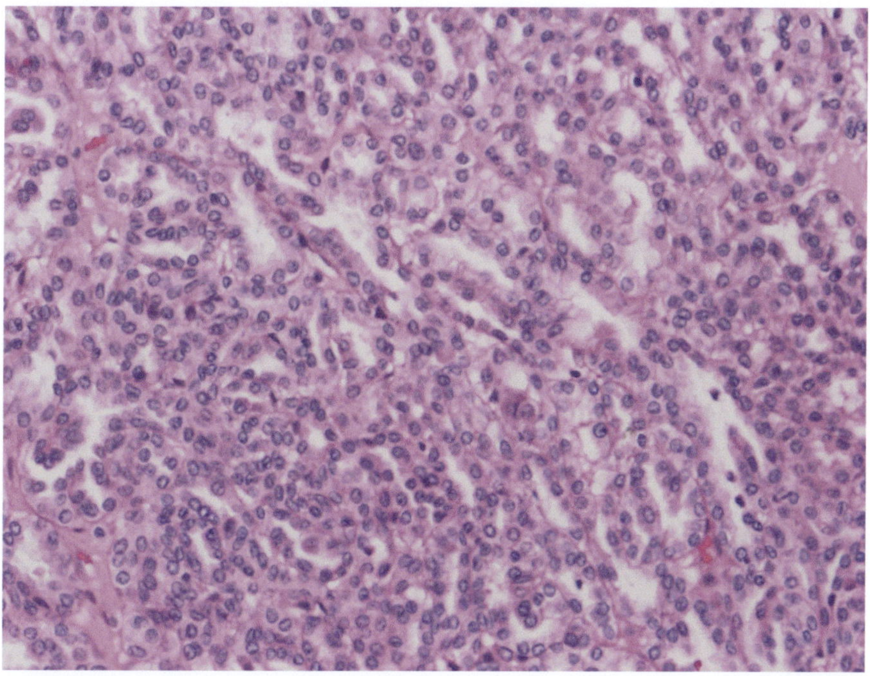

Fig. 1.5 Papillary type I pathology. Small basophilic cells with scant pale cytoplasm arranged in a single layer on the papillary basement membrane

Molecular Biology: Consequences of MET Activation

As discussed in the sporadic kidney cancer section, the HGF/Met pathway is responsible for various critical cellular functions that may contribute to cancer survival, invasion, and metastasis when altered [13]. HGF is primarily secreted by mesenchymal cells; it is the only known ligand for Met and acts in a paracrine fashion [67]. The Met protein product is a heterodimer with an entirely extracellular α-subunit and a β-subunit with three separate components: an extracellular region, a transmembrane component, and an intracellular TK domain. When HGF binds, Met is autophosphorylated at multiple tyrosine residues. The Y1313 residue in the TK domain is important for binding of phosphoinositide kinase-3 (PI3K), whereas Y1349 and Y1356 are involved in the activation of the multisubstrate-docking site, both important sites of regulation and targeting for therapy [68] (Fig. 1.2).

The HGF/Met signaling pathway regulates a large number of downstream signaling pathways, some of them critical in carcinogenesis. The RAS/mitogen-activated protein kinase (MAPK) pathway is activated via Grb2 binding of the multisubstrate-docking site of Met; this pathway mediates cell scattering and proliferation signals [69]. The PI3K pathway can be activated either downstream via RAS or directly recruited to the multisubstrate-docking site via phosphorylation of Gab1 and has been implicated in cell motility and remodeling of the extracellular matrix. PI3K also triggers activation of the AKT pathway, which is related to cell survival [70].

Hereditary Leiomyomatosis and Renal Cell Carcinoma

HLRCC was first described in 2001, with affected members at risk for both kidney cancer and extrarenal manifestations [71, 72]. Patients with HLRCC develop uterine leiomyoma (fibroids), cutaneous leiomyoma, and an aggressive variant of type II pRCC. Uterine leiomyomas are a highly penetrant manifestation of HLRCC with a lifetime risk of 98 % in some series [28]. Affected female patients tend to present with uterine fibroids at a young age, often necessitating surgical intervention by the third or fourth decade of life; approximately 57 % of female patients with uterine fibroids undergo hysterectomy by the age of 30 due to complications related to the fibroids. Cutaneous leiomyomas are also frequently seen in affected patients, with an estimated lifetime risk of >90 %. In contrast, kidney cancer is seen in only 15–30 % of affected individuals, with a median age at presentation of approximately 44 years [28]. In the initial population when this entity was characterized, 4 out of 11 patients with kidney cancer presented with unilateral solitary renal masses with a type II pRCC histology that had already metastasized at the time of diagnosis [71]. Once metastatic, HLRCC is uniformly lethal with an often poor clinical course. Approximately 7.8 % of patients affected by HLRCC develop primary adrenal nodules consistent with macronodular adrenal hyperplasia [73].

Genetics

HLRCC is inherited in an autosomal dominant fashion and was linked to mutations in a gene on chromosome 1q subsequently identified as the *fumarate hydratase* gene [72]. Fumarate hydratase is a tricarboxylic acid cycle (TCA) enzyme that catalyzes the conversion of fumarate to malate. Patients with HLRCC have a germline inactivating mutation or deletion of *FH*, with a second, somatic alteration in renal tumors leading to loss of fumarate hydratase activity and disruption of the TCA cycle.

Pathology

HLRCC-associated renal tumors generally present as a single solid or solid-cystic mass, but bilateral multifocal tumors are not uncommonly seen. These tumors usually have a prominent papillary pattern, although a variety of architectural patterns have been described. In a study of 40 HLRCC-associated renal tumors from patients with a known germline *FH* mutation, 25 cases had a papillary architecture, 8 cases were tubulopapillary, 2 cases were tubular, 1 case was solid, and 4 cases demonstrated a mixed pattern. Renal tumors associated with HLRCC have a characteristic appearance on histopathologic evaluation, demonstrating a large nucleus with a very prominent inclusion like orangiophilic or eosinophilic nucleolus and a clear perinuclear halo [74]. Uterine leiomyomas in HLRCC patients tend to present at a younger age than in the general population and are usually multiple [75]. In a study of 19 HLRCC patients with uterine leiomyomas, the authors found increase atypia, increased cellularity, and tumor nuclei with large orangiophilic nucleoli with a perinuclear halo, features reminiscent of HLRCC-associated RCC; however, these leiomyomas are generally benign and do not metastasize (Fig. 1.6).

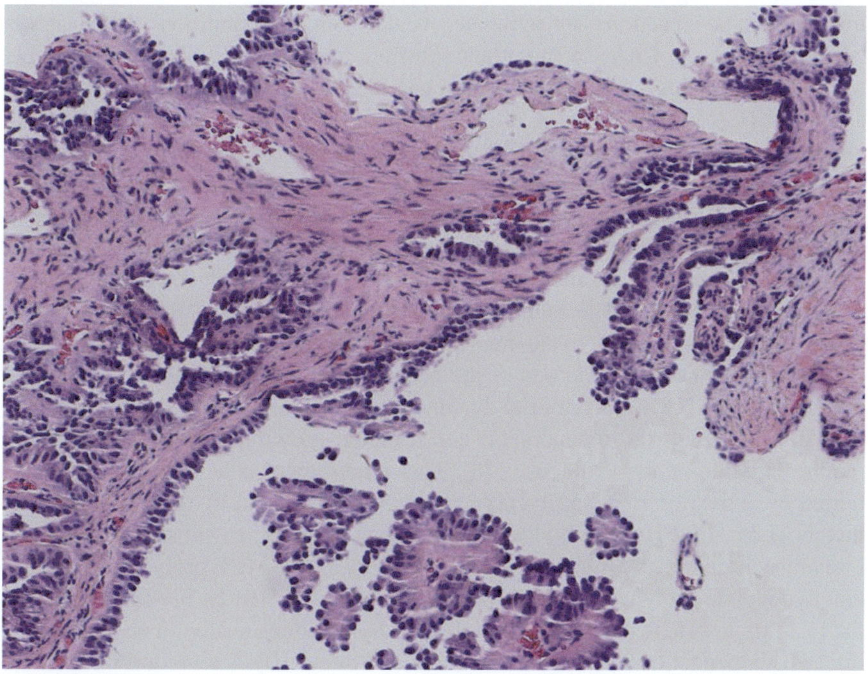

Fig. 1.6 Papillary type 2, HLRCC pathology. High-grade eosinophilic cells with pseudostratified nuclei on papillary cores, often with voluminous cytoplasm. Part of resected cyst with solid component and cyst wall lined by tumor

There are no standard IHC markers that are diagnostic for HLRCC-associated kidney tumors, but several are under evaluation. FH-deficient tumor cells accumulate intracellular fumarate, which covalently modifies cysteine residues in cellular proteins to S-(2-succinyl) cysteine (2SC). The utility of antibodies against 2SC as a diagnostic immunohistochemistry marker for HLRCC is under evaluation [57]. In one study, 2SC was undetectable in normal tissues and tumor types not associated with HLRCC, while in patients with confirmed HLRCC, strong 2SC staining accurately predicted this genetic alternation. This was confirmed by another study where tumors from HLRCC kidney and other types of kidney cancers were stained for 2SC [76]. HLRCC-associated renal tumors demonstrated strong and diffuse nuclear and cytoplasmic staining for 2SC; in contrast, ccRCC (184/184), high-grade unclassified RCC (93/97), and type II non-HLRCC pRCC (35/45) did not stain for 2SC. Although 2SC staining shows promise as an ancillary tool in the differentiation of HLRCC from other high-grade RCC, it remains an investigational tool with no commercially available antibody or assay. Furthermore, additional validation studies are needed, limiting the clinical utility of 2SC staining at the current time.

Molecular Biology: Consequences of Fumarate Hydratase Inactivation

Glucose is an important source of cellular energy (ATP) but also contributes carbon units for macromolecule synthesis, essential for supporting cell growth and proliferation. Following entry into the cell, glucose is converted by a series of cytoplasmic enzymatic reactions to pyruvate. Under aerobic conditions, pyruvate is converted to acetyl CoA, an important substrate for the mitochondrial TCA cycle and electron transport chain. Inactivation of FH leads to dysregulation of the mitochondrial TCA cycle, depriving affected cells of an efficient means of converting glucose to ATP. The cells adapt by utilizing a process called aerobic glycolysis, whereby ATP is synthesized by the conversion of pyruvate to lactate, albeit much less efficiently. This glycolytic shift, also known as the Warburg effect, was initially described in the 1920s by Otto Warburg, who observed that tumor cells consumed significantly more glucose and produced excessive amounts of lactic acid compared to normal cells [77]. While many tumors utilize aerobic glycolysis, largely in an effort to divert the TCA cycle intermediates toward macromolecule synthesis, FH-deficient tumors provide one of the best examples of an obligatory glycolytic shift necessitated by mitochondrial dysfunction as originally proposed by Warburg. In order to sustain the bioenergetic needs of the growing cell, HLRCC tumors require large amounts of glucose [78]. This requirement is at least partially supported by activation of a proglycolytic phenotype mediated by hypoxia-inducible factors. Loss of FH activity leads to accumulation of its substrate, fumarate. Fumarate competitively inhibits a group of enzymes called HIF prolyl hydroxylases that hydoxylate prolyl residues on the alpha subunits of HIF. In FH-deficient cells, the inability to efficiently hydroxylate HIF prolyl residues results in an inability of the VHL-dependent E3 ligase to recognize and target HIF for ubiquitin-mediated degradation. This results in transcriptional activation of a variety of proteins including vascular endothelial growth factor (VEGF), glucose transporter 1 (Glut 1), and several glycolytic enzymes critical for sustaining aerobic glycolysis. However, crossbreeding conditional *FH*(–/–)mice with *HIF1* or *HIF2* "knockout" mice failed to rescue the animals from the *FH*(–/–) renal phenotype, suggesting that there is at least one HIF-independent pathway for HLRCC tumorigenesis [79, 80]. Recent reports have demonstrated that one consequence of fumarate accumulation in FH-deficient cells is the posttranslational succination of several proteins, including KEAP1 [57]. KEAP1 is an important regulator of NRF2, serving as the client binding unit of an E3 ligase system that serves to target NRF2 for ubiquitination and subsequent degradation. Succinated KEAP1 is unable to bind NRF2, thereby leading to the accumulation and nuclear translocation of the latter and resulting in the transcriptional activation of several factors critical for cell survival in the setting of oxidative stress [81] (Fig. 1.3).

FH-deficient tumors have been studied from the metabolic point of view, in a bid to explore altered metabolism as a therapeutic target. These tumors have a high proliferative rate and exaggerated bioenergy requirements with a high demand for macromolecules for sustaining growth. In normal cells, glucose and glutamine are the main source of carbon and nitrogen molecules in the construction of macromolecules such as lipids, proteins, and nucleotides. In *FH* tumor cells, the entry of glucose into the TCA cycle is limited; glutamine serves instead as the major source of intermediates for macromolecule synthesis by a process known as glutaminolysis. In this process glutamine is converted to glutamate by glutaminase; subsequently, glutamate enters the TCA cycle as α-ketoglutarate via a process called reductive carboxylation [82, 83]. Attempts to disrupt glutamine utilization are being explored in preclinical models, with at least one small-molecule inhibitor of glutaminase currently in phase 1 evaluation. FH-deficient cells also appear and overexpress genes involved in heme synthesis and degradation, including heme oxygenase 1 (HMOX1), utilizing this pathway to generate NADH [84]. Knockdown experiments have demonstrated that inhibition of HMOX1 is synthetically lethal in FH-deficient cells, suggesting that strategies that target this gene and/or the hem biosynthesis/degradation pathway may have therapeutic relevance in HLRCC-associated tumors. HLRCC tumor dependency of this escape pathway was confirmed by short hairpin RNA silencing of HMOX1 in *FH*-deficient cells and the observation of reduced growth [85].

Management of Localized Disease

Sporadic pRCC

In general, most guideline suggests that localized sporadic pRCC should be managed in a similar fashion to sporadic ccRCC [86, 87]. The available treatment options include: active surveillance, radical nephrectomy (open or minimally invasive), partial nephrectomy (open or minimally invasive), or ablative techniques.

Nephron-sparing surgery (NSS) has gained acceptance as a standard of care option for renal masses ≤4 cm in size in the USA in the past decade [86]. This is based on several factors, including a higher risk of CKD in patients undergoing radical nephrectomy (RN), similar oncologic outcomes between partial and radical nephrectomy for tumors less than 7 cm, concerns about contralateral recurrence, and the fact that 20 % of renal masses are benign tumors. Several studies have demonstrated that partial nephrectomy is both technically feasible and oncologically sound for renal masses less than 7 cm [88, 89]. In a randomized controlled trial for patients with T1a–bN0M0 renal masses comparing NSS versus RN, the oncologic outcome was similar. The 10-year progression rates were 4.1 % (95 % CI: 1.7–6.5) after NSS and 3.3 % (95 % CI: 1.2–5.4) after RN, with no statistically significant difference between the two surgical approaches [90].

Reports comparing renal function outcomes of patients undergoing partial versus radical nephrectomy found that radical nephrectomy patients are more likely to have proteinuria and a serum creatinine >2 [91]. Renal function following radical nephrectomy was also evaluated in another study where estimated glomerular filtration (GFR) was used as a marker [92]. In this series the authors found approximately 26 % of patients undergoing renal surgery already have CKD, as defined by GFR <60 ml/min/1.73 m^2. Furthermore, 3-year probability of development of moderate CKD (GFR <45 ml/min/1.73 m^2) was 5 % for partial nephrectomy and 36 % for radical nephrectomy. Radical nephrectomy remained an independent risk factor for development of new-onset CKD even after controlling for other confounding factors. There is strong evidence that CKD is associated with increased risk of cardiovascular events, hospitalization, and death [93].

Radical nephrectomy should still be considered for patients with tumors that are judged by the surgeon not to be amenable to partial nephrectomy due to location, size, body habitus, prior surgeries, or comorbidities. There is strong evidence suggesting that although partial nephrectomy reduces the incidence of moderate renal dysfunction, overall survival still favors radical nephrectomy [90, 94]. In a prospective randomized study that evaluated 541 patients with a solitary T1a–bN0M0 renal mass, at 9.3 years of follow-up, the overall survival was 81.1 % for patients undergoing radical nephrectomy and 75.7 % for those receiving partial nephrectomy (HR 1.5, 95 % CI: 1.03–2.16) [94]. It is important to note that this study was comprised predominately of patients with ccRCC (59.7 % in RN group, 66 % in NSS group), and the results will need further validation in the pRCC population.

A variety of different techniques can be used to perform NSS: enucleation of the tumor, resection of the tumor with a small margin of normal tissue, and resection of tumor with a wide margin. In a large retrospective study of sporadic ccRCC patients, simple tumor enucleation had similar progression-free survival and cancer-specific survival rates when compared to standard radical and partial nephrectomy with a margin of normal kidney tissue [95]. Although there is some controversy about the impact of a positive surgical margin (PSM) following nephron-sparing surgery, PSM is a relatively rare occurrence (2–5 %). In a large retrospective study evaluating 1,344 patients undergoing 1,390 partial nephrectomies, Yossephowitch et al. found no significant difference between patients with PSM and patients without PSM when evaluating for 10-year freedom from local disease recurrence and metastatic progression ($p = 0.97$ and 0.18, respectively) [96]. However, when Khalifeh et al. studied 943 patients who underwent robotic assisted NSS, patients with PSM had higher local recurrence and metastatic rates ($p < 0.001$) [97]. In patients with sporadic RCC, the ability to maximally spare normal renal tissue with enucleation is highly valued. However the same is not true in patients with HLRCC, where any residual tumor can result in rapid progression and metastasis. It is important in HLRCC patients to obtain a wide margin during NSS and ensure the entire tumor is removed with no positive surgical margin.

Active surveillance is a viable option in some patients who have small renal masses and are elderly, with significant competing comorbidity, or do not desire surgery. Patients on active surveillance are monitored via serial abdominal imaging (CT, MR, or ultrasound) with the intention of intervention if there are signs of progression during follow-up. In a large active surveillance series, in patients with incidentally detected, asymptomatic, small renal masses (median size, 2.1 cm; range, 0.4–4 cm), the growth rate was estimated to be 0.13 cm/year and progression to metastatic disease was rare (1–3 %) [98]. This approach should be undertaken with caution in the pRCC patient cohort, as some type II pRCC can be aggressive and progress quickly. A renal mass biopsy may be helpful in patients with concerns for nccRCC and can aid in decision making for management with active surveillance.

Ablative therapies are not well studied and there is no randomized controlled trial comparing ablation to partial nephrectomy. In general ablation can be performed via percutaneous or laparoscopic approaches, with a variety of energy sources such as radio-frequency ablation, cryoablation, microwave ablation, high-intensity focused ultrasound ablation, and laser ablation. There are limitations to ablative techniques, such as the presence of multiple or bilateral tumors, large tumor size, and location close to the renal hilum and ureter. While a population-based study comparing ablation and partial nephrectomy in patients with small renal masses showed increased risk of death from kidney cancer and local recurrence in the former, other studies show no difference in cancer-specific survival or overall survival [99–101]. Long-term data is lacking for ablative therapies for renal masses, and the gold standard treatment remains partial nephrectomy.

As discussed in the epidemiology section, there is conflicting data in the literature regarding the prognostic significance of papillary histology. The existing studies provided conflicting data; two studies showed patients with ccRCC had lower cancer-specific survival when compared with pRCC, while two other studies showed histology had no impact on cancer-specific survival [10, 20, 21, 102].

HPRC

Physicians managing patients with HPRC are faced with a unique set of challenges: patients affected by HPRC are at risk for developing over 3,000 tumors in each kidney and may require multiple surgical procedures, increasing the risk for development of CKD. Patients with HPRC should be followed closely with abdominal imaging, and a partial nephrectomy should be done when the largest tumor is greater than 3 cm [66, 103–105]. The primary goal for surgical treatment of HPRC patients (and other patients with bilateral multifocal tumors) is to prevent metastasis while maximizing renal preservation and delaying dialysis. Secondary goals are to maximize the amount of time between surgeries while minimizing the number of interventions. Investigators at the NCI have reported on their experience in the management of bilateral multifocal kidney cancer patients of a variety of etiologies [106]. There are several general principles that are followed: enucleation to minimize normal renal parenchyma loss, avoidance of aggressive hilar dissection, off-clamp partial nephrectomy, use of minimally invasive technique when feasible, and reconstruction of normal anatomy to allow future reoperations [107]. pRCC tumors are often surrounded by a pseudocapsule, increasing the difficulty of enucleation when compared to ccRCC [41]. Based on the NCI experience, for patients with bilateral multifocal renal masses who undergo repeat or salvage renal surgery, only 3 % of patients required long-term dialysis [105]. Overall metastasis-free survival was 88 % and RCC-specific survival was 97 % at a median follow-up of 16 years [104]. A total of 128 patients were included in this study, while the majority of these had von Hippel-Lindau disease and 6 (5 %) patients had HPRC.

HLRCC

Kidney cancer associated with HLRCC behaves in a very aggressive manner with a propensity for metastasis even when the tumors are small, and patients with HLRCC kidney cancer often present with nodal metastasis [2, 107] (Fig. 1.1b). As a result, early intervention when any solid renal masses are discovered is critical. HLRCC-associated kidney cancer presents several unique surgical challenges: small cysts may contain lining that are infiltrated with tumor cells that are not easily see with conventional imaging, tumors can be difficult to find on intraoperative ultrasound, borders of the tumor are often ill-defined and irregular, and spillage of HLRCC tumor often results in seeding (Fig. 1.1c, d).

To combat these challenges, a careful partial nephrectomy with a wide surgical margin and diligent assessment of intraoperative frozen section to ensure complete removal of the tumor by a competent pathologist is critical in surgical management. Preoperative recognition of HLRCC is important in avoiding many pitfalls seen in the surgical management of HLRCC and can be accomplished in many cases with careful attention to history and physical findings, with appropriate genetic evaluation when indicated. While not validated by prospective studies, regional lymph node dissection when suspicious nodes are present is the current practice at the

NCI. Inclusion of regional lymph dissection is based on the observation that HLRCC- associated tumors tend to spread lymphatically and removal of these nodes may provide a therapeutic benefit. Unpublished data from the NCI suggest lymph node dissection may lower the risk of metastatic disease in patients with HLRCC. The feasibility of minimally invasive approach to this tumor entity is still being actively investigated.

Management of Metastatic Disease

General Outcomes

Over the past decade, several new therapeutic options for the management of patients with advanced RCC have been evaluated and successfully introduced into clinical practice. However, the clinical benefit seen with these molecular targeted agents is largely restricted to patients with the clear cell variant of RCC [108] (Table 1.1). There are currently no systemic agents of proven benefit for patients with metastatic pRCC, and most die from disease-related causes. Agents targeting the VEGF or mTOR pathways as well as other small molecules directed against pathways thought to be important in cancer are associated with modest clinical activity at best, and outcome in pRCC patients appears to be inferior to that seen in patients with advanced ccRCC. This is exemplified by a recent retrospective analysis of 2,215 metastatic RCC patients (1963 with ccRCC, and 252 with nccRCC) treated with first-line anti-VEGF or anti-mTOR agents. The study evaluated overall survival and time to treatment failure [12]. Median overall survival of the entire cohort was 20.9 months, with a median overall survival of 22.3 (95 % CI 20.7–23.5) months for ccRCC and 12.8 (95 % CI 11–16.1) months for nccRCC ($p<0.0001$). In a subgroup analysis, pRCC patients had a median overall survival of 14 (95 % CI 10.0–17.1) months, and when compared to ccRCC patients, the adjusted HR for death was 1.57 (95 % CI 1.27–1.94; $p<0.0001$).

Table 1.1 Summary of selected trials in papillary RCC

Agent	*N*	Median PFS (months)	Median OS (months)	Overall response rate (ORR)	Ref.
Erlotinib	45	<6	27	11 %	Gordon, *JCO*
Sunitinib	61	6	<18	12 %	Ravaud, *Ann Onc*
Sunitinib	27	1.6	12.6	0 %	Tannir, *Eur Urol*
Everolimus (RAPTOR)	92	3.7	21.1	–	Escudier, *ECCO*
Everolimus	49	52	–	10 %	Koh, *Ann Onc*
Everolimus vs. sunitinib (ESPN)	68 (27 pRCC)	4.1 vs. 6.1	NR vs. 10.5	0 % vs. 12 %	Tannir, *ASCO* 2014
Everolimus vs. sunitinib (ASPEN)	108 (71 pRCC)	5.6 vs. 8.3	13 vs. 32	9 % vs. 18 %	Armstrong, *ASCO* 2015

Most national and international treatment guidelines do not identify a standard treatment option for the majority of patients with metastatic pRCC, instead recommending participation in an appropriate clinical trial [109]. These recommendations take into account expert opinion as well as data from several retrospective analyses and phase 2 clinical trials that have evaluated the efficacy of VEGF-targeted tyrosine kinase inhibitors (TKI) and mTOR inhibitors in this patient population. Results from selected trials are discussed below.

Sunitinib has been the subject of several phase 2 trials in patients with pRCC ([110–112], Table 1.1), most demonstrating modest activity with a median PFS generally <6 months in the first-line setting. Tannir et al. conducted a phase 2 clinical trial of sunitinib in 57 nccRCC patients with metastatic disease, including 27 patients with pRCC [110]. The median progression-free survival for pRCC patients was 1.6 months (95 % CI 1.4–5.4), with no objective responses. Twelve pRCC patients had stable disease while 13 had progressive disease as their best response. The phase 3 global advance renal cell carcinoma (ARCC) trial was conducted to evaluate the overall survival of untreated, poor-risk, metastatic RCC patients when treated with interferon alpha versus temsirolimus [113]. In a cohort of 626 patients, the authors found significant longer overall survival (HR for death 0.73; 95 % CI: 0.58–0.92, $p = 0.008$) and progression-free survival ($p < 0.001$) in patients who received temsirolimus when compared to patients who received interferon alone, with a post hoc subgroup analysis demonstrating that the benefit extended to patients with papillary histology. The results of this trial provided the basis for the use of mTOR agents in the management of metastatic pRCC. In a subset analysis by Figlin et al., baseline levels of PTEN and HIF1-α were correlated with overall survival, progression-free survival, or objective response rate [114]. The authors found no correlation in PTEN and HIF1-α levels and survival; the baseline levels did not predict response to temsirolimus.

Escudier et al. conducted an open-label, phase 2 clinical trial evaluating the efficacy of everolimus as first-line agent in type I and type 2 metastatic pRCC [115]. A total of 92 patients were enrolled, and central pathology review confirmed papillary histology in 76 % of the patients (59 % with type 2, 33 % with type 1). The per-protocol cohort (centrally confirmed papillary histology) had a 6-month progression-free survival of 34.1 %, demonstrating a modest effect of everolimus in pRCC patients.

Several groups have undertaken a head-to-head comparison of sunitinib and everolimus in the first-line setting in patients with nccRCC. Results from a randomized phase 2 crossover study comparing the activity of sunitinib versus everolimus, an mTOR inhibitor, in patients with nccRCC were reported in abstract form. This trial was designed to study the efficacy of sunitinib and everolimus both in the first-line and second-line setting, with crossover from the sunitinib group to everolimus group and vice versa. Seventy-three patients were enrolled, and 68 patients were found eligible including 27 patients with pRCC. In the first-line setting, the overall response rate (ORR) for all patients was 12 % with sunitinib (one patient had pRCC) and 0 % with everolimus. Median PFS in the first-line setting with sunitinib was 6.1 months (95 % CI 4.7, 10.8) and 4.1 months with everolimus (95 % CI: 2.7, 7.4;

$p = 0.25$). 38 patients of all histologies went on to receive second-line therapy, 19 patients with each agent. Median progression-free survival was 1.8 months (95 % CI: 1.5, NA) in the sunitinib group and 4.3 months with everolimus (95 % CI: 1.4, NA). This study was stopped prematurely based on an interim analysis that revealed that everolimus was not better than sunitinib as a first-line agent for metastatic nccRCC. There was no subgroup analysis done on this trial for pRCC patients. More recently, an international study (ASPEN) randomized untreated metastatic non-clear cell RCC patients to everolimus or sunitinib [116]. A total of 108 patients were enrolled, 66 % of whom had metastatic pRCC. The median progression-free survival in pRCC patients was 5.6 months for patients who received everolimus and 8.3 months for patients who received sunitinib. Overall response rate was 9 % for patients who received everolimus and 18 % for patients who received sunitinib ($p = 0.16$; predefined $p < 0.2$ boundary value for statistically significance). Sunitinib also resulted in higher rate of >grade 4 treatment related toxicity when compared to everolimus, 65 % vs. 47 %, respectively.

Erlotinib is an oral small-molecule epidermal growth factor receptor (EGFR) tyrosine kinase inhibitor that is FDA approved for use in patients with EGFR-mutant non-small cell lung carcinoma. Gordon et al. conducted a phase 2 clinical trial with this agent in patients with advanced or metastatic pRCC who had received no prior immunotherapy or chemotherapy [117]. In 45 evaluable patients, ORR was 11 % (95 % CI 3–24 %), and the disease control rate was 64 %. Only 29 % of patients remained progression-free at 6 months; however, for reasons that are not entirely clear, median overall survival was 27 months (95 % CI 13–36 months), surprisingly higher than historical controls. It is unlikely that this seemingly high OS was a result of erlotinib treatment, and this agent is not typically used as a single agent in patients with pRCC.

As a result of heightened awareness of the heterogeneity of pRCC, and with the identification of several relevant genetic and molecular alterations in pRCC subgroups, there has been a greater focus over the last few years on developing more personalized, mechanism-based approaches for treating these tumors. One area of considerable interest is evaluation of inhibitors of the Met pathway, based on the identification of germline *MET* mutations in patients with the hereditary form of type 1 pRCC and the recognition that somatic *MET* mutations are present in a small proportion of patients with sporadic pRCC. Additionally, it has been argued that gain of chromosome 7, a relatively common event in type 1 pRCC, might represent an alternative mechanism of Met activation in tumors with wild-type *MET*. To test the validity of Met as a clinically relevant target in pRCC, a phase 2 trial of foretinib, a multi-kinase inhibitor with activity against Met as well as VEGF-receptor 2, AXL, and RON was undertaken. A total of 74 patients were enrolled to one of two alternative dosing regimens (a daily dosing regimen and an intermittent dosing regimen). Ten patients demonstrated an objective response (ORR 10/74, 13.5 %), with no significant differences between dosing regimens in terms of efficacy or adverse events. The median progression-free survival for the entire cohort was 9.3 months, considerably higher than that seen in historical controls [118]. An exhaustive biomarker analysis was undertaken as part of this study to explore whether *MET* status could outcome. Interestingly, patients with a germline mutation in *MET* (i.e., patients with HPRC) were found to have a very high response rate; five out of ten HPRC patients had a partial response (PR) (ORR 50 %), with an additional four patients demonstrating significant tumor regression without meeting criteria for Response Evaluation Criteria in Solid Tumors (RECIST) PR. In contrast, only 5 out of 57 patients without a germline *MET* mutation demonstrated a PR (ORR 9 %). With the limited data available, there was no clear correlation between outcome and the presence of a somatic *MET* mutation, *MET* amplification, or gain of chromosome 7. These data indicate that Met inhibition is associated with clinical activity in pRCC patients. However, several points are worth noting. First, while tumors with activating *MET* mutations appear to be highly sensitive to Met inhibition, the response rate in those without this alteration is modest. Second, although the median PFS in this study compared quite favorably with historic controls, such comparisons are fraught with bias and must be interpreted cautiously. One potential source of bias is the inclusion of patients with bilateral, multifocal tumors (without evidence of distant extrarenal spread) in this study; the natural history of these tumors is different from that of metastatic disease and these patients are not usually included in most systemic therapy studies. Third, the agent studied has activity against a variety of tyrosine kinases other than Met, and it is possible that some of the activity seen may be attributable to "off-target" effects. Lastly, the toxicity profile of the agent is very reminiscent of that seen with other VEGFR inhibitors and the dosing of the agent was largely limited by these toxicities. It has been suggested that this may have led to suboptimal Met inhibition and has prompted interest in more selective Met inhibitors that could theoretically be dosed to achieve maximal inhibition of this pathway. This hypothesis is the subject of ongoing clinical investigation and at least two selective Met inhibitors, INC280 (NCT02019693) and volitinib (NCT02127710), are currently in phase 2 trials in patients with advanced papillary RCC.

The identification of well-defined metabolic alterations in a subgroup of pRCC has generated considerable enthusiasm for exploring clinically relevant metabolic targets. A variety of approaches are currently in preclinical evaluation. Investigators at the National Cancer Institute have sought to exploit the dependence of FH-deficient pRCC on a high glucose flux. A combination of bevacizumab, a monoclonal antibody to VEGF, and erlotinib was developed as a possible approach to treating patients with HLRCC by constraining glucose delivery to tumors. The interim results of a phase II study of this combination (NCT01130519) in patients with HLRCC-associated or sporadic pRCC were recently presented in abstract form [119]. A total of 41 patients with up to two lines of prior VEGF-pathway directed therapy were enrolled in two independent cohorts, with cohort 1 consisting of HLRCC patients ($n=20$) and cohort 2 of sporadic papillary RCC patients ($n=21$). The regimen was associated with remarkable efficacy in patients with HLRCC, with an ORR of 65 % (PR in 13/20 pts). Most patients in this cohort enjoyed some clinical benefit, with the majority of non-responders demonstrating stable disease >6 months. In the sporadic pRCC cohort, 6 out of 21 patients (29 %) had a PR. The median PFS for the entire study population was 12.8 months (95 % CI 7.47–26.3), with a PFS of 24.4 months (95 % CI 12.8 – NR) in cohort 1 and 7.4 months (95 % CI 3.73–10.2) in cohort 2. This regimen is being further evaluated as a possible standard of care option in pRCC and efforts are afoot to identify those patients with sporadic disease who are most likely to respond.

Conclusion

Papillary renal cell carcinoma represents a heterogeneous group of entities. While the majority of pRCC occurs in sporadic form, two well-studied hereditary forms of pRCC represent unique surgical and therapeutic challenges as well as an opportunity to better understand the molecular alterations in pRCC. HPRC is a rare entity that results in bilateral multifocal type I papillary kidney tumor, while HLRCC is an aggressive, type II papillary kidney tumor that requires early surgical intervention and rigorous surveillance.

Localized papillary RCC is managed surgically, with nephron-sparing surgery used when appropriate, particularly in patients with bilateral, multifocal disease. HPRC patients will likely experience multiple kidney surgeries in their lifetime and therefore require techniques that will maximally preserve renal function and ability to perform reoperative surgery. HLRCC patients harbor tumors that have metastatic potential even with a small primary; they require either a radical nephrectomy or diligent nephron-sparing operations that result in removal of the entire tumor and a negative surgical margin.

There is no current standard of care systemic therapy for metastatic pRCC, and survival for these patients remains poor even with the recent availability of targeted agents for the treatment of other forms of RCC. While inhibitors of the mTOR and VEGF pathway have demonstrated activity in pRCC, better agents are needed in this patient population. Deeper understanding of the genetic and metabolic basis of HPRC and HLRCC has led to several exciting clinical approaches and will likely contribute to the evolving standard of care in pRCC patients.

References

1. Chow WH, Dong LM, Devesa SS. Epidemiology and risk factors for kidney cancer. Nat Rev Urol. 2010;7:245–57.
2. Linehan WM, Ricketts CJ. The metabolic basis of kidney cancer. Semin Cancer Biol. 2013;23:46–55.
3. Ishikawa I, Kovacs G. High incidence of papillary renal cell tumours in patients on chronic haemodialysis. Histopathology. 1993;22:135–9.
4. Gontero P, Ceratti G, Guglielmetti S, et al. Prognostic factors in a prospective series of papillary renal cell carcinoma. BJU Int. 2008;102:697–702.
5. Ikezawa E, Kondo T, Hashimoto Y, et al. Clinical symptoms predict poor overall survival in chronic-dialysis patients with renal cell carcinoma associated with end-stage renal disease. Jpn J Clin Oncol. 2014;44:1096–100.
6. Pavlovich CP, Grubb 3rd RL, Hurley K, et al. Evaluation and management of renal tumors in the Birt-Hogg-Dube syndrome. J Urol. 2005;173:1482–6.
7. Pavlovich CP, Walther MM, Eyler RA, et al. Renal tumors in the Birt-Hogg-Dube syndrome. Am J Surg Pathol. 2002;26:1542–52.

8. Steffens S, Janssen M, Roos FC, et al. Incidence and long-term prognosis of papillary compared to clear cell renal cell carcinoma – a multicentre study. Eur J Cancer. 2012;48:2347–52.
9. Ronnen EA, Kondagunta GV, Ishill N, et al. Treatment outcome for metastatic papillary renal cell carcinoma patients. Cancer. 2006;107:2617–21.
10. Leibovich BC, Lohse CM, Crispen PL, et al. Histological subtype is an independent predictor of outcome for patients with renal cell carcinoma. J Urol. 2010;183:1309–15.
11. Motzer RJ, Hutson TE, Tomczak P, et al. Overall survival and updated results for sunitinib compared with interferon alfa in patients with metastatic renal cell carcinoma. J Clin Oncol. 2009;27:3584–90.
12. Kroeger N, Xie W, Lee JL, et al. Metastatic non-clear cell renal cell carcinoma treated with targeted therapy agents: characterization of survival outcome and application of the International mRCC Database Consortium criteria. Cancer. 2013;119:2999–3006.
13. Su D, Singer EA, Srinivasan R. Molecular pathways in renal cell carcinoma: recent advances in genetics and molecular biology. Curr Opin Oncol. 2015;27:217–23.
14. Siegel RL, Miller KD, Jemal A. Cancer statistics. CA Cancer J Clin. 2015;65:5–29.
15. Ferlay J, Parkin DM, Steliarova-Foucher E. Estimates of cancer incidence and mortality in Europe in 2008. Eur J Cancer. 2010;46:765–81.
16. Lipworth L, Tarone RE, Lund L, McLaughlin JK. Epidemiologic characteristics and risk factors for renal cell cancer. Clin Epidemiol. 2009;1:33–43.
17. Sankin A, Cohen J, Wang H, Macchia RJ, Karanikolas N. Rate of renal cell carcinoma subtypes in different races. Int Braz J Urol Off Braz Soc Urol. 2011;37:29–32; discussion 3–4.
18. Chow WH, Shuch B, Linehan WM, Devesa SS. Racial disparity in renal cell carcinoma patient survival according to demographic and clinical characteristics. Cancer. 2013;119:388–94.
19. Olshan AF, Kuo TM, Meyer AM, Nielsen ME, Purdue MP, Rathmell WK. Racial difference in histologic subtype of renal cell carcinoma. Cancer Med. 2013;2:744–9.
20. Keegan KA, Schupp CW, Chamie K, Hellenthal NJ, Evans CP, Koppie TM. Histopathology of surgically treated renal cell carcinoma: survival differences by subtype and stage. J Urol. 2012;188:391–7.
21. Patard JJ, Leray E, Rioux-Leclercq N, et al. Prognostic value of histologic subtypes in renal cell carcinoma: a multicenter experience. J Clin Oncol. 2005;23:2763–71.
22. Antonelli A, Tardanico R, Balzarini P, et al. Cytogenetic features, clinical significance and prognostic impact of type 1 and type 2 papillary renal cell carcinoma. Cancer Genet Cytogenet. 2010;199:128–33.
23. Pignot G, Elie C, Conquy S, et al. Survival analysis of 130 patients with papillary renal cell carcinoma: prognostic utility of type 1 and type 2 subclassification. Urology. 2007;69:230–5.
24. Lee JH, Choi JW, Kim YS. The value of histologic subtyping on outcomes of clear cell and papillary renal cell carcinomas: a meta-analysis. Urology. 2010;76:889–94.
25. Luciani LG, Cestari R, Tallarigo C. Incidental renal cell carcinoma-age and stage characterization and clinical implications: study of 1092 patients (1982–1997). Urology. 2000;56:58–62.
26. Hollingsworth JM, Miller DC, Daignault S, Hollenbeck BK. Rising incidence of small renal masses: a need to reassess treatment effect. J Natl Cancer Inst. 2006;98:1331–4.
27. Gold PJ, Fefer A, Thompson JA. Paraneoplastic manifestations of renal cell carcinoma. Semin Urol Oncol. 1996;14:216–22.
28. Menko FH, Maher ER, Schmidt LS, et al. Hereditary leiomyomatosis and renal cell cancer (HLRCC): renal cancer risk, surveillance and treatment. Familial Cancer. 2014;13:637–44.
29. Reuter VE. The pathology of renal epithelial neoplasms. Semin Oncol. 2006;33:534–43.
30. Friend J, Su D, Thimmapuram R, et al. Malignant ascites as a manifestation of advanced papillary renal cell cancer (pRCC). 2015.
31. Vikram R, Ng CS, Tamboli P, et al. Papillary renal cell carcinoma: radiologic-pathologic correlation and spectrum of disease. Radiographics. 2009;29:741–54; discussion 55–7.
32. Saleh L, Juneman E, Movahed MR. The use of gadolinium in patients with contrast allergy or renal failure requiring coronary angiography, coronary intervention, or vascular procedure. Catheter Cardiovasc Interv: Off J Soc Card Angiography. 2011;78:747–54.

33. Pretorius ES, Wickstrom ML, Siegelman ES. MR imaging of renal neoplasms. Magn Reson Imaging Clin N Am. 2000;8:813–36.
34. Fujimoto H, Wakao F, Moriyama N, Tobisu K, Sakamoto M, Kakizoe T. Alveolar architecture of clear cell renal carcinomas (< or = 5.0 cm) show high attenuation on dynamic CT scanning. Jpn J Clin Oncol. 1999;29:198–203.
35. Wang JH, Min PQ, Wang PJ, et al. Dynamic CT evaluation of tumor vascularity in renal cell carcinoma. AJR Am J Roentgenol. 2006;186:1423–30.
36. Herts BR, Coll DM, Novick AC, et al. Enhancement characteristics of papillary renal neoplasms revealed on triphasic helical CT of the kidneys. AJR Am J Roentgenol. 2002;178:367–72.
37. Kim JK, Kim TK, Ahn HJ, Kim CS, Kim KR, Cho KS. Differentiation of subtypes of renal cell carcinoma on helical CT scans. AJR Am J Roentgenol. 2002;178:1499–506.
38. Yamada T, Endo M, Tsuboi M, et al. Differentiation of pathologic subtypes of papillary renal cell carcinoma on CT. AJR Am J Roentgenol. 2008;191:1559–63.
39. Wang ZJ, Coakley FV, Fu Y, et al. Renal cyst pseudoenhancement at multidetector CT: what are the effects of number of detectors and peak tube voltage? Radiology. 2008;248:910–6.
40. Roy C, Sauer B, Lindner V, Lang H, Saussine C, Jacqmin D. MR Imaging of papillary renal neoplasms: potential application for characterization of small renal masses. Eur Radiol. 2007;17:193–200.
41. Mancilla-Jimenez R, Stanley RJ, Blath RA. Papillary renal cell carcinoma: a clinical, radiologic, and pathologic study of 34 cases. Cancer. 1976;38:2469–80.
42. Delahunt B, Eble JN. Papillary renal cell carcinoma: a clinicopathologic and immunohistochemical study of 105 tumors. Mod Pathol: Off J U S Can Acad Pathol. 1997;10:537–44.
43. Amin MB, Corless CL, Renshaw AA, Tickoo SK, Kubus J, Schultz DS. Papillary (chromophil) renal cell carcinoma: histomorphologic characteristics and evaluation of conventional pathologic prognostic parameters in 62 cases. Am J Surg Pathol. 1997;21:621–35.
44. Langner C, Wegscheider BJ, Ratschek M, Schips L, Zigeuner R. Keratin immunohistochemistry in renal cell carcinoma subtypes and renal oncocytomas: a systematic analysis of 233 tumors. Virchows Arch Int J Pathol. 2004;444:127–34.
45. Zhou M, Roma A, Magi-Galluzzi C. The usefulness of immunohistochemical markers in the differential diagnosis of renal neoplasms. Clin Lab Med. 2005;25:247–57.
46. Xia QY, Rao Q, Shen Q, et al. Oncocytic papillary renal cell carcinoma: a clinicopathological study emphasizing distinct morphology, extended immunohistochemical profile and cytogenetic features. Int J Clin Exp Pathol. 2013;6:1392–9.
47. Srigley JR, Delahunt B, Eble JN, et al. The International Society of Urological Pathology (ISUP) Vancouver classification of renal neoplasia. Am J Surg Pathol. 2013;37:1469–89.
48. Argani P, Netto GJ, Parwani AV. Papillary renal cell carcinoma with low-grade spindle cell foci: a mimic of mucinous tubular and spindle cell carcinoma. Am J Surg Pathol. 2008;32:1353–9.
49. Furge KA, Chen J, Koeman J, et al. Detection of DNA copy number changes and oncogenic signaling abnormalities from gene expression data reveals MYC activation in high-grade papillary renal cell carcinoma. Cancer Res. 2007;67:3171–6.
50. Schmidt L, Junker K, Nakaigawa N, et al. Novel mutations of the MET proto-oncogene in papillary renal carcinomas. Oncogene. 1999;18:2343–50.
51. Albiges L, et al. "Distinct MET alterations to induce a common phenotype and to define a MET-driven subset of papillary RCC: Results from the Cancer Genome Atlas (TCGA) Kidney Renal Papillary (KIRP) Working Group." J Clin Oncol (Meeting Abstracts) May 2015;33:15_suppl 4521
52. Durinck S, Stawiski EW, Pavia-Jimenez A, et al. Spectrum of diverse genomic alterations define non-clear cell renal carcinoma subtypes. Nat Genet. 2015;47:13–21.
53. Ooi A, Dykema K, Ansari A, et al. CUL3 and NRF2 mutations confer an NRF2 activation phenotype in a sporadic form of papillary renal cell carcinoma. Cancer Res. 2013;73:2044–51.
54. Huh CG, Factor VM, Sanchez A, Uchida K, Conner EA, Thorgeirsson SS. Hepatocyte growth factor/c-met signaling pathway is required for efficient liver regeneration and repair. Proc Natl Acad Sci U S A. 2004;101:4477–82.

55. Lager DJ, Huston BJ, Timmerman TG, Bonsib SM. Papillary renal tumors. Morphologic, cytochemical, and genotypic features. Cancer. 1995;76:669–73.
56. Kobayashi A, Kang MI, Okawa H, et al. Oxidative stress sensor Keap1 functions as an adaptor for Cul3-based E3 ligase to regulate proteasomal degradation of Nrf2. Mol Cell Biol. 2004;24:7130–9.
57. Bardella C, El-Bahrawy M, Frizzell N, et al. Aberrant succination of proteins in fumarate hydratase-deficient mice and HLRCC patients is a robust biomarker of mutation status. J Pathol. 2011;225:4–11.
58. Pena-Llopis S, Vega-Rubin-de-Celis S, Liao A, et al. BAP1 loss defines a new class of renal cell carcinoma. Nat Genet. 2012;44:751–9.
59. Sato Y, Yoshizato T, Shiraishi Y, et al. Integrated molecular analysis of clear-cell renal cell carcinoma. Nat Genet. 2013;45:860–7.
60. Shuch B, Vourganti S, Ricketts CJ, et al. Defining early-onset kidney cancer: implications for germline and somatic mutation testing and clinical management. J Clin Oncol. 2014;32:431–7.
61. Cancer Genome Atlas Research N. Comprehensive molecular characterization of clear cell renal cell carcinoma. Nature. 2013;499:43–9.
62. Zbar B, Tory K, Merino M, et al. Hereditary papillary renal cell carcinoma. J Urol. 1994;151:561–6.
63. Schmidt LS, Nickerson ML, Angeloni D, et al. Early onset hereditary papillary renal carcinoma: germline missense mutations in the tyrosine kinase domain of the met proto-oncogene. J Urol. 2004;172:1256–61.
64. Schmidt L, Junker K, Weirich G, et al. Two north American families with hereditary papillary renal carcinoma and identical novel mutations in the MET proto-oncogene. Cancer Res. 1998;58:1719–22.
65. Lubensky IA, Schmidt L, Zhuang Z, et al. Hereditary and sporadic papillary renal carcinomas with c-met mutations share a distinct morphological phenotype. Am J Pathol. 1999;155:517–26.
66. Ornstein DK, Lubensky IA, Venzon D, Zbar B, Linehan WM, Walther MM. Prevalence of microscopic tumors in normal appearing renal parenchyma of patients with hereditary papillary renal cancer. J Urol. 2000;163:431–3.
67. Nakamura T, Sakai K, Nakamura T, Matsumoto K. Hepatocyte growth factor twenty years on: much more than a growth factor. J Gastroenterol Hepatol. 2011;26 Suppl 1:188–202.
68. Ma PC, Maulik G, Christensen J, Salgia R. c-Met: structure, functions and potential for therapeutic inhibition. Cancer Metastasis Rev. 2003;22:309–25.
69. Zhang YW, Vande Woude GF. HGF/SF-met signaling in the control of branching morphogenesis and invasion. J Cell Biochem. 2003;88:408–17.
70. Hennessy BT, Smith DL, Ram PT, Lu Y, Mills GB. Exploiting the PI3K/AKT pathway for cancer drug discovery. Nat Rev Drug Discov. 2005;4:988–1004.
71. Launonen V, Vierimaa O, Kiuru M, et al. Inherited susceptibility to uterine leiomyomas and renal cell cancer. Proc Natl Acad Sci U S A. 2001;98:3387–92.
72. Tomlinson IP, Alam NA, Rowan AJ, et al. Germline mutations in FH predispose to dominantly inherited uterine fibroids, skin leiomyomata and papillary renal cell cancer. Nat Genet. 2002;30:406–10.
73. Shuch B, Ricketts CJ, Vocke CD, et al. Adrenal nodular hyperplasia in hereditary leiomyomatosis and renal cell cancer. J Urol. 2013;189:430–5.
74. Merino MJ, Torres-Cabala C, Pinto P, Linehan WM. The morphologic spectrum of kidney tumors in hereditary leiomyomatosis and renal cell carcinoma (HLRCC) syndrome. Am J Surg Pathol. 2007;31:1578–85.
75. Sanz-Ortega J, Vocke C, Stratton P, Linehan WM, Merino MJ. Morphologic and molecular characteristics of uterine leiomyomas in hereditary leiomyomatosis and renal cancer (HLRCC) syndrome. Am J Surg Pathol. 2013;37:74–80.

76. Chen YB, Brannon AR, Toubaji A, et al. Hereditary leiomyomatosis and renal cell carcinoma syndrome-associated renal cancer: recognition of the syndrome by pathologic features and the utility of detecting aberrant succination by immunohistochemistry. Am J Surg Pathol. 2014;38:627–37.
77. Warburg O. On the origin of cancer cells. Science. 1956;123:309–14.
78. Shuch B, Linehan WM, Srinivasan R. Aerobic glycolysis: a novel target in kidney cancer. Expert Rev Anticancer Ther. 2013;13:711–9.
79. Pollard PJ, Spencer-Dene B, Shukla D, et al. Targeted inactivation of fh1 causes proliferative renal cyst development and activation of the hypoxia pathway. Cancer Cell. 2007;11: 311–9.
80. Pollard P, Briere J, Alam N, et al. Accumulation of Krebs cycle intermediates and over-expression of HIF1alpha in tumours which result from germline FH and SDH mutations. Hum Mol Genet. 2005;14:2231–9.
81. Kobayashi A, Kang M, Watai Y, et al. Oxidative and electrophilic stresses activate Nrf2 through inhibition of ubiquitination activity of Keap1. Mol Cell Biol. 2006;26:221–9.
82. Srinivasan R, Ricketts CJ, Sourbier C, Linehan WM. New strategies in renal cell carcinoma: targeting the genetic and metabolic basis of disease. Clin Cancer Res. 2015;21:10–7.
83. Mullen A, Wheaton W, Jin E, et al. Reductive carboxylation supports growth in tumour cells with defective mitochondria. Nature. 2012;481:385–8.
84. Frezza C, Zheng L, Folger O, et al. Haem oxygenase is synthetically lethal with the tumour suppressor fumarate hydratase. Nature. 2011;477:225–8.
85. Na HK, Surh YJ. Oncogenic potential of Nrf2 and its principal target protein heme oxygenase-1. Free Radic Biol Med. 2014;67:353–65.
86. Campbell SC, Novick AC, Belldegrun A, et al. Guideline for management of the clinical T1 renal mass. J Urol. 2009;182:1271–9.
87. Ljungberg B, Bensalah K, Canfield S, et al. EAU guidelines on renal cell carcinoma: 2014 update. Eur Urol. 2015;67:913–24.
88. Leibovich BC, Blute M, Cheville JC, Lohse CM, Weaver AL, Zincke H. Nephron sparing surgery for appropriately selected renal cell carcinoma between 4 and 7 cm results in outcome similar to radical nephrectomy. J Urol. 2004;171:1066–70.
89. Lee CT, Katz J, Shi W, Thaler HT, Reuter VE, Russo P. Surgical management of renal tumors 4 cm. or less in a contemporary cohort. J Urol. 2000;163:730–6.
90. Van Poppel H, Da Pozzo L, Albrecht W, et al. A prospective, randomised EORTC intergroup phase 3 study comparing the oncologic outcome of elective nephron-sparing surgery and radical nephrectomy for low-stage renal cell carcinoma. Eur Urol. 2011;59:543–52.
91. Lau WK, Blute ML, Weaver AL, Torres VE, Zincke H. Matched comparison of radical nephrectomy vs nephron-sparing surgery in patients with unilateral renal cell carcinoma and a normal contralateral kidney. Mayo Clin Proc. 2000;75:1236–42.
92. Huang WC, Levey AS, Serio AM, et al. Chronic kidney disease after nephrectomy in patients with renal cortical tumours: a retrospective cohort study. Lancet Oncol. 2006;7:735–40.
93. Go AS, Chertow GM, Fan D, McCulloch CE, Hsu CY. Chronic kidney disease and the risks of death, cardiovascular events, and hospitalization. N Engl J Med. 2004;351:1296–305.
94. Scosyrev E, Messing EM, Sylvester R, Campbell S, Van Poppel H. Renal function after nephron-sparing surgery versus radical nephrectomy: results from EORTC randomized trial 30904. Eur Urol. 2014;65:372–7.
95. Minervini A, Serni S, Tuccio A, et al. Simple enucleation versus radical nephrectomy in the treatment of pT1a and pT1b renal cell carcinoma. Ann Surg Oncol. 2012;19:694–700.
96. Yossepowitch O, Thompson RH, Leibovich BC, et al. Positive surgical margins at partial nephrectomy: predictors and oncological outcomes. J Urol. 2008;179:2158–63.
97. Khalifeh A, Kaouk JH, Bhayani S, et al. Positive surgical margins in robot-assisted partial nephrectomy: a multi-institutional analysis of oncologic outcomes (leave no tumor behind). J Urol. 2013;190:1674–9.

98. Jewett MA, Mattar K, Basiuk J, et al. Active surveillance of small renal masses: progression patterns of early stage kidney cancer. Eur Urol. 2011;60:39–44.
99. Choueiri TK, Schutz FA, Hevelone ND, et al. Thermal ablation vs surgery for localized kidney cancer: a Surveillance, Epidemiology, and End Results (SEER) database analysis. Urology. 2011;78:93–8.
100. Chang X, Zhang F, Liu T, et al. Radio frequency ablation versus partial nephrectomy for clinical T1b renal cell carcinoma: long-term clinical and oncologic outcomes. J Urol. 2015;193:430–5.
101. Whitson JM, Harris CR, Meng MV. Population-based comparative effectiveness of nephron-sparing surgery vs ablation for small renal masses. BJU Int. 2012;110:1438–43; discussion 43.
102. Cheville JC, Lohse CM, Zincke H, Weaver AL, Blute ML. Comparisons of outcome and prognostic features among histologic subtypes of renal cell carcinoma. Am J Surg Pathol. 2003;27:612–24.
103. Herring JC, Enquist EG, Chernoff A, Linehan WM, Choyke PL, Walther MM. Parenchymal sparing surgery in patients with hereditary renal cell carcinoma: 10-year experience. J Urol. 2001;165:777–81.
104. Singer EA, Vourganti S, Lin KY, et al. Outcomes of patients with surgically treated bilateral renal masses and a minimum of 10 years of follow-up. J Urol. 2012;188:2084–8.
105. Bratslavsky G, Linehan WM. Long-term management of bilateral, multifocal, recurrent renal carcinoma. Nat Rev Urol. 2010;7:267–75.
106. Shuch B, Singer EA, Bratslavsky G. The surgical approach to multifocal renal cancers: hereditary syndromes, ipsilateral multifocality, and bilateral tumors. Urol Clin N Am. 2012;39:133–48, v.
107. Metwalli AR, Linehan WM. Nephron-sparing surgery for multifocal and hereditary renal tumors. Curr Opin Urol. 2014;24:466–73.
108. Jonasch E, Motzer RJ. Ten years of progress in renal cell carcinoma. J Natl Compr Cancer Netw: JNCCN. 2012;10:690–3.
109. NCCN Clinical Practice Guidelines in Oncology: Kidney cancer, version 2.2014: Fort Washington: National Comprehensive Cancer Network, Inc; 2014.
110. Tannir NM, Plimack E, Ng C, et al. A phase 2 trial of sunitinib in patients with advanced non-clear cell renal cell carcinoma. Eur Urol. 2012;62:1013–9.
111. Tannir NM, Wong YN, Kollmannsberger CK, et al. Phase 2 trial of linifanib (ABT-869) in patients with advanced renal cell cancer after sunitinib failure. Eur J Cancer. 2011;47:2706–14.
112. Kejzman D, et al. "Patients with metastatic papillary renal cell carcinoma (RCC) who may benefit from sunitinib therapy (tx): Results from an international metastatic RCC database." J Clin Oncol. 2014;32 (suppl 4; abstr 486).
113. Hudes G, Carducci M, Tomczak P, et al. Temsirolimus, interferon alfa, or both for advanced renal-cell carcinoma. N Engl J Med. 2007;356:2271–81.
114. Figlin RA, de Souza P, McDermott D, et al. Analysis of PTEN and HIF-1alpha and correlation with efficacy in patients with advanced renal cell carcinoma treated with temsirolimus versus interferon-alpha. Cancer. 2009;115:3651–60.
115. Escudier BJ, et al. "Open-label, phase II raptor study of everolimus (EVE) for papillary mRCC: Efficacy in type 1 and type 2 histology." J Clin Oncol. 2014;32 (suppl 4; abstr 410).
116. Armstrong AJ, et al. "ASPEN: A randomized phase II trial of everolimus versus sunitinib in patients with metastatic non-clear cell renal cell carcinoma." J Clin Oncol 2013;31(15).
117. Gordon MS, Hussey M, Nagle RB, et al. Phase II study of erlotinib in patients with locally advanced or metastatic papillary histology renal cell cancer: SWOG S0317. J Clin Oncol. 2009;27:5788–93.
118. Choueiri TK, Vaishampayan U, Rosenberg JE, et al. Phase II and biomarker study of the dual MET/VEGFR2 inhibitor foretinib in patients with papillary renal cell carcinoma. J Clin Oncol. 2013;31:181–6.

119. Srinivasan R, Su D, Stamatakis L, et al. Mechanism based targeted therapy for Hereditary Leiomyomatosis and Renal Cell Cancer (HLRCC) and sporadic papillary renal cell carcinoma: interim results from a phase 2 study of Bevacizumab and Erlotinib. 2014.
120. Linehan S, et al. The genetic basis of kidney cancer: a metabolic disease. Nat Rev Urol. 2010;7(5):277–85. PMID 20448661.

Renal Medullary Carcinoma

2

Sachin Pai and Marc R. Matrana

Introduction

Renal medullary carcinoma (RMC) is a newly recognized, rare, and aggressive form of kidney cancer, which was first described in a case series by Davis in 1995 [1]. All patients in Davis' initial series were less than 40 years old, black, and nearly all had sickle cell trait. This new entity was quickly designated the seventh sickle cell nephropathy (the other six are gross hematuria, papillary necrosis, nephrotic syndrome, renal infarction, inability to concentrate urine, and pyelonephritis [2]). Since the original report, over 150 additional cases have been reported, and clear clinical and epidemiological associations noted in the original report have been confirmed.

Overall, RMC continues to be poorly understood and prognosis is dismal. New data is slowly emerging to suggest some potential genetic and molecular features of this unusual and typically devastating kidney disease, which hopefully will lead to better therapy options.

S. Pai, MD
Ochsner Medical Oncology Fellowship Program, Ochsner Clinic Foundation, 1514 Jefferson Hwy, New Orleans, LA, USA

M.R. Matrana, MD, MSc (✉)
Hematology/Oncology Section, The Gayle and Tom Benson Cancer Center, Ochsner Medical Center, New Orleans, LA, USA

Ochsner Clinical School, The University of Queensland School of Medicine, 1514 Jefferson Hwy, New Orleans, LA, USA
e-mail: mamatrana@ochsner.org

L. Pagliaro (ed.), *Rare Genitourinary Tumors*,
DOI 10.1007/978-3-319-30046-7_2

Epidemiology

Patients diagnosed with RMC tend to be young. In one of the largest series reporting RMC, patients presented at 5–32 years of age. In the same series, 82 % of patients were African American, following rates reported in other sources (rarely RMC has been reported in Hispanic/Brazilian patients and even a few Caucasians). Virtually all patients with RMC have sickle cell trait or uncommonly sickle cell disease. A male/female ratio of 2:1 has been observed in adults, although in children the male predominance is even greater.

Clinical Presentation/Features

RMC patients tend to present with symptoms and are usually found to have a renal mass on imaging. The right kidney is more often (>75 %) affected than the left [3]. Metastasis is very common at presentation, with the regional lymph nodes, adrenal glands, lung, liver, inferior vena cava, and peritoneum being the most common sites [4].

Symptoms/Signs

The clinical presentation of RMC varies, with pain and hematuria being the most common. Presentation may sometimes be very subtle with hematuria detected on routine evaluation or incidentally detected renal mass on kidney imaging. A right-sided renal mass in a sickle cell trait patient must alert an astute clinician to consider the possibility of RMC. RMC being a very aggressive malignancy, the initial presentation can often be due to metastatic disease. Unusual metastatic patterns like spread to the scalp have been recorded in RMC [5, 6].

Imaging

Ultrasound is one of the first investigations to evaluate hematuria but may fail to show the lesion [7]. When renal ultrasound detects the lesion, it typically shows an infiltrative, right-sided renal tumor with necrosis, caliectasis, and perhaps regional adenopathy. CT and MRI are used to better define the anatomy as well as stage and resectability of the tumor [8]. In one case report, Tc-99m methylene diphosphonate bone scintigraphy incidentally detected RMC in a sickle cell trait patient [9].

Tissue Diagnosis

Fine needle aspiration examination may show poorly differentiated cancer; however, immunohistochemical studies can be helpful in distinguishing renal medullary carcinoma from other poorly differentiated kidney tumors, except for collecting duct carcinoma [10]. Definitive diagnosis is usually by biopsy, mostly excisional, and will have the features described below.

Pathology

Pathologically, the tumors are malignant epithelial tumors, which arise from collecting duct epithelium. They tend to be solitary, gray-white masses with macroscopic necrosis and hemorrhage. Microscopically, these tumors tend to be infiltrative, with poorly differentiated carcinoma of solid sheets and poorly formed vacuoles seen, although much heterogeneity exists between specimens. Other histological features seen include solid, reticular, tubular, trabecular, cribriform, and micropapillary architecture. Sarcomatoid morphology has also been described. There is usually evidence of active inflammatory cell infiltrate, with neutrophils and lymphocytes predominating. Immunoprofiles of these tumors tend to show positive expression for cytokeratin AE1/AE3, low molecular weight cytokeratin, vimentin, HIF, and VEGF. Variable expression of high molecular weight cytokeratin has been noted as well [11, 12]. The presence of rhabdoid features and the absence of INI1 expression are markers of aggressive behavior of the tumor [13]. Ultrastructural analysis showed tumor cells contain large intracytoplasmic vesicles lined by long slender microvilli with condensed fibrillary electron-dense deposits [14].

Davis and colleagues who did the seminal work on describing the pathogenesis found RMC to have overlapping features with collecting duct carcinoma [1]. Given its unique association with sickle cell anemia, the World Health Organization classification considers it as a distinct entity [15]. Other researchers have suggested that RMC might represent an aggressive variant of collecting duct tumor. It is also noted that the morphologic features show some overlaps with those seen in collecting duct carcinoma and high-grade urothelial tumors of the renal pelvis. Sarcomatoid and yolk sac tumor like morphology have been described as well. Sickle cell erythrocytes are a frequent finding within the tumor and adjacent renal tissue (Figs. 2.1 and 2.2).

Genetics and Molecular Features

A case series studied nine tumors for genetic gains and losses using comparative genomic hybridization (CGH), and eight showed no changes and one showed loss of chromosome 22. However, balanced translocations have been reported in RMC which may cause negative CGH [16]. Molecular signature of renal medullary carcinoma, clustered closely with urothelial (transitional cell) carcinoma of the renal pelvis, rather than renal cell carcinoma (RCC), may explain RMC's tendency to respond in some cases to regimens that are used in bladder cancer [17].

BCR-ABL rearrangement was reported in a single case report [18]. Another study however found that ABL gene was amplified in all three cases evaluated;

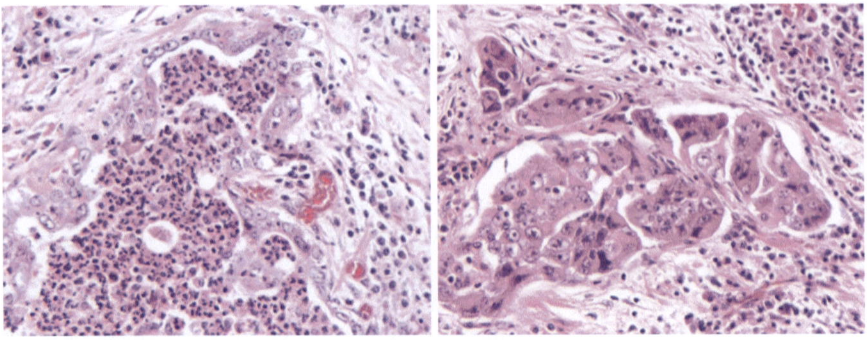

Figs. 2.1 and 2.2 Representative pathology samples of typical renal medullary carcinoma. Note the reticular architecture associated with marked desmoplasia and inflammatory infiltrates. Cells have a high nuclear-to-chromatin ratio and prominent nucleoli, large vesicular nuclei, and varying amounts of eosinophilic cytoplasm. Mitoses can be readily seen. Sickle cells are identified in blood vessels in and/or near tumor

ABL protein increased in two of three cases, but no evidence of BCR-ABL translocation was detected [19]. Topoisomerase II has been shown to be overexpressed in RMC, and the degree of topoisomerase II α overexpression has been associated with aggressive cancer and shortened survival [20].

Genetically, the loss of INI1, a factor in the ATP-dependent chromatin-modifying complex, is seen in some renal medullary carcinoma as well as renal rhabdoid tumors. The absence of INI1 expression does not appear to be predictive of rhabdoid histopathology but is associated with aggressive behavior in renal medullary carcinoma [13]. Deep sequencing of medullary kidney cancer will be needed to determine which gene or genes are critical for initiation, progression, and metastasis and much work needs to be done.

Clinical Course

As noted earlier, RMC tends to be aggressive, frequently presents in advanced stage, and responds poorly to both targeted therapies and most traditional chemotherapy agents. Mean survival time of less than 1 year is seen in most cases. There is typically poor response to most traditional therapies, especially targeted therapies that have become mainstays in other forms of kidney cancer.

Management

Given the rarity of this disease, there are no well-designed randomized clinical trials which can guide treatment decisions. Localized disease can be treated by surgery alone, and it is widely accepted that operable disease should be surgically resected. There have been a few case reports of long-term survival following complete resection of operable disease [21–23]. The role of neoadjuvant therapy to control micrometastatic disease or downstage tumors prior to surgery or the need for adjuvant therapy following surgical removal is not known.

Tannir et al. presented a series of 22 patients with RMC from four major institutions at the 2011 ASCO GU Symposium. The authors of this study found that targeted therapy has low efficacy when given as monotherapy. They noted that currently cytotoxic chemotherapy remains the mainstay of treatment, but this modality provides only modest short-term palliation, with most patients dying within a year of diagnosis [24]. Radiation may be used sparingly mostly for palliation as these tumors have not been shown to be particularly radiosensitive. Each of these strategies is discussed in detail below.

Chemotherapy

Selection of chemotherapy is based on limited experience from anecdotal case reports and small case series. The role of adjuvant therapy after surgery is not clear. There is no evidence to guide treatment decision regarding whether or not to give systemic chemotherapy following a complete resection of disease, but given that RMC typically presents with advanced disease, the question of adjuvant therapy following a complete resection is usually not an issue.

Combination chemotherapy has been favored in treating metastatic or otherwise inoperable RMC although the observed response to chemotherapy has been dismal in most cases. Cisplatin, carboplatin, gemcitabine, and paclitaxel have been found to be active compounds in RMC [25]. In one small study of three patients, the dose dense regimen of methotrexate, vinblastine, doxorubicin, and cisplatin (MVAC) was used. In this study all three patients were able to tolerate multiple cycles of MVAC and achieved at least a partial response and longer survival than predicted from the historical controls [26]. Another case report showed similar results [27].

Albadine et al. showed overexpression of topoisomerase II alpha in 11 of 13 (85 %) RMC cases which could explain the reason for activity against topoisomerase inhibitors like Adriamycin [28]. Schaeffer et al. then reported results of whole-genome expression of four RMC tumors that showed increases of topoisomerase II in all cases. They further reported a case of metastatic RMC in which a complete response was achieved for 9 months using topoisomerase II inhibitor therapy [29].

Partial responses to combination cisplatin and gemcitabine have been reported [30].

Targeted Therapy

There have been attempts to use targeted therapy with little prolonged success [31].

Tannir et al. found that targeted therapy has low efficacy when used as monotherapy [32]. A phase 2 study evaluating sunitinib in advanced non-clear cell renal cell carcinoma included six patients with RMC. In that series, four of the six patients had partial response/stable disease by RECIST criteria with a median PFS 3.1 months (CI 95 %) [33]. However, two patients in another case series from Brazil showed no response to sunitinib [13].

In a recent report, a patient was found to have decreased expression of ribonucleotide reductase M1 (RRM1) and phosphatase and tensin homolog (PTEN) on molecular analysis. Based on findings of PTEN deficiency, this patient was treated with everolimus (an MTOR inhibitor) maintenance after an induction chemotherapy regimen of paclitaxel, cisplatin, and gemcitabine. His tumor responded to induction therapy, and he went into complete remission and remained in remission for 7 months and was alive about 14 months from his diagnosis and was asymptomatic with minimal disease on last follow-up [34].

Kondagunta et al. conducted a phase 2 trial of bortezomib in metastatic RCC. One patient in this trial received intravenous bortezomib at 1.3 mg/m^2 on a twice-weekly schedule for 2 weeks followed by a 1 week treatment break, continuing for a total of 7 months of bortezomib therapy. The patient achieved a complete remission and remained free of disease after more than 27 months of follow-up [35].

Radiotherapy

There is little data about the use of radiotherapy in RMC. A few reports suggest some responsiveness to RMC metastases of the central nervous system (CNS). Walsh et al. published a case of a young man who was diagnosed with metastatic RMC and who sustained a complete response to systemic chemotherapy but later developed brain metastases and leptomeningeal disease. This patient had a partial response to brain irradiation [36]. Schaeffer et al. described a case of a 35-year-old man with metastatic RMC who had a PR after seven cycles of PGC who experienced relapse in the brain after 6 months of therapy. The patient had brain irradiation and salvage chemotherapy resulting in an initial excellent response that lasted 9 months [29]. Other cases of radiotherapy for RMC CNS have had mixed or poor response.

Karaman et al. and Stahlschmidt et al. published cases in which they used adjuvant abdominal radiation following surgical resection and chemotherapy both with little success [37, 38]. There are a few published reports of palliative radiation for bone metastases from RMV, and some of these have reported a reduction in pain and/or some decrease in the size of lesions [19]. Avery et al. noted no response to lung irradiation in a patient with RMC pulmonary metastases [16]. Although the evidence is mixed, it appears that RMC is radiosensitive in many cases (Figs. 2.3, 2.4, and 2.5).

Other Possible Therapies

The use of interferon alpha and IL-2 has been uniformly unsuccessful in RMC, but to date, there have been no reports of newer targeted immunotherapies such as PD-1 or PD-L1 antibodies. Given some similarities between RMC and urothelial cancers and given the fact that early data suggests response of urothelial to PD-1- and PD-L1-targeted immunotherapies, it seems reasonable that these newer therapies might be tried in metastatic RMC.

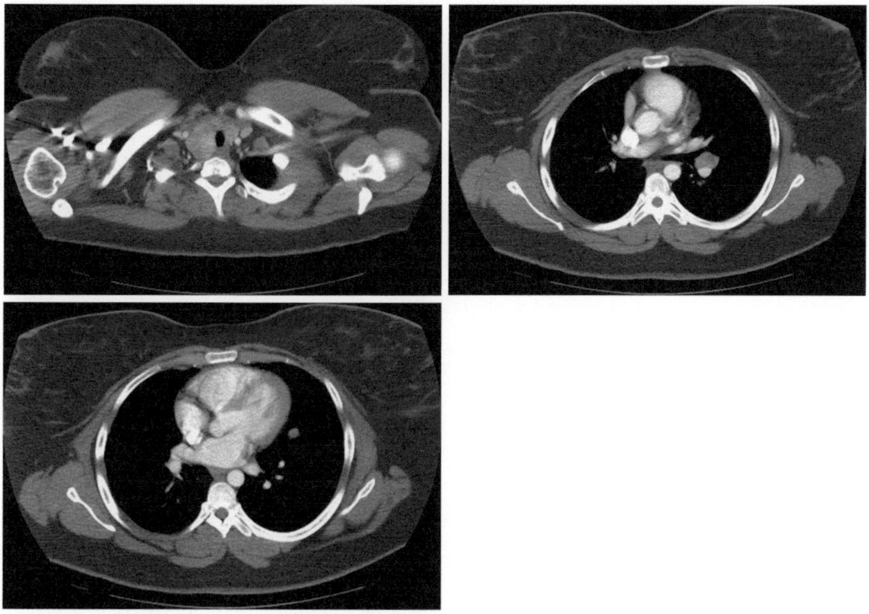

Figs. 2.3, 2.4, and 2.5 Typical radiographic findings of metastatic disease with nodules seen in the lung parenchyma and a prominent paratracheal mass

Table 2.1 Selected renal medullary carcinoma case series

Series with citation	Number of patients	Age range (in years)	Percentage with sickle cell hemoglobinopathy	Right side preponderance (percentage)	Survival range (in months)
Davis [1]	34	11–39	97	74	1–12
Avery [16]	6	24–36	100	66	1–7
Swartz [40]	40	5–32	100	75	1–15
Simpson [19]	95	5–40	98	74	1–24
Watanabe [23]	7	8–69	100	71	0–96
Hakimi [41]	9	13–31	100	89	4–16
Silvino [42]	5	23–30	100	N/A	1–26
Tannir [43]	20	N/A	95 (5 % not tested)	N/A	7–18

Rearrangement of the ALK receptor tyrosine kinase has been reported in renal medullary carcinoma as well. Mariño-Enríquez et al. identified a novel ALK oncoprotein in which the cytoskeletal protein vinculin (VCL) was fused to the ALK kinase domain in a case of RMC harboring a t(2;10)(p23;q22) translocation. Their report suggests a rationale for studying the treatment of RMC with targeted ALK inhibitors [39] (Tables 2.1 and 2.2).

Table 2.2 Clinical features of renal medullary carcinoma

Typical patient characteristics	
Younger patients	Patients tend to present in adolescence or early adulthood
Racial predominance	African Americans are most predominantly affected by RMC
Gender predominance	Males are much more common affected than females
Sickle cell association	Most patients with RMC carry sickle cell trait or rarely have sickle cell disease
Tumor characteristics	
Right-sided predominance	Tumors tend to originate in the right kidney more often than the left
Pathology	RMC is malignant epithelial tumor that arises from collecting duct epithelium
	Have features that overlap with collecting duct tumors
	Microscopically, RMC tend to be infiltrative, with poorly differentiated carcinoma of solid sheets and poorly formed vacuoles, although much heterogeneity exists between specimens
	There is usually evidence of active inflammatory cell infiltrate
Typical clinical course	
Aggressive course	RMC typically presents in advanced stages and behaves aggressively
Response to therapy	There is limited response to targeted therapies and generally weak response to traditional chemotherapy regions
Prognosis	Prognosis is poor, with most patients with metastatic disease surviving less than 1 year

Conclusion

Although rare, RMC has garnered interest among oncologists, as well as physicians who treat sickle cell disease. There are currently no open clinical trials aimed solely at RMC, but a handful of trials seek to enroll patients with various forms of non-clear cell kidney cancer. As the molecular drivers of RMC are further elucidated in the laboratory, new treatment options should emerge.

References

1. Davis CJ, Mostofi FK, Sesterhenn IA. Renal medullary carcinoma: the seventh sickle cell nephropathy. Am J Surg Pathol. 1995;19:1–11.
2. Berman LB. Sickle cell nephropathy. JAMA. 1974;228:1279.
3. Sathyamoorthy K, Teo A, Atallah M. Renal medullary carcinoma in a patient with sickle-cell disease. Nat Clin Pract Urol. 2006;3:279–83.
4. Patel K, Livni N, Macdonald D. Renal medullary carcinoma, a rare cause of hematuria in sickle cell trait. Br J Haematol. 2005;132:1.
5. Johnson RP, et al. Renal medullary carcinoma metastatic to the scalp. Am J Dermatopathol. 2011;33(1):e11–3.
6. Nava VE, Mullin BR, Schuldenfrei JA. Renal medullary carcinoma metastatic to forehead. Am J Dermatopathol. 2011;33(7):757.

7. Wesche WA, et al. Renal medullary carcinoma: a potential sickle cell nephropathy of children and adolescents. Pediatr Pathol Lab Med. 1998;18(1):97–113.
8. Blitman NM, et al. Renal medullary carcinoma: CT and MRI features. AJR Am J Roentgenol. 2005;185(1):268–72.
9. Brown JM, Berkey BD, Brooks JA. Discovery of a renal medullary carcinoma in an adolescent male with sickle cell trait by Tc-99m methylene disphosponate bone scintigraphy. Clin Nucl Med. 2008;33(12):896–900.
10. Assad L, et al. Cytologic features of renal medullary carcinoma. Cancer. 2004;105(1):28–34.
11. Yan BC, Mackinnon AC, Al-Ahmadie HA. Recent developments in the pathology of renal tumors: morphology and molecular characteristics of select entities. Arch Pathol Lab Med. 2009;133:1026–32.
12. Srigley JR, Delahunt B. Uncommon and recently described renal carcinomas. Mod Pathol. 2009;22 Suppl 2:S2–23.
13. Cheng JX, et al. Renal medullary carcinoma: rhabdoid features and the absence of INI1 expression as markers of aggressive behavior. Mod Pathol. 2008;21(6):647–52.
14. Wartchow EP, et al. Renal medullary carcinoma: ultrastructural studies may benefit diagnosis. Ultrastruct Pathol. 2008;32(6):252–6.
15. Srigley JR, Moch H. Carcinoma of the collecting ducts of Bellini. In: Eble JN, Sauter G, Epstein JI, et al., editors. World Health Organization classification of tumors pathology & genetics: tumors of the urinary system and male genital organs. Lyons: IARC; 2004. p. 33–4.
16. Avery RA, et al. Renal medullary carcinoma: clinical and therapeutic aspects of a newly described tumor. Cancer. 1996;78(1):128–32.
17. Yang XJ, et al. Gene expression profiling of renal medullary carcinoma. Cancer. 2004;100(5):976–85.
18. Stahlshmidt J, et al. Renal medullary carcinoma: prolonged remission with chemotherapy, immunohistochemical characterisation and evidence of bcr/abl rearrangement. Med Pediatr Oncol. 1999;33(6):551–7.
19. Simpson L, et al. Renal medullary carcinoma and Abl gene amplification. J Urol. 2005;173(6):1883–8.
20. Linehan WM. Genetic basis of kidney cancer: role of genomics for the development of disease-based therapeutics. Genome Res. 2012;22(11):2089–100.
21. Khan A, Thomas N, Costello B, et al. Renal medullary carcinoma: sonographic, computed tomography, magnetic resonance and angiographic findings. Eur J Radiol. 2000;35:1–7.
22. Selby DM, Simon C, Foley JP, et al. Renal medullary carcinoma: can early diagnosis lead to long-term survival? J Urol. 2000;163:1238.
23. Watanabe IC, Billis A, Guimaraes MS, et al. Renal medullary carcinoma: report of seven cases from Brazil. Mod Pathol. 2007;20:914–20.
24. Tannir NM, Lim ZD, Rao P, et al. Outcome of patients with renal medullary carcinoma (RMC) treated in the era of targeted therapies (TT): a multicenter experience. GU ASCO Symposium, Orlando, 18 Feb 2011.
25. Gangireddy V, et al. Response of metastatic renal medullary carcinoma to carboplatin and Paclitaxel chemotherapy. Clin Genitourin Cancer. 2012;10(2):134–9.
26. Rathmell WK, Monk JP. High-dose-intensity MVAC for advanced renal medullary carcinoma: report of three cases and literature review. Urology. 2008;72(3):659–63.
27. Amjad AI, et al. Renal medullary carcinoma: case report of an aggressive malignancy with near-complete response to dose-dense methotrexate, vinblastine, Doxorubicin, and Cisplatin chemotherapy. Case Rep Oncol Med. 2014;2014:615895.
28. Albadine R, et al. Topoisomerase II α status in renal medullary carcinoma: immuno-expression and gene copy alterations of a potential target of therapy. J Urol. 2009;182(2):735–40.
29. Schaeffer EM, Guzzo TJ, Furge KA, et al. Renal medullary carcinoma: molecular, pathological and clinical evidence for treatment with topoisomerase-inhibiting therapy. BJU Int. 2010;106(1):62–5.
30. Maroja Silvino MC, Venchiarutti Moniz CM, Munhoz Piotto GH, et al. Renal medullary carcinoma response to chemotherapy: a referral center experience in Brazil. Rare Tumor. 2013;5(3):e44.

31. Shetty A, Matrana MR. Renal medullary carcinoma: a case report and brief review of the literature. Ochsner J. 2014;14(2):270–5.
32. Tannir NM, Lim ZD, Bekele BN, et al. Outcome of patients with renal medullary carcinoma (RMC) treated in the era of targeted therapies (TT): a multicenter experience. J Clin Oncol. 2011;29(Suppl 7):abstract 386.
33. Tannir NM, et al. A phase 2 trial of sunitinib in patients with advanced non–clear cell renal cell carcinoma. Eur Urol. 2012;62(6):1013–9.
34. Lipkin JS, et al. Therapeutic approach guided by genetic alteration: use of MTOR inhibitor in renal medullary carcinoma with loss of PTEN expression. Cancer Biol Ther. 2015;16(1):28–33.
35. Kondagunta GV, Drucker B, Schwartz L, et al. Phase II trial of bortezomib for patients with advanced renal cell carcinoma. J Clin Oncol. 2004;22(18):3720–5.
36. Walsh AM, Fiveash JB, Reddy AT, et al. Response to radiation in renal medullary carcinoma. Rare Tumors. 2011;3(3):e32.
37. Karaman S, Celkan T, Kuruoglu S, et al. Renal medullary carcinoma case presenting with abdominal mass. Turk J Cancer. 2005;35:96–8.
38. Stahlschmidt J, Cullinane C, Roberts P, Picton SV. Renal medullary carcinoma: prolonged remission with chemotherapy, immunohistochemical characterisation and evidence of bcr/abl rearrangement. Med Pediatr Oncol. 1999;33:551–7.
39. Mariño-Enríquez A, Ou WB, Weldon CB, Fletcher JA, Pérez-Atayde AR. ALK rearrangement in sickle cell trait-associated renal medullary carcinoma. Genes Chromosom Cancer. 2011;50(3):146–53.
40. Swartz MA, et al. Renal medullary carcinoma: clinical, pathologic, immunohistochemical, and genetic analysis with pathogenetic implications. Urology. 2002;60(6):1083–9.
41. Hakimi AA, et al. Renal medullary carcinoma: the bronx experience. Urology. 2007;70(5):878–82.
42. Silvino MCM, et al. Renal medullary carcinoma response to chemotherapy: a referral center experience in Brazil. Rare Tumors. 2013;5(3):44.
43. Tannir NM, Lim ZD, Bekele BN, Johnson ED, Tamboli P, Vaishampayan UN, Plimack ER, Rathmell K, Jonasch E. Outcome of patients (pts) with renal medullary carcinoma (RMC) treated in the era of targeted therapies (TT): a multicenter experience. J Clin Oncol. 2011;29(suppl 7):abstr 386.

Translocation Renal Cell Carcinomas 3

Jad Chahoud, Gabriel G. Malouf, and Nizar M. Tannir

Introduction

Translocation renal cell carcinoma (tRCC) is a rare kidney cancer subtype, first added to the 2004 WHO RCC classification based on morphologic features and genetics [1]. tRCCs are defined by translocations involving MiT family genes including *TFE3*, *TFEB*, and *MiTF*. First, the TFE3 family translocation carcinomas are characterized by translocations involving *TFE3* gene and leading to overexpression of the chimeric fusion protein that disrupts transcription regulation. The hallmark of this group is a fusion of *TFE3* gene to various targets that include *PRCC* in t(X;1)(p11.2;q21), *ASPSCR1* in t(X;17)(p11.2;q25), *SFPQ* in t(X;1)(p11.2;p34), *NONO* in inv (X)(p11.2;q12), *CLTC* in t(X;17)(p11;q23), *LUC7L3* on 17q (17q21.33), and *MED15* on (22q11.2) [2–6]. The two most common Xp11 tRCCs are those bearing the t(X;1)(p11.2;q21), which fuses the *PRCC* and *TFE3* genes, and the t(X;1)(p11.2;p34), which fuses the *SFPQ* gene. The second, less common group is the MiT/TFEB family, t(6;11)(p21;q22), that harbors multiple specific *Alpha-TFEB*, *KHDRBS-TFEB*, or *CLTC-TFEB* gene fusions which induce the overexpression of transcription factor EB (TFEB) [5, 7, 8]. A third family was recently

J. Chahoud, MD
Department of Internal Medicine, The University of Texas Health Science Center, University of Texas Medical School at Houston, Houston, TX 77030, USA
e-mail: Jad.M.Chahoud@uth.tmc.edu

G.G. Malouf, MD, PhD
Department of Medical Oncology, Groupe Hospitalier Pitié-Salpêtrière, Hopitaux de Paris, Faculty of Medicine Pierre et Marie Curie, Institut Universitaire de Cancérologie GRC5, University Paris 6, Paris, France
e-mail: gabriel.malouf@aphp.fr

N.M. Tannir, MD (✉)
Department of Genitourinary Medical Oncology, The University of Texas MD Anderson Cancer Center, Houston, TX 77030, USA
e-mail: ntannir@mdanderson.org

L. Pagliaro (ed.), *Rare Genitourinary Tumors*,
DOI 10.1007/978-3-319-30046-7_3

described by Durinck et al. consisting of the *ACTG1-MiTF* fusion gene [8]. Argani et al. proposed nuclear immunohistochemical staining for TFE3 and TFEB as an indicator of abnormal overexpression of these proteins in tRCCs as these proteins are not usually expressed in normal tissue, but this method remains highly nonspecific [9]. Since the genetic alterations in these tumors are different from those reported in conventional RCCs, their clinical features, epidemiology, biological behavior, prognostic factors, and treatment paradigms may be different. This chapter addresses in detail the aforementioned aspects of tRCC.

Epidemiology and Clinical Presentation

The first published case of Xp11 tRCC was reported in a 17-month-old child by Tomlinson et al. [10]. It is estimated that the majority of pediatric RCCs are Xp11 tRCCs, whereas conventional clear cell RCCs make up about less than 5 % of RCCs in children [11]. Although tRCC is rare in adults, it estimated to represent 15 % of RCCs in patients younger than 45 years [12–14]. The reported overall incidence of tRCC ranges between 1 and 6 % according to previously published studies, few of which used morphology and *TFE3* expression alone to screen for tRCC cases [15–17]. However, the frequency in adults may be underestimated, due to morphological overlap with more common adult RCC subtypes, such as conventional clear cell RCC and papillary RCC. One single-institution study assessed 443 consecutive nephrectomies performed for RCC in adults and found that 1.6 % were Xp11 tRCC by cytogenetic or TFE3 immunohistochemical analysis [17]. Also, Zhong et al. assessed 120 consecutive RCCs older than 18 years of age by FISH for *TFE3* rearrangements and showed an estimated incidence for Xp11 tRCC of at least 4.2 % [16]. In North America, a case series demonstrated that tRCCs are more frequent in female patients (male-to-female ratio (1:3.6)) and in those of African-American descent [14, 18]. While in the European continent, we know even less about the epidemiology of these tumors. Notably, 15 % of tRCC occurs in patients who had received cytotoxic chemotherapy during childhood [19]. Although a history of prior treatment for primary malignancies has been reported by several publications as a risk factor for tRCC [20–22], it is not clear yet whether RCC in these settings results from specific therapeutic regimens that promote its carcinogenesis or if underlying genetic predisposition is involved [23]. Indications for the antecedent chemotherapy included acute promyelocytic leukemia, acute myeloid leukemia, Wilms' tumor, systemic lupus erythematosus, and conditioning regimen of bone marrow transplant for Hurler's syndrome [19]. The interval between chemotherapy and time of diagnosis ranged between 4 and 13 years. All of the reported cases included in the review by Argani et al. were pediatric patients and had received either a DNA topoisomerase II inhibitor and/or an alkylating agent [19]. Although they have differing mechanisms of action, both cytotoxic agents break DNA, which may initiate repair or recombination mechanisms that permit a chromosome translocation to occur [19].

On the other hand, the t(6;11) RCCs are less common than the Xp11 tRCCs [24]. They have recently been accepted by the 2013 International Society of Urological

Pathology Vancouver classification of renal neoplasia as a subtype of the MiT family of tRCC. The distinctive clinicopathologic features of these neoplasms were first described in 2001, and till this date, approximately 50 cases only have been reported in the literature [25]. While the original reported cases were in children and young adults, it was clear that these neoplasms will also present in adults. In fact, the reported ages ranged between 3 and 68 years, with respective mean and median age of 31 years and 43, representing a much younger age in comparison with conventional clear cell and papillary RCC of adults [25]. Similar to the Xp11 tRCC, a subset of cases occurred in patients who had received cytotoxic chemotherapy for other disorders [26]. Pediatric patients maintain a favorable short-term prognosis, even though the majority of cases present with an advanced tumor stage at time of diagnosis. Meanwhile, reports indicate that tRCCs arising in adults are more aggressive and produce an unfavorable outcome, with the majority showing nodal spread at time of diagnosis [18, 27]. The prognosis and outcome will be discussed in detail under section "X.7. Prognosis and Outcome." A large cohort of TFE3 and TFEB RCC was evaluated by Malouf et al. [28]. Their results strongly indicated that age and lymph node stage should be considered as prognostic factors in patients with tRCC. They noted a bimodal distribution of patients according to age, with two peaks at 16 and 36 years. The only clinicopathological difference between patients younger and those older than 25 years was the presence of distant metastasis, with mediastinal lymph nodes representing the most common site of metastasis. In their study, the two patients with *ASPSCR1-TFE3* fusion had more aggressive disease compared to others with *PRCC*, *CLTC*, or *SFPQ* fusion genes. These results corroborate previous reports about the poor prognosis of *ASPSCR1-TFE3* fusion RCC subtype [17, 18]. Moreover, gender may have a role, since males seem to experience metastasis twice as frequently as females which is also consistent with previous reports describing a more aggressive disease course in adult males [18, 27].

Gross and Microscopic Features

The typical gross appearance of Xp11 tRCC often reveals a tan-yellow necrotic and hemorrhagic tumor, grossly confused with conventional clear cell RCC. The typical microscopic pattern is a combination of both clear cells and papillary architecture where abundant psammoma bodies can be noted. Areas with a solid growth pattern are rarely observed. It is of great importance to always consider Xp11 tRCC in the differential of renal tumors in adolescents and young adults, as multiple reports have described a wide spectrum of microscopic presentations seen in this type of tumors that can mimic other types of RCC. For example, Xp11 tRCCs can alternatively show solid or nested growth with clear to granular eosinophilic cytoplasm. Certain distinctive morphologies are associated with specific gene fusions. The *ASPL-TFE3* gene fusion is associated with extensive psammomatous calcification, large tumor cells with voluminous abundant cytoplasm, vesicular chromatin, discrete cell borders, and prominent nucleoli [29–31]. On the other hand, the *PRCC-TFE3* gene fusion typically has tumor cells with less cytoplasm, a more nested growth pattern, and absent or few psammoma bodies [32–34]. Other fusion gene-associated typical morphology is yet to be clarified, as there are no sufficient reports describing their features. One case reported an Xp11 tRCC in a young adult that presented with multilocular cystic RCC-like and microscopic features consistent with a single layer of clear cells, small areas with a papillary pattern, psammomatous calcification, and grade 3 nuclear atypia. Also, immunohistochemical analysis confirmed labeling for TFE3 protein [35]. Two large, clinicopathologic studies evaluated, respectively, 28 [18] and 31 cases [36] of Xp11.2 tRCCs and reported, respectively, 50 % and 62 % frequency of identified psammoma bodies. However, psammoma bodies, a feature that is rarely observed in conventional clear cell RCC, are not specific nor pathognomonic of tRCC as it has occasionally been seen in papillary RCC [9, 18, 27].

Immunohistochemistry

Translocation RCC tend to demonstrate an immunoreactivity pattern that differs from conventional clear cell RCC. We will discuss separately the variable Xp11 and t(6,11) tRCC presenting patterns of immunoreactivity.

First, Xp11 RCCs express both of the clear cell and papillary RCC markers: CD10, a cell membrane metal-lopeptidase whose expression is localized to the proximal tubular brush border, and RCC antigen marker, also a proximal brush border antigen, which is fairly specific and sensitive for RCC. This is in contrast with cases of chromophobe RCC where these markers are not expressed [37]. Moreover, the largest study evaluating patients with t(6,11) reported that RCC marker antigen and CD10 each labeled 10 out of the 14 evaluated cases [25]. Xp11 tRCCs mostly expressed PAX2 and PAX8, which are lineage-restricted transcription factors known to be expressed in the renal and Müllerian systems in most clear cell and papillary RCCs [38–40]. On the other hand, t(6,11) RCCs were only positive for PAX8 in 14 of 23 cases (59 %) in the same study referenced above [25].

Both Xp11 and t(6,11) RCCs underexpress epithelial markers such as cytokeratin and epithelial membrane antigen (EMA). However, cathepsin-K may be useful as a specific marker for these carcinomas. The cathepsin-K has been proven to be mediated by overexpression of *MiTF* in osteoclasts [23]. A study by Martignoni et al. reported the expression of cathepsin-K in six out of ten confirmed Xp11 tRCCs. In contrast, none of the conventional clear cell RCCs (210 cases), papillary RCCs (40 cases), chromophobe RCCs (25 cases), oncocytomas (30 cases), or adjacent nonneoplastic renal tissue showed immunoreactivity for cathepsin-K [41]. Therefore, this marker is considered highly specific and may be useful to rule in the suspected diagnosis of an Xp11 tRCC, even though the sensitivity is less than that of TFE3. The immunohistochemical marker that combines the highest sensitivity and specificity for the Xp11 tRCC is strong nuclear *TFE3* immunoreactivity. In one study, the sensitivity was 97.5 % (39 of 40 positive control tumors) and specificity was 99.6 % (6 of 1,476 negative controls) [42]. Nuclear labeling for *TFE3* is specific to Xp11.2 translocations, keeping in mind that immunostaining of *TFE3* is nuclear and should be obvious at low-power magnification with absence cytoplasmic labeling of tumor cells and nuclear labeling in adjacent normal kidney. Also, previous reports have shown that 83 % of the t(6; 11) RCCs labeled diffusely for cathepsin-K, while 12 of 13 cases labeled for HMB-45, though the labeling was much less extensive, and cytokeratin Cam 5.2 was expressed in 8 of 13 cases (62 %) [25]. Rarely, Xp11 tRCCs with typical morphology express melanocytic markers such as Melan-A and HMB-45. Even though IHC might be helpful in few instances, this test remains of low sensitivity and predictive value, and the diagnosis of Xp11.2 translocation RCC may be made only genetically [43].

Cytogenetic and Molecular Features

Xp11 and t(6,11) RCCs are characterized, respectively, by translocations involving the genes for transcription factors E3 (*TFE3*) and EB (*TFEB*). TFE3 and TFEB are members of the microphthalmia transcription factor-transcription factor E (MiTF/TFE) family of basic helix-loop-helix leucine zipper (bHLH-zip) [9, 18, 44]. The *TFEB* gene is known to fuse with the *Alpha* gene, the *CLTC* gene, and *KHDBRS2* gene. On the other hand, the *TFE3* gene (Xp11.2) has been found to rearrange with a minimum of seven different partners: *PRCC* (1q21), *ASPSCR1* (17q25), *SFPQ* (1p34), *NONO* (Xq12), *LUC7L3* (17q21.33), *MED15* (22q11.2), and *CLTC* (17q23) [5, 6, 9, 16–18, 44]. Also, t(X;3)(p11;q23) and t(X;19)(p11.2;q13.1s) have been reported without a defined gene partner. Moreover, the *TFEB* gene rearranges with *Alpha*, leading to a translocation that preserves the full-length *TFEB* coding region [27]. All TFE3 fusion proteins contain the bHLH-LZ and transcriptional activation domains of *TFE3*, but the breakpoints of those translocations differ according to the *TFE3* partner [7]. Little is known about whether additional genetic alterations are associated with tRCC. Malouf et al. were the first to shed light on this in their study evaluating single-nucleotide polymorphism array profiling and LINE-1 methylation [45]. This study found cytogenomic and epigenetic heterogeneity in tRCCs cases. Interestingly, these included alterations common in clear cell RCC (e.g., 3p loss) and papillary RCC (e.g., trisomy 7 and/or 17). They also found that adults, in comparison with patients younger than 18 years, displayed distinct genomic and epigenetic aberrations, exemplified by lower LINE-1 methylation and frequent 17q partial gain. Their data showed the significant inverse correlation between the degree of genomic alterations and the LINE-1 methylation levels, similar to previously reported data in other tumor types [46]. The partial 17q gain was frequent in tumors from adult men and was associated with a poor outcome. Of interest, 17q gains are rare in clear cell RCC and papillary RCC, in contrast to trisomy 7 and 17, which are very frequent in papillary RCC [47]. A larger study should evaluate, whether adults with tRCC without a 17q gain have a different prognosis than adults with the 17q gain. It is notable that cases with 17q gain also had gene expression patterns consistent with activation of T-helper cells and the CTLA-4 signaling pathway. Their study did not evaluate for intratumoral heterogeneity with respect to the presence of 17q and other chromosomal abnormalities, which might be helpful to understand whether 17q is an initiating event or acquired during tumor progression [48]. Another study by Malouf et al. evaluated genome-wide analysis to assess for the genomic abnormalities of tRCC [5]. Their results reported that first, the *MiTF/TFE* was the most frequent recurrent translocation identified. The landscape of mutations for tRCC differs from those of other RCC types which are characterized by mutations of *VHL*, *PBRM1*, or *BAP1*, yet no recurrent mutations were identified. Second, the spectrum of *TFE3/TFEB* fusion transcripts in adults was different compared to historical series, and they identified two novel partners of *TFE3*, *LUC7L3* and *KHSRP*. Third, transcriptomic profiling of tRCC revealed that the majority of cases belonged to the ccB transcriptomic group, and ingenuity pathway analysis revealed TGF-β1 and PI3K complex activations. This highlights the interest of inhibiting the TGFβ1 and PI3K pathways, as these may represent potential therapeutic options for patients with tRCC. Lastly, 75 % of the evaluated tRCC cases had mutations in chromatin remodeling genes, specifically, mutations in *INO80D* chromatin remodeling gene, a mutation never previously reported in cancer. It is interesting to note that knockdown of *INO80D* controls the amplitude of the S phase and decreased cell proliferation in HCR-59 cell line bearing *LUC7L3-TFE3* translocation [49]. This may render the *INO80D* mutations a marker of an aggressive phenotype of tRCC.

Prognosis and Outcome

Xp11.2 tRCCs occur primarily, but not exclusively, in children and young adults and are believed to be rather indolent in this subgroup, even when presenting with a locally advanced disease and regional lymph node involvement, without hematogenous spread. Based on a literature review, over 90 % of these patients remained disease-free at last follow-up having a median of 4.4 years and a mean of 6.3 years [14]. In contrast, the tumor tends to be more aggressive in adults with widespread systemic metastases [43, 49]. Overall, survival is similar to that of patients with clear cell RCC and significantly worse than that of patients with papillary RCC. In a case series of 15 Xp11 tRCC treated with vascular endothelial growth factor (VEGF)-targeted therapy, the median PFS and OS of the entire cohort were 7.1 months and 14.3 months, respectively [50]. Malouf et al. described outcomes in 54 patients with tRCC, at diagnosis two-thirds of patients had localized disease and a third presented with distant metastasis [28]. All but one patient underwent nephrectomy with regional lymphadenectomy. Overall, the 35 patients with localized disease had complete surgical resection; in addition, one patient with lung metastasis underwent wedge lung resection. No perioperative death occurred and no patients received neoadjuvant chemotherapy. Of the 36 patients who underwent complete resection, 8 had recurrence. Multivariate analysis showed that solely lymph node involvement was independently associated with recurrence-free survival (RFS) [28]. Median RFS was 8.7 months in lymph node-positive cases and was not reached in lymph node-negative cases. After a median follow-up of 19.2 months, median overall survival (OS) of patients with distant metastasis was

22.2 months. OS at 1 and 3 years was 61.1 % (95 % CI 42.3–88.3) and 14.3 % (95 % CI 4–51.5), respectively [28]. Median OS of patients without distant metastasis was not reached. OS at 1 and 3 years was 100 % and 70.6 % (95 % CI 51.9–95.9), respectively. Based on the multivariate analysis, lymph node involvement and age were independently associated with poor OS [28]. In a smaller case series, mean survival after diagnosis was 18 months with a range of 10–24 months [27]. Another adult series, with at least 1 year of follow-up, reported that five of six patients developed hematogenous spread, and two patients died within 1 year of diagnosis [18].

On the other hand, the t(6;11) RCCs are more indolent neoplasms than the Xp11 tRCCs. Of the approximately 50 cases in the published literature, only four have developed metastases, leading to patient death in three cases. The majority of neoplasms presented at low stage (pT1 or pT2) and had a slow disease progression of disease. Like the Xp11 tRCC, these neoplasms have demonstrated the capacity to recur late (up to 20 years after diagnosis), thus the importance of long-term follow-up for tRCC patients. Furthermore, Ellis et al. recently reviewed the literature on Xp11 tRCC with the *ASPSCR1-TFE3* and *PRCC-TFE3* gene fusions [33]. Using a multivariate analysis, they concluded that only advanced stage (specifically distant metastasis) and older age at diagnosis were independent predictor of overall survivor [33]. The association of older age with a worse outcome is supported by the abovementioned genetic data by Malouf et al., who found more chromosome 17q gain in adult Xp11 tRCCs compared with pediatric cases [45]. *ASPSCR1-TFE3* RCCs were significantly more associated with locoregionally advanced presentation at diagnosis and distant metastasis (24 of 32 cases, 75 %) than were *PRCC-TFE3* RCC (5 of 14 cases, 36 %), while most of the previous patients remained disease-free without adjuvant therapy. Hence, locally advanced stage may not predict adverse outcomes. However, all patients who presented with distant metastases had *ASPSCR1-TFE3* RCC, and these patients have poor outcomes [33]. A considerable clinical heterogeneity in the cases was reported, as some patients with advanced disease died rapidly, whereas others followed a more indolent course. Another interesting finding was that nonmetastatic patients with node positive tended to have a worse outcome when they had a *PRCC-TFE3* RCC than if they had an *ASPSCR1-TFE3* RCC, though that reported difference was not statistically significant [33]. Moreover, a partial 17q gain is frequent in tumors from adult patients, particularly in men, and this genetic lesion might be used as marker of aggressive disease and poor outcomes [45]. Interestingly, tRCC patients with 3p loss (clear cell RCC-like profile) had worse outcomes compared to those without 3p loss [45].

Treatment

The optimal therapy for the Xp11.2 tRCCs remains to be determined, as clinical trials have been mainly conducted in patients with clear cell histology. In this section, we will discuss some of the largest studies that reported outcomes in concordance with different therapeutic options. Choueiri et al. [50] published one of the largest studies reporting targeted therapy for adult patients with metastatic translocation Xp11 RCC. They retrospectively reviewed 15 patients with metastatic Xp11 RCC, of whom 10, 3, and 2 received sunitinib, sorafenib, and monoclonal anti-VEGF antibodies, respectively. The median follow-up period was 19.1 months, the median age of the patients was 41 years, and the female-to-male ratio was 4:1. Five patients had received prior systemic therapy, none of them experienced disease response at that time, 12 patients had received a prior nephrectomy, and 9 patients were intermediate risk as per Memorial Sloan-Kettering Cancer Center (MSKCC) score [50]. When treated with VEGF-targeted therapy, three patients achieved a partial response, seven patients had stable disease, and five patients developed progressive disease. Three patients who developed disease progression after initial VEGF-targeted therapy subsequently received temsirolimus, and all were found to develop progressive disease at their first restaging evaluation [50]. The median PFS and OS of the entire cohort were 7.1 months and 14.3 months, respectively. These results demonstrated that VEGF-targeted therapy can provide benefit for adults with metastatic Xp11.2 RCC, as evidenced by a response rate of 20 % and a median PFS of 7.1 months [50]. However, it was impossible for the authors to make definitive conclusions regarding the best VEGF-targeted agent for patients with this disease since responses occurred with three different drugs, and the studied sample was small.

Another recent multicenter study from several French centers by Malouf et al. [51] reported on 21 patients with metastatic Xp11.2 RCC who were treated with VEGF- and mTOR-targeted therapies. Fifteen had metastases at presentation and six developed distant metastasis within 1 year of nephrectomy (range 2–9 months). The median age of the patients was 34 years, and the female-to-male ratio was 1:1. All 21 patients had received a nephrectomy, while 9 patients had a prior systemic therapy with cytokine. As per the MSKCC score, 15 patients were intermediate and 6 were high risk [51]. Patients treated with sunitinib were found to have a median PFS of 8.2 months if they received prior therapy similar to that for clear cell RCC and a median PFS of 11 months if they were previously treatment-naive [51]. Patients treated with sorafenib had a median PFS of 6 months, whereas for patients treated with temsirolimus it was 3 months. Seven patients (33 %) experienced objective responses, with a median follow-up of 19 months, the estimated median OS was 27 months (range 12–43 months) [51]. All the patients treated with sunitinib and one patient treated with temsirolimus achieved responses. The efficacy data reported by Malouf et al. are somewhat better than those reported by Choueiri et al., which could be explained by the fact that the French series did not restrict their study to adults, with five patients (24 %) aged <18 years [50, 51]. As it has been shown in previous reports, adults with Xp11.2 RCC tend to have a more aggressive disease course than their pediatric counterparts. The mechanism of efficacy of VEGF-targeted therapy in patients with Xp11.2 RCC is largely unknown. VEGF-targeted agents demonstrated efficacy in two of the largest published experiences in the treatment of this subgroup of RCC, comprised of retrospective series of 15 and 21 metastatic patients. All patients who progressed on VEGF-targeted therapy and were switched over in the French series to an mTOR inhibitor achieved stable disease. One patient even had a partial response lasting 15 months. This highlights the importance of maintaining some form of targeted therapy in patients with Xp11 translocation mRCC progressing on VEGF-targeted therapy. The mTOR inhibitors temsirolimus and everolimus target the PI3K/AKT/mTOR signaling pathways. A recent study interestingly found that transcriptomic profiling of tRCC and ingenuity pathway analysis revealed TGF-β1 and PI3K complex activations in the majority of tRCC cases [5], though inhibiting the TGFβ1 and PI3K pathways may present other potential therapeutic options. Nevertheless, the abovementioned two studies had a retrospective design with inherent potential biases that preclude a definitive statement regarding whether VEGF-targeted agents should be the preferred therapy for patients with advanced stage Xp11.2 RCC. At the present time, there is no standard treatment protocol for patients with tRCC. For future research, further genetic and epigenetic studies are needed to prioritize the discovery of more effective targeted therapies.

References

1. Cubilla A, Dillner J, Schellhammer P, et al. Tumors of the penis. World Heal Organ Classif Tumour Pathol Genet Tumour Urin Syst Male Genet Organ. 2004;65:281–298. doi:10.1016/j.urology.2004.09.048.
2. Argani P, Lui MY, Couturier J, Bouvier R, Fournet J-C, Ladanyi M. A novel CLTC-TFE3 gene fusion in pediatric renal adenocarcinoma with t(X;17)(p11.2;q23). Oncogene. 2003;22(34):5374–8. doi:10.1038/sj.onc.1206686.
3. Argani P, Antonescu CR, Couturier J, et al. PRCC-TFE3 renal carcinomas: morphologic, immunohistochemical, ultrastructural, and molecular analysis of an entity associated with the t(X;1)(p11.2;q21). Am J Surg Pathol. 2002;26(12):1553–66. http://www.ncbi.nlm.nih.gov/pubmed/12459622. Accessed June 21, 2015.
4. Argani P, Antonescu CR, Illei PB, et al. Primary renal neoplasms with the ASPL-TFE3 gene fusion of alveolar soft part sarcoma: a distinctive tumor entity previously included among renal cell carcinomas of children and adolescents. Am J Pathol. 2001;159(1):179–92. doi:10.1016/S0002-9440(10)61684-7.
5. Malouf GG, Su X, Yao H, et al. Next-generation sequencing of translocation renal cell carcinoma reveals novel RNA splicing partners and frequent mutations of chromatin-remodeling genes. Clin Cancer Res. 2014;20(15):4129–40. doi:10.1158/1078-0432.CCR-13-3036.
6. Classe M, Malouf G, Grégoire V, Villers A, Leroy X. Is molecular analysis the key for translocation renal cell carcinoma?: an extensive study of 23 cases. 27th Eur Congr Pathol. 2015:OFP – 07. https://www1.esp-congress.org/guest/AbstractView?ABSID=10350. Accessed 24 Sept 2015.
7. Argani P, Laé M, Hutchinson B, et al. Renal carcinomas with the t(6;11)(p21;q12): clinicopathologic features and demonstration of the specific alpha-TFEB gene fusion by immunohistochemistry, RT-PCR, and DNA PCR. Am J Surg Pathol. 2005;29(2):230–40. http://www.ncbi.nlm.nih.gov/pubmed/15644781. Accessed June 21, 2015.
8. Durinck S, Stawiski EW, Pavía-Jiménez A, et al. Spectrum of diverse genomic alterations define non-clear cell renal carcinoma subtypes. Nat Genet. 2015;47(1):13–21. doi:10.1038/ng.3146.
9. Argani P, Ladanyi M. Translocation carcinomas of the kidney. Clin Lab Med. 2005;25(2):363–78. doi:10.1016/j.cll.2005.01.008.
10. Tomlinson GE, Nisen PD, Timmons CF, Schneider NR. Cytogenetics of a renal cell carcinoma in a 17-month-old child. Evidence for Xp11.2 as a recurring breakpoint. Cancer Genet Cytogenet. 1991;57(1):11–7. http://www.ncbi.nlm.nih.gov/pubmed/1684532. Accessed June 22, 2015.

11. Geller JI, Ehrlich PF, Cost NG, et al. Characterization of adolescent and pediatric renal cell carcinoma: a report from the children's oncology group study AREN03B2. Cancer. 2015;121(14):2457–64. doi:10.1002/cncr.29368.
12. Altinok G, Kattar MM, Mohamed A, Poulik J, Grignon D, Rabah R. Pediatric renal carcinoma associated with Xp11.2 translocations/TFE3 gene fusions and clinicopathologic associations. Pediatr Dev Pathol. 2005;8(2):168–80. doi:10.1007/s10024-004-9106-3.
13. Bruder E, Passera O, Harms D, et al. Morphologic and molecular characterization of renal cell carcinoma in children and young adults. Am J Surg Pathol. 2004;28(9):1117–32. http://www.ncbi.nlm.nih.gov/pubmed/15316311. Accessed June 22, 2015.
14. Geller JI, Argani P, Adeniran A, et al. Translocation renal cell carcinoma: lack of negative impact due to lymph node spread. Cancer. 2008;112(7):1607–16. doi:10.1002/cncr.23331.
15. Sukov WR, Hodge JC, Lohse CM, et al. TFE3 rearrangements in adult renal cell carcinoma. Am J Surg Pathol. 2012;36(5):1. doi:10.1097/PAS.0b013e31824dd972.
16. Zhong M, De Angelo P, Osborne L, et al. Dual-color, break-apart FISH assay on paraffin-embedded tissues as an adjunct to diagnosis of Xp11 translocation renal cell carcinoma and alveolar soft part sarcoma. Am J Surg Pathol. 2010;34(6):757–66. doi:10.1097/PAS.0b013e3181dd577e.
17. Komai Y, Fujiwara M, Fujii Y, et al. Adult Xp11 translocation renal cell carcinoma diagnosed by cytogenetics and immunohistochemistry. Clin Cancer Res. 2009;15(4):1170–6. doi:10.1158/1078-0432.CCR-08-1183.
18. Argani P, Olgac S, Tickoo SK, et al. Xp11 translocation renal cell carcinoma in adults: expanded clinical, pathologic, and genetic spectrum. Am J Surg Pathol. 2007;31(8):1149–60. doi:10.1097/PAS.0b013e318031ffff.
19. Argani P, Laé M, Ballard ET, et al. Translocation carcinomas of the kidney after chemotherapy in childhood. J Clin Oncol. 2006;24(10):1529–34. doi:10.1200/JCO.2005.04.4693.
20. Dhall D, Al-Ahmadie HA, Dhall G, Shen-Schwarz S, Tickoo SK. Pediatric renal cell carcinoma with oncocytoid features occurring in a child after chemotherapy for cardiac leiomyosarcoma. Urology. 2007;70(1):178.e13–5. doi:10.1016/j.urology.2007.03.055.
21. Rais-Bahrami S, Drabick JJ, De Marzo AM, et al. Xp11 translocation renal cell carcinoma: delayed but massive and lethal metastases of a chemotherapy-associated secondary malignancy. Urology. 2007;70(1):178.e3–6. doi:10.1016/j.urology.2007.03.037.
22. Schafernak KT, Yang XJ, Hsueh W, Leestma JL, Stagl J, Goldman S. Pediatric renal cell carcinoma as second malignancy: reports of two cases and a review of the literature. Can J Urol. 2007;14(6):3739–44. http://www.ncbi.nlm.nih.gov/pubmed/18163925. Accessed June 22, 2015.
23. Sausville JE, Hernandez DJ, Argani P, Gearhart JP. Pediatric renal cell carcinoma. J Pediatr Urol. 2009;5(4):308–14. doi:10.1016/j.jpurol.2009.04.007.
24. Argani P, Hawkins A, Griffin CA, et al. A distinctive pediatric renal neoplasm characterized by epithelioid morphology, basement membrane production, focal HMB45 immunoreactivity, and t(6;11)(p21.1;q12) chromosome translocation. Am J Pathol. 2001;158(6):2089–96. doi:10.1016/S0002-9440(10)64680-9.
25. Smith NE, Illei PB, Allaf M, et al. t(6;11) renal cell carcinoma (RCC): expanded immunohistochemical profile emphasizing novel RCC markers and report of 10 new genetically confirmed cases. Am J Surg Pathol. 2014;38(5):604–14. doi:10.1097/PAS.0000000000000203.
26. Argani P. MiT family translocation renal cell carcinoma. Semin Diagn Pathol. 2015;32(2):103–13. doi:10.1053/j.semdp.2015.02.003.
27. Meyer PN, Clark JI, Flanigan RC, Picken MM. Xp11.2 translocation renal cell carcinoma with very aggressive course in five adults. Am J Clin Pathol. 2007;128(1):70–9. doi:10.1309/LR5G1VMXPY3G0CUK.
28. Malouf GG, Camparo P, Molinié V, et al. Transcription factor E3 and transcription factor EB renal cell carcinomas: clinical features, biological behavior and prognostic factors. J Urol. 2011;185(1):24–9. doi:10.1016/j.juro.2010.08.092.
29. Salles PGO, Soto M. Kidney carcinoma associated with Xp11.2 translocation/TFE3 (ASPL-TFE3) gene fusion. Int Braz J Urol. 2005;31(3):251–4. http://www.ncbi.nlm.nih.gov/pubmed/15992428. Accessed June 24, 2015.

30. Mansouri D, Dimet S, Couanet D, et al. Renal cell carcinoma with an Xp11.2 translocation in a 16-year-old girl: a case report with cytological features. Diagn Cytopathol. 2006;34(11):757–60. http://www.ncbi.nlm.nih.gov/pubmed/17121199. Accessed June 24, 2015.
31. Schinstine M, Filie AC, Torres-Cabala C, Abati A, Linehan WM, Merino M. Fine-needle aspiration of a Xp11.2 translocation/TFE3 fusion renal cell carcinoma metastatic to the lung: report of a case and review of the literature. Diagn Cytopathol. 2006;34(11):751–6. http://www.ncbi.nlm.nih.gov/pubmed/17121198. Accessed June 24, 2015.
32. Weterman MJ, van Groningen JJ, Jansen A, van Kessel AG. Nuclear localization and transactivating capacities of the papillary renal cell carcinoma-associated TFE3 and PRCC (fusion) proteins. Oncogene. 2000;19(1):69–74. doi:10.1038/sj.onc.1203255.
33. Ellis CL, Eble JN, Subhawong AP, et al. Clinical heterogeneity of Xp11 translocation renal cell carcinoma: impact of fusion subtype, age, and stage. Mod Pathol. 2014;27(6):875–86. doi:10.1038/modpathol.2013.208.
34. Kuroda N, Mikami S, Pan C-C, et al. Review of renal carcinoma associated with Xp11.2 translocations/TFE3 gene fusions with focus on pathobiological aspect. Histol Histopathol. 2012;27(2):133–40. http://www.ncbi.nlm.nih.gov/pubmed/22207547. Accessed June 20, 2015.
35. Suzigan S, Drut R, Faria P, et al. Xp11 translocation carcinoma of the kidney presenting with multilocular cystic renal cell carcinoma-like features. Int J Surg Pathol. 2007;15(2):199–203. doi:10.1177/1066896906295891.
36. Camparo P, Vasiliu V, Molinie V, et al. Renal translocation carcinomas: clinicopathologic, immunohistochemical, and gene expression profiling analysis of 31 cases with a review of the literature. Am J Surg Pathol. 2008;32(5):656–70. doi:10.1097/PAS.0b013e3181609914.
37. Argani P, Hicks J, De Marzo AM, et al. Xp11 translocation renal cell carcinoma (RCC): extended immunohistochemical profile emphasizing novel RCC markers. Am J Surg Pathol. 2010;34(9):1295–303. doi:10.1097/PAS.0b013e3181e8ce5b.
38. Daniel L, Lechevallier E, Giorgi R, et al. Pax-2 expression in adult renal tumors. Hum Pathol. 2001;32(3):282–7. doi:10.1053/hupa.2001.22753.
39. Mazal PR, Stichenwirth M, Koller A, Blach S, Haitel A, Susani M. Expression of aquaporins and PAX-2 compared to CD10 and cytokeratin 7 in renal neoplasms: a tissue microarray study. Mod Pathol. 2005;18(4):535–40. doi:10.1038/modpathol.3800320.
40. Nonaka D, Chiriboga L, Soslow RA. Expression of pax8 as a useful marker in distinguishing ovarian carcinomas from mammary carcinomas. Am J Surg Pathol. 2008;32(10):1566–71. doi:10.1097/PAS.0b013e31816d71ad.
41. Martignoni G, Pea M, Gobbo S, et al. Cathepsin-K immunoreactivity distinguishes MiTF/TFE family renal translocation carcinomas from other renal carcinomas. Mod Pathol. 2009;22(8):1016–22. doi:10.1038/modpathol.2009.58.
42. Argani P, Lal P, Hutchinson B, Lui MY, Reuter VE, Ladanyi M. Aberrant nuclear immunoreactivity for TFE3 in neoplasms with TFE3 gene fusions: a sensitive and specific immunohistochemical assay. Am J Surg Pathol. 2003;27(6):750–61. http://www.ncbi.nlm.nih.gov/pubmed/12766578. Accessed June 26, 2015.
43. Klatte T, Streubel B, Wrba F, et al. Renal cell carcinoma associated with transcription factor E3 expression and Xp11.2 translocation: incidence, characteristics, and prognosis. Am J Clin Pathol. 2012;137(5):761–8. doi:10.1309/AJCPQ6LLFMC4OXGC.
44. Macher-Goeppinger S, Roth W, Wagener N, et al. Molecular heterogeneity of TFE3 activation in renal cell carcinomas. Mod Pathol. 2012;25(2):308–15. doi:10.1038/modpathol.2011.169.
45. Malouf GG, Monzon FA, Couturier J, et al. Genomic heterogeneity of translocation renal cell carcinoma. Clin Cancer Res. 2013;19(17):4673–84. doi:10.1158/1078-0432.CCR-12-3825.
46. Aoki Y, Nojima M, Suzuki H, et al. Genomic vulnerability to LINE-1 hypomethylation is a potential determinant of the clinicogenetic features of multiple myeloma. Genome Med. 2012;4(12):101. doi:10.1186/gm402.
47. Hagenkord JM, Gatalica Z, Jonasch E, Monzon FA. Clinical genomics of renal epithelial tumors. Cancer Genet. 2011;204(6):285–97. doi:10.1016/j.cancergen.2011.06.001.
48. Alvarez K, Kash SF, Lyons-Weiler MA, et al. Reproducibility and performance of virtual karyotyping with SNP microarrays for the detection of chromosomal imbalances in formalin-

fixed paraffin-embedded tissues. Diagn Mol Pathol. 2010;19(3):127–34. doi:10.1097/PDM.0b013e3181d527c5.
49. Stephens PJ, Greenman CD, Fu B, et al. Massive genomic rearrangement acquired in a single catastrophic event during cancer development. Cell. 2011;144(1):27–40. doi:10.1016/j.cell.2010.11.055.
50. Choueiri TK, Lim ZD, Hirsch MS, et al. Vascular endothelial growth factor-targeted therapy for the treatment of adult metastatic Xp11.2 translocation renal cell carcinoma. Cancer. 2010;116(22):5219–25. doi:10.1002/cncr.25512.
51. Malouf GG, Camparo P, Oudard S, et al. Targeted agents in metastatic Xp11 translocation/TFE3 gene fusion renal cell carcinoma (RCC): a report from the Juvenile RCC Network. Ann Oncol. 2010;21(9):1834–8. doi:10.1093/annonc/mdq029.

Primitive Neuroectodermal Tumors and Other Sarcomas of the Kidney

4

Leonardo D. Borregales, Arun Z. Thomas, Mehrad Adibi, Jose A. Karam, and Christopher G. Wood

Abbreviations

AML	Angiomyolipoma
CSS	Cancer-specific survival
ESFT	Ewing sarcoma family of tumors
EWS	Ewing sarcoma gene
FLI1	Friend leukemia integration 1
FS	Fibrosarcoma
HMB-45	Human melanoma black 45
HPC	Hemangiopericytoma
IHC	Immunohistochemical
LMS	Leiomyosarcoma
LPS	Liposarcoma
MFH	Malignant fibrous histiocytoma
OS	Overall survival
PNET	Primitive neuroectodermal tumor
PRSS	Primary renal synovial sarcoma
RCC	Renal cell carcinoma
RMS	Rhabdomyosarcoma
sRCC	Sarcomatoid renal cell carcinoma

L.D. Borregales, MD • A.Z. Thomas, MD • M. Adibi, MD • J.A. Karam, MD
C.G. Wood, MD, FACS (✉)
Department of Urology, The University of Texas MD Anderson Cancer Center, 1515 Holcombe Blvd., Houston, TX 77030, USA
e-mail: cgwood@mdanderson.org

L. Pagliaro (ed.), *Rare Genitourinary Tumors*,
DOI 10.1007/978-3-319-30046-7_4

Introduction

In 2015, an estimated 11,930 patients in the United States were diagnosed with soft tissue sarcomas [1]. Primary genitourinary tract sarcomas account for 2 % of all soft tissue sarcomas and 1–2 % of genitourinary malignancies [2]. Sarcomas represent up to 3 % (range, 0.8–2.7 %) of renal malignancies in adults, with the highest incidence in the sixth decade of life [3]. Leiomyosarcoma is the most common histological type of renal sarcomas (50–60 %), followed by liposarcoma (15 %), hemangiopericytoma (9 %), fibrosarcoma (7 %), malignant fibrous histiocytoma or undifferentiated pleomorphic sarcoma (6 %), and rhabdomyosarcoma (3 %) [4]. Renal primitive neuroectodermal tumors (PNETs) are particularly rare, with fewer than 200 reported cases, and account for less than 2 % of renal malignancies.

Genitourinary sarcomas can cause high rates of morbidity and death. The literature highlights the aggressive nature of these tumors, with a 5-year cancer-specific survival (CSS) rate of 56 % for genitourinary sarcomas and worse outcomes for renal sarcomas (5-year CSS rate, 29 %) [5]. There is no standardized treatment for renal sarcomas, and evidence from the literature to help clinicians manage these malignancies is limited. Here, we summarize the clinical knowledge about the major clinicopathological characteristics, outcomes, and management of primary renal PNETs and other rare types of kidney sarcomas, including leiomyosarcoma, liposarcoma, hemangiopericytoma, fibrosarcoma, malignant fibrous histiocytoma, rhabdomyosarcoma, and primary renal synovial sarcoma.

Primitive Neuroectodermal Tumor

PNETs are neural crest malignancies that arise from the neuroectoderm and are classified as central or peripheral depending on where the tumors originate in the nervous system. Peripheral PNETs occasionally originate in unusual sites such as the chest wall, paraspinal region, bones, ovaries, uterus, testes, and, rarely, urinary tract [6]. Genitourinary PNETs are very rare; fewer than 200 case reports have documented PNETs in the bladder, prostate, ureter, and kidneys [7–10]. Most of our knowledge about PNETs comes from case reports; only seven case series have been published, and these series involved fewer than 200 patients [11]. Based on these studies, the clinical presentation and course of renal PNETs differ significantly from the natural history of renal cell carcinomas (RCCs). Compared with RCCs, renal PNETs are more commonly associated with patients younger than 20 years and with large tumors at presentation. Although rare, patients with PNETs have a poor prognosis despite multimodal therapy, with high rates of early recurrence and dismal cancer-specific survival [12]. This chapter will focus primarily on renal PNETs, which are the most common genitourinary PNETs described in the literature [13].

History and First Description of Renal PNETs

The first report of a PNET originating in the ulnar nerve was described by Stout in 1918 [7]. In 1921, similar tumors were reported in adolescent patients presenting with disabling pain in the extremities. These tumors were noted to differ histologically from classic osteogenic sarcomas and were vaguely named round cell sarcomas. These new tumors were highly sensitive to radiation therapy but had high recurrence rates and tended to progress rapidly. Later, these tumors were referred to as Ewing sarcoma [14]. With the advancements of molecular characterization, similarities in histological and chromosomal abnormalities were found between PNETs and Ewing sarcomas; thus PNETs were reclassified as part of the Ewing sarcoma family of tumors (ESFT). Both malignancies are small round cell tumors that occur in the bone and soft tissue of young patients [14]. Additionally, they share distinctive chromosomal anomalies and originate from the same stem cell precursor [15].

In a 1975 case series of four patients with peripheral PNETs, Seemayer and colleagues first documented a renal PNET [16]. However, the first case report depicting the clinical and pathological characteristics of a renal PNET was published in 1994 when a 61-year-old man presented with classic symptoms of locally advanced RCC, including flank pain, a palpable abdominal mass, and severe weight loss and fatigue [6]. Mor and colleagues reported that the patient had a large solid mass that replaced the entire parenchyma of the kidney and metastatic lymphadenopathy with associated hydroureteronephrosis. On microscopic examination, the mass was characterized by clusters of small and medium round cells with irregular nuclei that were displayed in cords and embedded in fibrous tissue. On the basis of these results, the patient was thought to have an anaplastic, blastemal-predominant Wilms tumor and was treated with chemotherapy including doxorubicin, dactinomycin, vincristine, and cyclophosphamide [6]. Despite aggressive treatment, the authors reported a marked deterioration in the patient's condition with severe abdominal pain and compressive symptoms from a vertebral metastasis. Given the tumor's unresponsiveness to treatment and rapid progression, the National Wilms Tumor Study Pathology Center was consulted. Immunohistochemical (IHC) analysis revealed a characteristic pattern: the tumor stained positive for neuron-specific enolase and chromogranin A and negative for cytokeratin, vimentin, and synaptophysin. Although the patient was diagnosed with renal PNET and treated, the patient died within 6 months.

Epidemiology

PNETs infrequently are seen as an organ-derived neoplasm. Less than 15 % of PNETs originate in the abdomen, retroperitoneum, and pelvis [17]. While renal PNETs account for less than 1 % of renal tumors, representing an extremely rare entity [17], this incidence is likely underreported since just recent genetic advances in the tumor characterization have enabled us to distinguish PNETs from other round cell tumors.

Renal PNETs tend to occur in men (male/female, 1.5:1) [18]. In contrast to RCC and other sarcomas, renal PNETs are more common in young patients. In a systematic review of 79 patients, the median age was 20 years (range, 2 months to 73 years) [21], and recent reports described a median age of 28 years (interquartile range, 20–42 years), with almost a quarter of the patients aged 15 years or younger [13, 19]. One of the largest series concluded that PNETs occur with similar frequency in both kidneys [11].

Although PNETs have not been associated with a particular ethnicity, data on peripheral PNETs suggest that the disease occurs more frequently in white and Hispanic patients and less frequently in African Americans or Asian Americans [20]. Owing to the rarity of renal PNETs, no risk factors have been identified for this disease. Nonetheless, PNETs and Ewing sarcomas have similarities in non-modifiable risk factors, such as age, sex, and ethnicity, underlying a shared biology [19].

Biology and Possible Origin

The origin of renal PNETs has yet to be elucidated. Although theories regarding the histological origin of PNETs remain hypothetical, PNETs are presumed to originate from neural crest cells, given the morphological resemblance of PNETs to neuroblastoma [11]. Another theory suggests a mesenchymal stem cell origin, as PNETs commonly present as bone or soft tissue masses in the trunk or axial skeleton of children and young adults [21]. A less popular hypothesis is that PNETs originate from pluripotent germ cells; this theory is linked to the histogenesis of gonadal PNETs [19].

Mor and colleagues suggested that renal PNETs are caused by an aberrant migration of neural crest cells or the dedifferentiation of native neural elements on the basis of previous descriptions of neural elements found in other renal neoplasms such as Wilms tumors [5]. Similarly, Parham and colleagues proposed that embryonic neural crest cells migrate into the kidney and, with the appropriate environmental and genetic changes, undergo oncogenesis [19]. Although the nature of these changes was not described, the authors did suggest that the neural components of renal PNETs originate in the neural adrenergic fibers of the celiac plexus that innervate the kidney [19]. Studies have described an interaction of neural differentiation factors such as c-RET and the development of metanephros and subsequent nephrogenesis in rodents [22]. However, the specific implications of this neural differentiation factor for the development of renal PNETs have not been elaborated, and further research is needed to determine the cell of origin of renal PNETs.

Clinical Presentation

The most common symptoms of renal PNETs at presentation are flank pain (67.5 %), hematuria (33.8 %), and a palpable abdominal mass (33.8 %) [11]. This triad of symptoms, once typical for patients with advanced RCC, tends to be an often encountered scenario at presentation of renal PNETs, given the rapid natural progression of PNETs [23]. Risi et al. [7] showed in a systematic review of 116 patients with renal PNETs that 98 % of the patients had at least one of these three symptoms at presentation and 2 % each had dysuria, fever, weight loss, and fatigue. Although these symptoms are nonspecific, this triad may raise suspicions for an unusual histology such as PNETs.

Patients with renal PNETs tend to present with locally advanced or metastatic disease. In one of the largest single-institution case series, Thyavihally and colleagues found that of 16 patients with renal PNETs, 5 (31 %) had metastatic disease, with a median age of 27 years at presentation. Thyavihally and colleagues proposed that young patients with a renal mass and distant metastasis at presentation should be suspected of having renal PNETs [24]. Systematic studies have reported that at PNET diagnosis, approximately 20–50 % of patients have distant metastatic disease, with the regional lymph nodes, bone marrow, liver, and lungs being the most common metastatic sites [19].

Tumor thrombus extension has also been described in renal PNET. Cuesta Alcala and colleagues reported two patients presenting with atrial tumor thrombus extension at diagnosis [25]. Many other case series have also reported this finding. In a series of ten patients, Lee and colleagues reported that most patients had a large necrotic and hemorrhagic mass, eight patients had renal vein invasion, and four patients presented with inferior vena cava invasion [26]. Moreover, in a 2010 literature review, Xu and colleagues showed that of 103 patients, 49 % had tumor thrombus into the renal vein and 33 % had inferior vena cava involvement, exemplifying that tumor thrombus is not a rare phenomenon in PNETs and highlighting the importance of suspecting renal PNETs in young patients with renal masses and inferior vena cava involvement [27]. Although these findings raise a suspicion of PNETs, no clinical characteristics pathognomomonic of renal PNETs have been identified, and accurate diagnosis relies predominantly on the histopathological, IHC, and cytogenetic features of the disease [28].

Histology and IHC Findings

On gross examination, renal PNETs are usually large (commonly over 10 cm in diameter), gray, encapsulated masses with focal areas of tumor necrosis and hemorrhage [29]. On microscopic examination, renal PNETs exhibit small round cells arranged as perivascular Homer Wright rosettes or pseudorosettes [24]. These microscopic findings have also been described in neuroblastoma and extraskeletal Ewing sarcoma [30]. The most common microscopic findings for PNETs are densely cellular sheets of primitive, largely undifferentiated cells with round hyperchromatic nuclei and pale to lightly amphophilic cytoplasm [19]. Mitotic figures may be numerous, and intracytoplasmic glycogen can be detected on periodic acid-Schiff staining [31]. On electron microscopy, renal

PNETs demonstrate neurosecretory granules, microtubules, and multiple peripheral microfilaments [32].

Positive IHC staining for neuron-specific enolase facilitates the diagnosis of PNETs but is not pathognomonic [6]. Renal PNETs stain positive most commonly for glycoprotein CD99, a product of the *CD99* gene located on the short arm of chromosomes X and Y [33]. CD99 is a distinctive feature in peripheral PNETs and is present in approximately 90 % of the cases. In a 1997 series of four patients aged between 4 and 20 years, tumor tissue samples from all four patients stained positive for CD99 [22]. Despite the fact that 90 % of PNETs/ESFTs stain positive for CD99, this marker is not pathognomonic for these tumor, as CD99 can be expressed in other round blue cell tumors [13]. Additionally, these tumors are commonly negative for markers such as pankeratin, cytokeratin, vimentin, S100 protein, and chromogranin A. Pomara and colleagues described the need for an extensive IHC panel to diagnose PNETs because there is not a specific marker for this disease, and depending on the technique, false-negative results could occur [32]. Furthermore, although relevant for the differential diagnosis, IHC results are not recommended as the sole means of diagnosis, as molecular fusion studies should be used to validate and confirm the diagnosis [32].

Molecular Analysis

While IHC analysis facilitates and increases the specificity of a diagnosis of renal PNETs, molecular analysis is recommended when an atypical renal mass is suspected to be a PNET. Cytogenetic studies such as karyotyping and fluorescence in situ hybridization are now required for identifying a Ewing sarcoma aberration commonly found in PNETs. The translocation of t(11:22)(q24:q12) with the fusion transcript between the Ewing sarcoma gene (*EWS*, 22q12) and the erythroblast transformation-specific oncogene (11q24) occurs in 88–95 % of PNET cases, and this translocation has been described as an important oncogenic step leading to a hybrid transcript and oncogenic chimeric protein [32, 34]. This unique genetic characteristic reclassified PNETs as part of the ESFT [35].

Antibodies against the Friend leukemia integration 1 (FLI1) transcription factor, present in some renal PNETs, also may aid in the molecular diagnosis of this entity [36]. In the largest systematic review of 116 patients with renal PNETs, Risi and colleagues found that 72 % of the patients had chromosomal translocation that resulted in the fusion gene *EWS-FLI1* on chromosome 11, and this finding was associated with the IHC expression of FLI1 protein ($p=0.03$) [7]. Some studies have suggested that the type of fusion may have prognostic significance and that patients carrying the *EWS-FLI1* translocation may have longer cancer-specific survival than those without this translocation [11]. However, Risi and colleagues found that cancer-specific survival did not differ significantly among their patients with or without this translocation [7].

Differential Diagnosis

The diagnosis of PNETs poses a significant challenge. Table 4.1 summarizes the most common clinicopathological characteristics of renal PNETs and differential diagnosis. Despite its distinctive small round cell histology, renal PNETs are difficult to distinguish from other primitive tumors such as blastemal-predominant Wilms tumors, embryonal rhabdomyosarcomas, neuroblastomas, small cell carcinomas, and synovial sarcomas [21]. Homer Wright rosettes are found more typically in PNETs than in these other tumor types; however, Homer Wright rosettes also occur in neuroblastoma [32].

To distinguish renal PNETs from these other entities, IHC and chromosomal findings, rather than clinical or radiological findings, are used. CD99 has been linked almost universally to all peripheral PNETs, with an incidence of approximately 90 %. Strong positive staining for CD99 protein on IHC analysis can help distinguish PNETs from other small round cell tumors [32]. Although frequently confused with blastemal-predominant Wilms tumors, PNETs usually stain negative for WT1 gene expression [19].

The diagnosis of PNEt also can be confirmed by demonstrating the reciprocal translocation between the long arms of chromosomes 11 and 22 t(11:22)(q24:q12) or the *EWS-FLI1* gene fusion with the help of fluorescence in situ hybridization techniques or reverse transcription polymerase chain reaction [37]. Although IHC and cytogenetic analysis are commonly recommended, further diagnostic analyses should be performed because the results of a single method do not exclude many of the tumor types in the differential diagnosis [9].

Imaging

The radiological findings for renal PNETs presented in the literature thus far, although nonspecific, as commonly present in locally advanced RCC, highlight four characteristics as the most common features of renal PNETs: tumor thrombus, multifocal necrosis, irregular septae and calcifications, and weak enhancement [38].

Tumor thrombus has been repeatedly described in patients with renal PNETs. Renal PNETs tend to be multifocal and diffuse, whereas RCC is characterized by central hemorrhage or necrosis. Wu and colleagues found that magnetic resonance imaging studies of a series of patients with renal PNETs showed peripheral necrosis and hemorrhages rather than central necrosis [39]. A similar observation has been documented for PNETs of the uterus and retroperitoneum [39].

Irregular septae and calcifications in both the necrotic and solid portions of the tumor have been reported in several series of patients with renal PNETs, and studies have reported similar findings for PNETs of the retroperitoneum [26]. Several reports of primary renal PNETs have described weak heterogeneous contrast enhancement on computed tomography studies. Despite typically large tumor masses, renal PNETs show very weak enhancement or do not enhance in arterial and delayed contrast phases, unlike RCC [26]. Although the radiological

Table 4.1 Characteristics of renal primitive neuroectodermal tumors (PNETs) and other sarcomas of the kidney

Tumor type	Clinical presentation	Radiological features	Pathological features	Positive antibodies (IHC)
PNET/EWS	Flank pain	Large tumor burden	Neurosecretory granules	CD99
	Palpable mass	Hypervascular	Rosettes on EM	Chromogranin A
	Hematuria	Necrotic and hemorrhagic parenchyma	Pseudorosettes on LM	Synaptophysin
	Weight loss	No renal vein involvement	Neuron-specific enolase	
		Largely calcified with moderate parenchymal infiltration		
Leiomyosarcoma	Similar to those of PNET/EWS	Well-delineated and multinodular	Smooth muscle morphology	Alpha-smooth muscle actin
	Rarely, presents as spontaneous rupture	Low parenchymal density with delayed enhancement	Fascicles of spindle cells	Vimentin
		Septum-like structures	Eosinophilic cytoplasm	Desmin
			5–10 mitoses per HPF	Calponin
				H-caldesmon
Liposarcoma	Similar to those of renal masses	Inner fat density −20 to −50 HU) with heterogeneous and dense septum	Classified based on histological subtypes: well-differentiated, dedifferentiated, pleomorphic, round cell and myxoid	HMB-45
Hemangiopericytoma	Paraneoplastic syndrome with secondary hypertension, hypoglycemia, and hypokalemia	Well-defined	Spindle cells alternating with small fascicles of cells	CD34 antibody
		Strongly enhanced solid mass with necrosis and occasionally calcifications	"Staghorn" perivascular distribution with moderate to high cellularity	Vimentin

Fibrosarcoma	Similar to those of renal masses	Nonspecific enhancing soft tissue mass with perinephric or retroperitoneal extension	Spindle cells organized in parallel rows intersecting each other at acute angles in a broken zigzag pattern	Vimentin
	Often presents as symptoms of adjacent organ invasion, e.g., GI tract obstruction			Proliferation-related Ki-67 antigen
Rhabdomyosarcoma	Similar to those of renal masses	Nonspecific large, heterogeneously enhancing neoplasm	Spindle cells with areas of small round blue cell tumor	Myogenin and MyoD1
Primary renal synovial sarcoma (PRSS)	Similar to those of renal masses	Large, well-defined mass extending into perinephric fat or renal pelvis with heterogeneous enhancement	Monophasic, composed solely of spindle cells; biphasic, composed of both epithelial and spindle cell components and poorly differentiated	CD99 and CD56
		Tendency for cystic development and air-fluid levels		
Malignant fibrous histiocytoma	Mimic pyelonephritis, with symptoms such as fever, chills, and dysuria	Large, lobulated soft tissue mass with central necrosis or myxoid materials	Four histological subtypes of MFH: storiform-pleomorphic, giant cell, myxoid, and inflammatory	Positive for CD34 and CD68 and is negative for cytokeratin

Data from references [2, 6, 51, 54, 55, 60, 75, 83, 89, 95, 96]

EWS Ewing sarcoma, *GI* gastrointestinal, *HU* Hounsfield units, *EM* electron microscopy, *LM* light microscopy, *HPF* high-power field, *IHC* immunohistochemical analysis, *HMB-45* human melanoma black 45, *MyoD1* myoblast determination protein 1 appearance of renal PNETs is nonspecific, the presence of these four characteristics should raise suspicion when one encounters a large renal mass with aggressive features.

Treatment

Only a few case studies have reported recurrence-free survival after treatment with surgery alone [40]. The preferred treatment for localized and locally advanced renal PNETs is radical nephrectomy combined with cytotoxic chemotherapy and radiation therapy [41]. The role of radiation therapy in renal PNETs, however, is not clearly defined. Most studies have differed on the indications for radiation therapy and the dosage, with a limited consensus only for patients with evidence of positive margins or other residual diseases or when the renal fascia is involved [24].

Radical nephrectomy, on the other hand, has been shown to be essential in local control, and most case series advocate early surgical resection to maximize survival [13, 21]. In a systematic review of 116 patients with renal PNETs, Risi and colleagues found that 89 % of the patients underwent surgical resection of the primary tumor, and 95 % of those underwent radical nephrectomy. The patients who underwent surgery had a 2-year overall survival (OS) rate of 80 % compared with 30 % for patients who did not undergo surgery ($p=0.017$) [13]. These results, however, were not adjusted for performance status or taken from a homogeneous cohort because of the rarity of the disease. In addition, in a series of 16 patients with renal PNETs, Thyavihally and colleagues found that patients with localized disease and negative margins after nephrectomy had significantly longer median OS (60 months) than patients who had locally advanced disease or distant metastasis (OS, 15 months) [24]. Unfortunately, up to 38 % of patients with renal PNETs present with a locally advanced mass that has invaded adjacent organs by the time of resection. Therefore, additional postoperative treatment is needed to diminish the risk of recurrence.

Although PNETs are generally chemosensitive [36], there is no consensus about the best adjuvant treatment for renal PNETs, and regimens are extrapolated from those used for other ESFTs [42]. A range of responses to cytotoxic chemotherapy, depending on differentiation and tumor extension, have been described, and standard therapies include doxorubicin plus cyclophosphamide; vincristine, doxorubicin, and cyclophosphamide with optional dactinomycin; or vincristine, doxorubicin, and cyclophosphamide alternating with ifosfamide plus etoposide [43]. These protocols are based on the Intergroup Ewing Sarcoma Study guidelines and on significantly improved survival outcomes in phase III clinical trials in patients with Ewing sarcoma/PNETs [44]. One study showed that alternating cycles of ifosfamide plus etoposide significantly improved 5-year recurrence-free survival compared with the standard treatment of doxorubicin plus cyclophosphamide (69 % versus 54 %, respectively) [34]. Studies have also demonstrated effective results in patients with refractory primary or recurrent disease with the addition of ifosfamide and etoposide to the standard regimes [45]. Fergany and colleagues found that adjuvant therapy with ifosfamide and etoposide along with cytoreductive nephrectomy had favorable results and may be recommended for those whom complete surgical excision was not guaranteed; in a case reported one patient with IVC thrombus and lung metastasis experienced complete response after 12 cycles of chemotherapy and 2-year disease-free survival [46].

The high response rates to adjuvant therapy in patients with metastatic PNETs have sparked interest in the possible role of presurgical therapy [13]. Studies have demonstrated that presurgical therapy is beneficial for patients with large unresectable masses or with distant metastasis [36]. Richey and colleagues reported that a patient with a PNET and metastases to the infradiaphragmatic and supradiaphragmatic lymph nodes experienced an 8-year response after induction and maintenance chemotherapy. Further, Richey et al. suggested that cytoreductive nephrectomy could limit tolerance for subsequent adjuvant therapy and advised that patients with PNETs and metastatic disease be treated with up-front chemotherapy [31].

The management of renal PNETs remains difficult. The rare incidence of PNETs precludes single-institution and large-scale prospective or randomized trials, and aggressive multimodal management that is based on previous case reports remains the standard of care. Careful interpretation of diagnostic results could clarify management strategies and define prognostic factors.

Leiomyosarcoma

Renal leiomyosarcoma (LMS) is the most common primary renal sarcoma, accounting for 50–60 % of cases (Table 4.2), but it is nevertheless rare [47, 48]. In one of the largest published series, Kendal reported that of 95,935 patients with kidney cancer identified in the Surveillance, Epidemiology, and End Results (SEER) database, only 112 patients had primary renal LMS (0.12 % of renal malignancies) [49]. In another series, Miller and colleagues identified only 27 patients from three high-volume cancer institutions in the United States during a 23-year period [50].

Compared with patients with renal PNETs, patients presenting with renal LMS tend to be older; most patients reported in the literature were older than 20 years, with a mean age at diagnosis in the sixth decade. LMS occurs more frequently in women (60 %), and right-sided renal masses are more common [50, 51].

Table 4.2 Most common malignant mesenchymal renal tumors

Tumor type	Percentage of renal sarcomas (%)
Leiomyosarcoma	50–60
Liposarcoma	15
Hemangiopericytoma	9
Fibrosarcoma	7
Rhabdomyosarcoma	5
Primary renal synovial sarcoma	5
Malignant fibrous histiocytoma	1

Data from Moudouni et al. [47]

The clinical presentation of renal LMS varies, but nearly all patients present with symptoms similar to those of RCC, including flank pain, a palpable abdominal mass, and hematuria. Other symptoms include fever of unknown origin, weight loss, and urinary frequency. Life-threatening conditions, such as spontaneous renal neoplasm rupture, have also been reported at presentation in a few cases [48, 52].

Renal LMS tends to be highly aggressive, with a median tumor size of 13.4 cm, and approximately 55 % of patients have direct tumor extension beyond the kidney capsule at initial presentation [50]. Metastasis to the lungs, liver, and bone is common at diagnosis, and the 3-year progression-free survival rate is as low as 10 % [50].

Primary renal LMS is thought to originate from renal blood vessels, the smooth muscle fibers of the renal pelvis, or the renal capsule [47, 53]. Macroscopically, primary renal LMSs are solid, gray-white, and well-circumscribed, with a soft consistency and a propensity for cystic degeneration [54]. Microscopically, renal LMSs have a typical smooth muscle morphology alternating with clusters of spindle cells with non-tapering nuclei and eosinophilic cytoplasm. Renal LMS tumors tend to have moderate to severe pleomorphism, cellular necrosis, and greater than five to ten mitotic cells per high-power field. These findings differentiate LMSs from benign leiomyomas [55]. Often LMSs exhibit a myxoid morphology; however, the prognostic implications of this feature remain unclear [50]. On IHC staining, LMS tissue expresses mesenchymal markers such as alpha-smooth muscle actin, vimentin, desmin, calponin, and h-caldesmon and typically is negative for epithelial markers such as cytokeratin or S100 protein [51, 56].

The differential diagnosis of primary renal LMS includes angiomyolipoma (AML), leiomyoma, and sarcomatoid RCC (sRCC). There are no pathognomonic criteria to distinguish between LMS and other histological types. Furthermore, similar smooth muscle tumors within the kidney, such as AML, may mimic the radiological and pathological findings of LMS.

AML is often included in the differential diagnosis of LMS. AML is found in the context of tuberous sclerosis disease in over 40 % of cases and is composed of mixed mature fat, smooth muscle, and thick-walled blood vessels [57]. Although considered benign, AML often resembles aggressive disease with local infiltration and may even present with lymph node invasion and local recurrence [57]. Specimens should be reviewed extensively for the combination of adipose tissue, abnormal blood vessels, and smooth muscle indicative of AML. Additionally, the diagnosis of AML is confirmed by high expression of human melanoma black 45 (HMB-45) on IHC analysis, whereas LMS has low HMB-45 expression [50]. Given the difficulty in diagnosing LMS, it is not surprising that renal LMS has a reported misdiagnosis rate of up to 50 % [49].

sRCC is an aggressive spindle cell tumor arising from the kidney that is commonly included in the differential diagnosis of LMS. Although rare, sRCC occurs more commonly than renal LMS, accounting for 4–32 % of all RCC [50, 58]. More importantly, sRCC has a distinctive malignant epithelial component that is reactive with epithelial markers on IHC staining and lacks the characteristic fascicular formation seen in AML [59].

Few distinctive radiological features have been associated with LMS. On renal angiography, LMS shows a vascular distribution with hypervascular and tortuous intrarenal vessels, but this finding is nonspecific [54]. Computed tomography studies of LMS typically show a well-delineated, multinodular mass of low parenchymal density with delayed enhancement along with high-density septum-like structures in the early contrast phase. On T2-weighted magnetic resonance imaging, the multinodular structures appear as low-signal intensity areas, and the septum-like structures appear as high-signal intensity areas [60, 61]. Nonetheless, a renal biopsy is recommended when LMS is suspected, since this last cannot be distinguished accurately from leiomyoma by radiological findings.

No standard treatment for LMS has been established. Radical nephrectomy has been the frontline therapy; however, prognosis is poor even with aggressive en bloc resection [62]. Only a few patients have survived long-term, and the CSS duration remains at 2 years after surgery alone [54].

The outcomes and prognostic factors have been study recently in an effort to address these concerns. In a study by Dominici and colleagues, favorable prognostic factors included tumor size less than 4 cm, low tumor grade, lack of nodal involvement, and radical surgery [63]. The investigators reported a 5-year OS rate of 29–36 %. In the largest series to date by Kendal et al., the major predictors for survival in patients with renal LMS were tumor stage and patient age at diagnosis. Results from this series reported a median OS of 25 months, a 5-year OS rate of 25 %, and a 5-year CSS rate of 60 % [49]. The lack of follow-up data from case reports prevents the estimation of accurate survival rates and outcomes [49].

In light of the poor survival data for patients with LMS, adjuvant therapy has been proposed to address micrometastatic disease and positive margins [64]. Objective response rates of 47 % have been observed in patients with locally advanced disease treated with adjuvant chemotherapy regimens consisting of dactinomycin, cyclophosphamide, and vincristine [64]. Furthermore, chemosensitivity testing in soft tissue sarcomas has shown promise and increasingly has been used to develop tumor sensitivity and resistance profiles for approved and experimental agents [65]. Despite these advancements, neither chemotherapy nor radiation therapy has consistently demonstrated objective response for renal LMS, and outcomes are heterogeneous [64]. Owing to the rarity of LMS, there are no open clinical trials aimed solely at any of these diseases.

Liposarcoma

Renal liposarcoma (LPS) is a rare malignancy derived from the mesenchymal tissue of the kidney parenchyma. Isolated renal LPS is uncommon and must be differentiated from LPS of retroperitoneal origin. Renal LPS most commonly arises from the renal pelvis; LPS originating from the renal capsule has been reported in only 18 cases [66], and few instances of LPS with concomitant extension of tumor thrombus into the renal vein have been reported [67].

Renal LPS usually presents in the fifth to sixth decades of life and is seen in patients with end-stage renal disease or a family history of polycystic kidney disease [68]. The clinical presentation is consistent with the classic triad of symptoms seen in patients with other kidney masses (flank pain, a palpable abdominal mass, and hematuria) along with weight loss.

The natural history of this entity depends largely on the degree of tumor differentiation. Well-differentiated LPS tends to progress slowly, while undifferentiated may present with large tumor invading adjacent organs. The most common sites of metastases are the lungs, lymph nodes, and liver, and case reports often describe disseminated intra-abdominal masses [66].

Macroscopically, primary renal LPS tumors are well differentiated and yellow and have a median diameter of 5 cm [68]. Microscopically, renal LPS is categorized as well-differentiated, dedifferentiated, pleomorphic, round cell, or myxoid. While well-differentiated renal LPS has recurrence rates of less than 30 % and virtually no distant metastasis, dedifferentiated LPS has the potential for metastasis. In a review by Singer and colleagues, patients with dedifferentiated retroperitoneal LPS had the most aggressive clinical course, with an 83 % local recurrence rate, a 30 % distant recurrence rate, and a 60 % higher risk of death than patients with well-differentiated tumors [69]. Another study found that the grade of tumor differentiation was the most significant predictor of survival [70]. LPS prognosis is associated with the degree of histological dedifferentiation, tumor size, and tumor stage [68]. Tissue and clinical data analysis to characterize treatments for LPS on the basis of histopathological characteristics could improve patient outcomes for this rare malignancy.

Early reports may have misdiagnosed LPS as AML, many LPS tumors have been described in the context of tuberous sclerosis syndrome, and revisions of early series revealed that the LPSs had identical morphological features to those of AML [71]. Because the management and survival outcomes differ between these two tumors, it is paramount to diagnose the disease correctly. For an accurate diagnosis of primary renal LPS, involvement of the renal parenchyma on imaging should be established to eliminate retroperitoneal soft tissue LPS abutting the kidney [72]. Furthermore, LPS tends to be a diagnosis of exclusion. LPS tissue typically is negative for IHC markers such as alpha-smooth muscle actin, HMB-45, desmin, and actin [73]. The absence of IHC staining for alpha-smooth muscle actin helps establish the diagnosis of LPS.

Unlike many other sarcomas, LPS can display significant neovascularization. On computed tomography studies, many LPSs exhibit inner fat density (−20 to −50 Hounsfield units), with heterogeneous and dense septae that can be used to distinguish LPSs from tumors with more homogeneous borders, such as AML and renal lipomas [2].

Radical surgery with or without adjuvant chemotherapy is the preferred treatment approach, and evidence of negative surgical margins remains the most significant prognostic factor [66]. Binder and colleagues reported that cytoreductive resection of retroperitoneal LPS should be used only in a palliative fashion for symptomatic patients since results showed that patients who underwent partial excision had survival rates similar to those who underwent only tumor biopsy [74].

Adjuvant chemotherapy and radiation therapy have been used for high-risk disease. Doxorubicin and ifosfamide, the most common agents used to treat LPS in advanced stages, have resulted in a median recurrence-free survival duration of over 9 months [75]. The combination of doxycycline and ifosfamide has also produced responses in the metastatic disease setting in patients with soft tissue sarcomas; however, cytotoxic chemotherapy has been minimally effective [76]. Radiation therapy also has shown minimal effectiveness; initial reports described renal LPS as highly radiation resistant [77]. However, for patients with positive resection margins, radiation therapy and cisplatin-based adjuvant therapy have been reported to improve overall survival [78].

Hemangiopericytoma

Hemangiopericytoma (HPC) is a rare soft tissue sarcoma that arises from the pericytes of the walls of capillaries. Pericytes normally surround capillaries and venules and regulate blood flow and capillary permeability [79]. The first HPC was reported by Stout and colleagues in 1942 when they described the presentation of an uncontrolled proliferation of pericytes enveloping a perivascular tumor [80]. HPC arises most commonly from the extremities, head or neck, meninges, and pelvis and very rarely from the kidney [81]. Since the initial report of renal HPC by Black and Heinemann in 1955 [82], approximately 50 cases of primary renal HPC have been reported.

This tumor typically presents in patients between the ages of 16 and 50 years; most patients are 30 years old or younger [83]. In contrast to other renal sarcomas, HPCs often are associated with paraneoplastic syndromes, including secondary hypertension, hypoglycemia, electrolyte abnormalities, and cachexia [84]. The hypertension is thought to be due to the overstimulation by endothelial cells for the production of renin. Many theories to account for the hypoglycemia have been proposed, but most researchers agree that it results from an excess of carbohydrate storage or increased tumor metabolism [85].

Macroscopically, primary renal HPCs are well-delineated, encapsulated, yellow tumors. Microscopically, HPC sections reveal spindle cells alternating with small fascicles of cells in a characteristic "staghorn" perivascular distribution with moderate to high cellularity [81, 86]. HPC has high levels of reactivity with CD34 antibody and vimentin, characteristic of cells of mesenchymal origin. Primary renal synovial sarcoma (PRSS) and sRCC are included in the differential diagnosis of HPC. IHC analysis often assists in confirming the diagnosis: HPC is negative for both cytokeratin and epithelial membrane antigen, but both PRSS and sRCC stain strongly positive for these markers [83].

On computed tomography imaging, renal HPC typically presents as a well-differentiated, strongly enhancing solid mass with necrosis and calcifications. Magnetic resonance imaging findings are generally nonspecific. Necrosis and hemorrhage appear as areas of low intensity or iso-intensity on T1-weighted imaging and high signal intensity on T2-weighted imaging [87]. In one series of renal HPCs, angiography revealed a common pattern during the arterial phase: displacement of the main arteries, large vessels surrounding the tumor, and a well-demarcated stain [88].

Although the clinical course of HPC has been poorly characterized, early reports suggest several prognostic factors. Enzinger and colleagues reported a 10-year OS rate as high as 80 % in patients with low-grade disease (defined as fewer than three mitotic bodies per high-power field), compared with less than 30 % in patients with 4 or more mitotic bodies per high-power field [89]. While HPC has a more indolent course than other primary renal sarcomas, increased mitotic figures, cellularity, hemorrhage, and necrosis may identify those with more aggressive behavior.

Surgical excision remains the main treatment for HPC. Associated symptoms usually disappear spontaneously after tumor excision [84]. Preoperative angiography may allow for clarification of the vascular anatomy when HPC is suspected and thus allow for a more complete resection. As with many sarcomas, complete excision with negative margins is associated with long-term disease-free survival [83].

Radiation therapy is not commonly used. Only seven patients were reported to have undergone postoperative radiation treatment; one of them survived 11 years, but the remainder had a mean OS of only 32 months [90].

Cytotoxic chemotherapy has been used in an adjuvant setting, and anthracyclines are the most common agents. However, survival remains poor for the majority of patients. The highly vascular nature of this tumor suggests a role for vascular endothelial growth factor receptor inhibitors for unresponsive disease. Lee and colleagues reported the use of pazopanib to treat several patients with metastatic HPCs: one patient achieved a partial response after 1 month of treatment, and two patients had stable disease during 8 months of treatment [86].

Fibrosarcoma

Renal fibrosarcoma originates from the mesenchymal tissue of the renal capsule and most frequently occurs in patients 40–70 years old. Because fibrosarcoma symptoms are similar to those of RCC, renal fibrosarcomas are often found incidentally in asymptomatic patients [91]. Advanced renal fibrosarcoma frequently invades the gastrointestinal tract, and patients sometimes present with upper gastrointestinal bleeding or obstruction [92].

On gross examination, renal fibrosarcomas tend to be large, encapsulated, and lobulated with a fleshy consistency [93]. Microscopically, fibrosarcomas are formed by various types of collagen and have a fascicular growth pattern. Renal fibrosarcomas typically show spindle cells organized in parallel rows intersecting at acute angles in a broken zigzag pattern. Cells have moderately eosinophilic cytoplasm and oval nuclei, with irregularly distributed chromatin [94]. Fibrosarcomas are not reactive to cytokeratin and desmin antibodies but are highly reactive to vimentin and proliferation-related Ki-67 antigen [94].

Fibrosarcoma is a diagnosis of exclusion that is based on histology and IHC analysis [95]. Multiple case reports and series have highlighted the challenges in differentiating fibrosarcoma, sRCC, and LMS with IHC analysis [96]. Retrospective

IHC analysis has shown that some reported cases of sRCC were actually primary renal fibrosarcoma. Cavaliere and colleagues presented such a case in a retrospective series of 17 patients with primary renal sarcomas [97]. The advances in IHC analysis, as well as the routine use of this tool, are improving the accurate diagnosis of fibrosarcomas.

Radical nephrectomy is the treatment of choice, and resection of the adrenal gland and surrounding lymph nodes is recommended owing to the aggressive behavior of fibrosarcomas [91]. The vague data reported thus far on this entity highlights the aggressive behavior and dismal prognosis. According to a review of renal sarcomas by Srinivas and colleagues, primary renal fibrosarcoma has the worst prognosis, with a 5-year CSS rate of less than 10 % [98]. Moreover, adjuvant therapy does not appear to improve survival, and long-term survival is rare: in a review of 21 cases, Pettirssen and colleagues found only two patients who survived over 10 years [99].

Malignant Fibrous Histiocytoma

Malignant fibrous histiocytoma (MFH) is a mesenchymal tumor that most commonly arises from the extremities or the retroperitoneum. In 2014, the World Health Organization redefined MFH as a pleomorphic undifferentiated sarcoma, a category that includes tumors with undefinable lines of differentiation [100]. Although fewer than 100 cases of renal MFH have been reported, this entity may be underdiagnosed, as accurate diagnosis remains challenging.

MFH of the kidney arises from the renal capsule and primarily occurs in patients in the fifth to sixth decades of life. The clinical presentation of MHS does not differ from other renal masses; however, an inflammatory variant may mimic pyelonephritis, with symptoms such as fever, chills, dysuria, and marked neutrophilic leukocytosis. Recent reports of renal MFH associated with renal calculi, although extremely rare, illustrate the possibility of a simultaneous presentation [101].

MFH is highly aggressive; most patients present with retroperitoneal invasion and/or extension into the renal vein and inferior vena cava [102]. MFH commonly metastasizes to the lungs (82 %) and lymph nodes (32 %) [103].

There are four histological subtypes of MFH: storiform-pleomorphic, giant cell, myxoid, and inflammatory. Storiform-pleomorphic, the most frequent form, consists of pleomorphic spindle cells arranged in sheets with an irregular whorled pattern [102]. MFH can be difficult to differentiate from other tumors such as LMS and sRCC. On IHC analysis, MFH stains positive for CD34 and CD68 and is negative for cytokeratin, unlike LMS and sRCC [95]. The diagnosis of MFH therefore relies heavily on IHC analysis and extensive tissue sampling to rule out carcinoma or epithelial components.

Previous studies reporting on MFH have described the radiological characteristics [104, 105]. On computer tomography studies, MFH often presents as a large, lobulated soft tissue mass with central necrosis or myxoid materials [105]. Less than 20 % of the cases are reported with calcifications. On MRI, MFH is exhibit as isointense on T1-weighted images and hyperintense on T2-weighted images. The myxoid and fibrous features are best observed on T2-weighted images. Heterogeneous enhancement is also seen on contrast-enhanced CT and MR images [104]. On certain occasions, MFH may present as a cystic lesion when extensive necrosis or hemorrhage is present.

Radical nephrectomy is the preferred treatment modality since MFH is commonly suspected to be RCC preoperatively. Despite aggressive surgical management, local recurrence occurs in up to 44 % of patients from 3 to 24 months after nephrectomy [106] and the 1-year CSS rate is less than 40 % after surgery alone [107]. The majority of patients with MFH present at an advanced stage, but long-term survival in patients with small renal MFHs who underwent only partial nephrectomy suggests the effectiveness of early treatment [108]. Adjuvant therapy with ifosfamide and doxorubicin is often given after resection, but no significant benefit has been shown, with recurrence reported between 3 and 24 months after adjuvant therapy [101, 109].

Rhabdomyosarcoma

Rhabdomyosarcoma (RMS) is a malignant mesenchymal tumor of embryonal origin that arises from striated skeletal muscle. Among soft tissue sarcomas, RMS is the most common sarcoma in children, accounting for 5–10 % of pediatric solid tumors but for only 1–3 % of all renal sarcomas. RMS has been categorized as one of the least frequent sarcomas of the kidney, on the basis of large series reports. Primary renal RMSs are highly aggressive with a poor prognosis despite aggressive management.

There are three histological subtypes of RMS: alveolar, embryonal, and pleomorphic [110]. The embryonal and alveolar subtypes are most commonly found in children. The alveolar subtype exhibits more aggressive behavior than the embryonal subtype. RMS stains positive for cytokeratin [112], and for myogenin and myoblast determination protein 1, two myogenic regulatory proteins expressed early in skeletal muscle differentiation [111]. The largest series of pediatric renal RMS, presented by the Intergroup RMS Study Group [108], included only six patients diagnosed with primary renal RMS between 1975 and 2005. All six patients presented with embryonal histology [112]. Lastly, Sola and colleagues described a case of a child with RMS with an unusual variant of embryonal histology known as botryoid. This particular variant is associated with favorable prognosis; the patient, despite having distant metastasis to the lungs, was free of recurrence 28 months after surgical resection and chemotherapy [113].

Renal RMSs have deregulated cell-cycle checkpoints, high genome instability, and v-myc avian myelocytomatosis viral oncogene homolog family amplification [114]. The signature genetic changes resulting in the paired box 3-forkhead box O1 fusion gene in alveolar RMS, produced from the translocation of chromosomes 2 and 13, have been strongly linked with the malignant phenotype in pediatric RMS [113, 114].

Primary renal RMS in adults has been described in fewer than 20 patients. The pleomorphic histology was the most common subtype [115], and all patients had a dismal prognosis. The most comprehensive report of adult renal RMS included eight patients with a 14-month OS rate of 50 % [112]. The authors emphasized the difficulty of distinguishing sarcomas of the kidney, such as RMS, from RCC and suggested that a previous history of sarcoma should be ruled out to eliminate the possibility of distant metastatic disease. Imaging studies and pathology should demonstrate that the tumor arises from renal parenchyma instead of from the retroperitoneum or adjacent structures. In addition, sRCC should be excluded if epithelial subcomponents of this entity stain positive for cytokeratin antibodies on IHC analysis [116].

Management of renal RMS consists of radical nephrectomy followed by adjuvant chemoradiation therapy. An aggressive excision is recommended, as evidence of negative margins is one of the most significant prognostic factors for survival. Lymph node dissection is also advised to help determine whether radiation therapy is needed [112]. Adjuvant systemic therapy with vincristine, dactinomycin, and cyclophosphamide has resulted in moderate responses after the first year of treatment [117].

Primary Renal Synovial Sarcoma (PRSS)

PRSS is a newly recognized, aggressive form of kidney sarcoma, previously known as embryonal sarcoma of the kidney. Fewer than 80 cases have been reported [118]. Synovial sarcomas usually occur adjacent to joints in the extremities, and only a few cases have been reported in other sites including the abdominal wall, retroperitoneum, and solid organs.

The clinical presentation of PRSS is similar to that of other sarcomas, with a peak incidence in the fourth to fifth decades of life [73]. A recent series has suggested that PRSS occurs more frequently in adolescents and young adults (mean age, 27 years; range, 15–43 years) [119]. Patients with PRSS typically present with advanced disease, and most patients (98 %) present with flank pain, an abdominal mass, and/or hematuria. This tumor characteristically develops cystic degeneration and, when the majority of the renal parenchyma is affected, patients present with secondary hypertension [120]. Although most patients with PRSS present with locally advanced disease, only 8–10 % of patients present with concurrent metastatic disease, with the most common site of metastasis being the lungs [121].

Macroscopically, PRSSs are rubbery, homogeneous masses, often exhibiting necrosis with focal and/or extended hemorrhage. Characteristically, these tumors are solid, cystic masses with a pseudocapsule [122]. PRSS tumors are classified as either monophasic (composed solely of spindle cells) or biphasic (composed of both epithelial and spindle cells and poorly differentiated). The monophasic subtype occurs more frequently and is associated with a more favorable prognosis than the biphasic subtype [123]. PRSS tissue consistently stains positive for markers such as BCL2 (B-cell chronic lymphocytic leukemia/lymphoma 2), vimentin, CD99 antigen, epithelial membrane antigen, and CD56 antigen and negative for S100, desmin, alpha- smooth muscle actin, hematopoietic progenitor cell antigen CD34, and WT1.

Genetic analysis of PRSS has shown that these tumors harbor unique, pathognomonic chromosomal abnormalities. PRSS are almost exclusively associated with gene fusion of the synovial sarcoma translocation gene on chromosome 18 to the synovial sarcoma X breakpoint 1, synovial sarcoma X breakpoint 2, or, rarely, the synovial sarcoma X breakpoint 4 genes on chromosome X [120]. These three typical chromosomal rearrangements were previously considered to represent embryonal sarcoma of the kidney until Argani and colleagues molecularly characterized PRSS [118]. Further studies have validated these genetic aberrations; thereby, molecular analysis by reverse transcription polymerase chain reaction is currently recommended to distinguish these tumors from poorly differentiated renal sarcomas [124].

The differential diagnosis of PRSS includes sRCC, primary renal PNET, and Wilms tumor. The distinction between the four should be made cautiously since agents used for Wilms tumor are not optimal for PNETs or PRSS. Renal PNETs typically stain positive for neuron-specific enolase, and approximately 50–70 % of PNETs express S100, while PRSS tissue is negative for both markers [125]. Core biopsy often reveals an epithelial component with stromal differentiation in Wilms tumor, which excluded PRSS. sRCC can be excluded by the expression of specific epithelial markers; if a sRCC has a predominantly mesenchymal component, paired box gene 8 is at least focally expressed. Genetic testing remains the most accurate diagnostic method [125].

PRSSs also have unique characteristics on radiological imaging. On computed tomography, these tumors are large, well-defined masses with heterogeneous enhancement and extend into the perinephric fat or renal pelvis [121]. PRSS frequently presents as a cystic mass with enhancing septa and solid components [119]. Hemorrhage, calcification, air-fluid levels, and septations are common [121, 126, 127].

Patients with metastatic PRSS have a poor prognosis. Although PRSSs tend to growth slow, they are characterized by high recurrence rates and hematogenous metastasis in the first year. In 2012, Iacovelli and colleagues studied 64 patients with PRSS who underwent radical nephrectomy [117]. The median disease-free survival was only 33 months, and 36 % of patients developed metastatic disease within the first year of follow-up [121]. Other studies have shown a poor prognosis for patients who developed metastasis after radical nephrectomy, with a median OS of 6 months [119].

There are no standard adjuvant systemic therapy regimens for PRSS. Combinations of anthracyclines with ifosfamide most commonly are used, as for other sarcomas [121]. Neoadjuvant systemic therapy with high-dose ifosfamide has resulted in moderate response rates in soft tissue synovial sarcomas [128]. Park and colleagues reported complete remission in a patient with metastatic PRSS treated with a combination of ifosfamide and doxorubicin [129]. In 13 patients with metastatic soft tissue synovial sarcomas treated with high-dose ifosfamide, Rosen et al. noted partial responses in nine patients and complete responses in four [130]. Because synovial sarcomas often respond favorably to high-dose chemotherapeutic agents, molecular analysis is valuable in identifying patients with suspected disease particularly for young patients with a poorly differentiated cystic renal mass.

Conclusion

Despite advances in IHC and molecular analysis and radiological characterization, the diagnosis of renal sarcomas remains difficult, and most diagnoses are made postoperatively. Prognosis is poor in most patients. Owing to the rarity of these tumors, adequate accrual for prospective clinical trials is not feasible. Collaborations among high-volume centers are necessary to better differentiate these malignancies and develop standard treatment regimens.

References

1. Siegel RL, Miller KD, Jemal A. Cancer statistics, 2015. CA Cancer J Clin. 2015;65(1):5–29.
2. Rodriguez Faba O, Martin Benito JL, Parra Muntaner L, Jalon Monzon A, Regadera Sejas J. Renal liposarcoma. Report of one case and bibliographic review. Arch Esp Urol. 2004;57(6):646–9.
3. Wang X, Xu R, Yan L, et al. Adult renal sarcoma: clinical features and survival in a series of patients treated at a high-volume institution. Urology. 2011;77(4):836–41.
4. Vogelzang NJ, Fremgen AM, Guinan PD, Chmiel JS, Sylvester JL, Sener SF. Primary renal sarcoma in adults. A natural history and management study by the American Cancer Society, Illinois Division. Cancer. 1993;71(3):804–10.
5. Dotan ZA, Tal R, Golijanin D, et al. Adult genitourinary sarcoma: the 25-year Memorial Sloan-Kettering experience. J Urol. 2006;176(5):2033–8; discussion 2038–9.
6. Mor Y, Nass D, Raviv G, Neumann Y, Nativ O, Goldwasser B. Malignant peripheral primitive neuroectodermal tumor (PNET) of the kidney. Med Pediatr Oncol. 1994;23(5):437–40.
7. Ap S. A tumor of the ulnar nerve. Proc N Y Pathol Soc. 1918;12:2–12.
8. Mohsin R, Hashmi A, Mubarak M, et al. Primitive neuroectodermal tumor/Ewing's sarcoma in adult uro-oncology: a case series from a developing country. Urol Ann. 2011;3(2):103–7.
9. Ellinger J, Bastian PJ, Hauser S, Biermann K, Muller SC. Primitive neuroectodermal tumor: rare, highly aggressive differential diagnosis in urologic malignancies. Urology. 2006;68(2):257–62.
10. Thetę N, Rastogi D, Arya S, et al. Primitive neuroectodermal tumour of the prostate gland: ultrasound and MRI findings. Br J Radiol. 2007;80(956):e180–3.
11. Aghili M, Rafiei E, Mojahed M, Zare M. Renal primitive neuroectodermal tumor: does age at diagnosis impact outcomes? Rare Tumor. 2012;4(1):e15.
12. Maccioni F, Della Rocca C, Salvi PF, et al. Malignant peripheral neuroectodermal tumor (MPNET) of the kidney. Abdom Imaging. 2000;25(1):103–6.
13. Risi E, Iacovelli R, Altavilla A, et al. Clinical and pathological features of primary neuroectodermal tumor/Ewing sarcoma of the kidney. Urology. 2013;82(2):382–6.
14. Ewing J. Diffuse endothelioma of bone. Proc N Y Pathol Soc. 1921;21:17–24.
15. Karpate A, Menon S, Basak R, Yuvaraja TB, Tongaonkar HB, Desai SB. Ewing sarcoma/primitive neuroectodermal tumor of the kidney: clinicopathologic analysis of 34 cases. Ann Diagn Pathol. 2012;16(4):267–74.
16. Seemayer TA, Thelmo WL, Bolande RP, Wiglesworth FW. Peripheral neuroectodermal tumors. Perspect Pediatr Pathol. 1975;2:151–72.

17. Sharifi Doloui D, Fakharian T, Yahyavi V, Nekooei S, Zivarifar HR, Ghafarzadegan K. Primitive neuroectodermal tumor with kidney involvement: a case report. Iran J Radiol Q J Publ Iran Radiol Soci. 2014;11(2):e4661.
18. Bing Z, Zhang P, Tomaszewski JE, Maclennan GT. Primary Ewing sarcoma/primitive neuroectodermal tumor of the kidney. J Urol. 2009;181(3):1341–2.
19. Parham DM, Roloson GJ, Feely M, Green DM, Bridge JA, Beckwith JB. Primary malignant neuroepithelial tumors of the kidney: a clinicopathologic analysis of 146 adult and pediatric cases from the National Wilms' Tumor Study Group Pathology Center. Am J Surg Pathol. 2001;25(2):133–46.
20. Jawad MU, Cheung MC, Min ES, Schneiderbauer MM, Koniaris LG, Scully SP. Ewing sarcoma demonstrates racial disparities in incidence-related and sex-related differences in outcome: an analysis of 1631 cases from the SEER database, 1973–2005. Cancer. 2009;115(15):3526–36.
21. Jimenez RE, Folpe AL, Lapham RL, et al. Primary Ewing's sarcoma/primitive neuroectodermal tumor of the kidney: a clinicopathologic and immunohistochemical analysis of 11 cases. Am J Surg Pathol. 2002;26(3):320–7.
22. Rodriguez-Galindo C, Marina NM, Fletcher BD, Parham DM, Bodner SM, Meyer WH. Is primitive neuroectodermal tumor of the kidney a distinct entity? Cancer. 1997;79(11):2243–50.
23. Friedrichs N, Vorreuther R, Poremba C, et al. Primitive neuroectodermal tumor (PNET) in the differential diagnosis of malignant kidney tumors. Pathol Res Pract. 2002;198(8):563–9.
24. Thyavihally YB, Tongaonkar HB, Gupta S, et al. Primitive neuroectodermal tumor of the kidney: a single institute series of 16 patients. Urology. 2008;71(2):292–6.
25. Cuesta Alcala JA, Solchaga Martinez A, Caballero Martinez MC, et al. Primary neuroectodermal tumor (PNET) of the kidney: 26 cases. Current status of its diagnosis and treatment. Arch Esp Urol. 2001;54(10):1081–93.
26. Lee H, Cho JY, Kim SH, Jung DC, Kim JK, Choi HJ. Imaging findings of primitive neuroectodermal tumors of the kidney. J Comput Assist Tomogr. 2009;33(6):882–6.
27. Xu N, Zheng Y, Zhang X, Gao Q, Peng Z. Inferior vena cava thrombus in renal primitive neuroectodermal tumor is not rare. J Natl Med Assoc. 2010;102(7):654–6.
28. Gupta S, Billadello L, Casalino DD. Renal primitive neuroectodermal tumor. J Urol. 2012;187(6):2211–2.
29. Patnaik N, Mishra K, Saini P, Agarwal N. Primitive neuroectodermal tumor of the kidney in a young male: case report and review of literature. Urol Ann. 2015;7(2):236–9.
30. Mandal PK, Mukherjee S, Roy S, Bhattacharyya NK. PNET of kidney: report of four cases. Indian J Med Paediatr Oncol Off J Indian Soc Med Paediatr Oncol. 2012;33(2):130–3.
31. Richey SL, Rao P, Wood CG, Patel S, Tannir NM. Metastatic extraosseous Ewing's sarcoma (EES)/primitive neuroectodermal tumor (PNET) of the kidney: 8-year durable response after induction and maintenance chemotherapy. Clin Genitourin Cancer. 2012;10(3):210–2.
32. Pomara G, Cappello F, Cuttano MG, et al. Primitive Neuroectodermal Tumor (PNET) of the kidney: a case report. BMC Cancer. 2004;4:3.
33. Franzetti GA, Laud-Duval K, Bellanger D, Stern MH, Sastre-Garau X, Delattre O. MiR-30a-5p connects EWS-FLI1 and CD99, two major therapeutic targets in Ewing tumor. Oncogene. 2013;32(33):3915–21.
34. Angel JR, Alfred A, Sakhuja A, Sells RE, Zechlinski JJ. Ewing's sarcoma of the kidney. Int J Clin Oncol. 2010;15(3):314–8.
35. Ginsberg JP, de Alava E, Ladanyi M, et al. EWS-FLI1 and EWS-ERG gene fusions are associated with similar clinical phenotypes in Ewing's sarcoma. J Clin Oncol Off J Am Soc Clin Oncol. 1999;17(6):1809–14.
36. Chu WC, Reznikov B, Lee EY, Grant RM, Cheng FW, Babyn P. Primitive neuroectodermal tumour (PNET) of the kidney: a rare renal tumour in adolescents with seemingly characteristic radiological features. Pediatr Radiol. 2008;38(10):1089–94.
37. Chea YW, Agrawal R, Poh A. Primitive neuroectodermal tumour of the kidney: radiologic-pathological correlations. Hong Kong Med J Xianggang Yi Xue Za Zhi/Hong Kong Acad Med. 2008;14(3):240–3.

38. Almeida MF, Patnana M, Korivi BR, Kalhor N, Marcal L. Ewing sarcoma of the kidney: a rare entity. Case Rep Radiol. 2014;2014:283902.
39. Wu CF, Wang LJ, Chen CS. Images in clinical urology. Magnetic resonance imaging of primitive neuroectodermal tumor of the kidney. Urology. 2000;55(2):284–5.
40. Wada Y, Yamaguchi T, Kuwahara T, Sugiyama Y, Kikukawa H, Ueda S. Primitive neuroectodermal tumour of the kidney with spontaneous regression of pulmonary metastases after nephrectomy. BJU Int. 2003;91(1):121–2.
41. Sun C, Du Z, Tong S, et al. Primitive neuroectodermal tumor of the kidney: case report and review of literature. World J Surg Oncol. 2012;10:279.
42. Kairouani M, Mokrim M, Mellas N, et al. Metastatic Ewing's sarcoma/PNET of kidney in 40 year old patient. Int J Surg Case Rep. 2012;3(6):215–7.
43. Ohgaki K, Horiuchi K, Mizutani S, Sato M, Kondo Y. Primary Ewing's sarcoma/primitive neuroectodermal tumor of the kidney that responded to low-dose chemotherapy with ifosfamide, etoposide, and doxorubicin. Int J Clin Oncol. 2010;15(2):210–4.
44. Grier HE, Krailo MD, Tarbell NJ, et al. Addition of ifosfamide and etoposide to standard chemotherapy for Ewing's sarcoma and primitive neuroectodermal tumor of bone. N Engl J Med. 2003;348(8):694–701.
45. El Weshi A, Memon M, Raja M, et al. VIP (etoposide, ifosfamide, cisplatin) in adult patients with recurrent or refractory Ewing sarcoma family of tumors. Am J Clin Oncol. 2004;27(5):529–34.
46. Fergany AF, Dhar N, Budd GT, Skacel M, Garcia JA. Primary extraosseous ewing sarcoma of the kidney with level III inferior vena cava thrombus. Clin Genitourin Cancer. 2009;7(3):E95–7.
47. Moudouni SM, En-Nia I, Rioux-Leclerq N, Guille F, Lobel B. Leiomyosarcoma of the renal pelvis. Scand J Urol Nephrol. 2001;35(5):425–7.
48. Moazzam M, Ather MH, Hussainy AS. Leiomyosarcoma presenting as a spontaneously ruptured renal tumor-case report. BMC Urol. 2002;2:13.
49. Kendal WS. The comparative survival of renal leiomyosarcoma. Can J Urol. 2007;14(1):3435–42.
50. Miller JS, Zhou M, Brimo F, Guo CC, Epstein JI. Primary leiomyosarcoma of the kidney: a clinicopathologic study of 27 cases. Am J Surg Pathol. 2010;34(2):238–42.
51. Deyrup AT, Montgomery E, Fisher C. Leiomyosarcoma of the kidney: a clinicopathologic study. Am J Surg Pathol. 2004;28(2):178–82.
52. Grasso M, Blanco S, Fortuna F, Crippa S, Di Bella C. Spontaneous rupture of renal leiomyosarcoma in a 45-year-old woman. Arch Esp Urol. 2004;57(8):870–2.
53. Narula V, Siraj F, Bansal A. Renal leiomyosarcoma with soft tissue metastasis: an unusual presentation. Can Urol Assoc J J Assoc Urologues Can. 2015;9(3–4):E139–41.
54. Sharma D, Pradhan S, Aryya NC, Shukla VK. Leiomyosarcoma of kidney: a case report with long term result after radiotherapy and chemotherapy. Int Urol Nephrol. 2007;39(2):397–400.
55. Weiss SW. Smooth muscle tumors of soft tissue. Adv Anat Pathol. 2002;9(6):351–9.
56. Rosai J, Damjanov I, Ackerman LV, Nola M. Rosai and Ackerman's surgical pathology review. Philadelphia: Mosby Elsevier; 2007.
57. Jinzaki M, Silverman SG, Akita H, Nagashima Y, Mikami S, Oya M. Renal angiomyolipoma: a radiological classification and update on recent developments in diagnosis and management. Abdom Imaging. 2014;39(3):588–604.
58. Merrill MM, Wood CG, Tannir NM, et al. Clinically nonmetastatic renal cell carcinoma with sarcomatoid dedifferentiation: natural history and outcomes after surgical resection with curative intent. Urol Oncol Sem Original Invest. 2015;33(4):166.e121–9.
59. Shuch B, Bratslavsky G, Linehan WM, Srinivasan R. Sarcomatoid renal cell carcinoma: a comprehensive review of the biology and current treatment strategies. Oncologist. 2012;17(1):46–54.
60. Ochiai K, Onitsuka H, Honda H, et al. Leiomyosarcoma of the kidney: CT and MR appearance. J Comput Assist Tomogr. 1993;17(4):656–8.

61. Ebara M, Ohto M, Watanabe Y, et al. Diagnosis of small hepatocellular carcinoma: correlation of MR imaging and tumor histologic studies. Radiology. 1986;159(2):371–7.
62. Davis R, Vaccaro JA, Hodges GF, Belville WD, Kiesling Jr V. Renal leiomyosarcoma: plea for aggressive therapy. Urology. 1992;40(2):168–71.
63. Dominici A, Mondaini N, Nesi G, Travaglini F, Di Cello V, Rizzo M. Cystic leiomyosarcoma of the kidney: an unusual clinical presentation. Urol Int. 2000;65(4):229–31.
64. Beccia DJ, Elkort RJ, Krane RJ. Adjuvant chemotherapy in renal leiomyosarcoma. Urology. 1979;13(6):652–4.
65. Lehnhardt M, Muehlberger T, Kuhnen C, et al. Feasibility of chemosensitivity testing in soft tissue sarcomas. World J Surg Oncol. 2005;3(1):20.
66. Ciccarello G, Mucciardi G, Morgia G, et al. A case of renal capsular liposarcoma with intracaval fat thrombus. Eur Urol. 2010;57(2):350–3.
67. Manini C, Pedalino M, Di Primio OG, et al. Renal liposarcoma clinical and pathological aspects. Case report and literature review. Urologia. 2010;77 Suppl 16:25–7.
68. Bader DA, Peres LA, Bader SL. Renal liposarcoma. Int Braz J Urol. 2004;30(3):214–5.
69. Singer S, Antonescu CR, Riedel E, Brennan MF. Histologic subtype and margin of resection predict pattern of recurrence and survival for retroperitoneal liposarcoma. Ann Surg. 2003;238(3):358–71.
70. Dalal KM, Antonescu CR, Singer S. Diagnosis and management of lipomatous tumors. J Surg Oncol. 2008;97(4):298–313.
71. Mayes DC, Fechner RE, Gillenwater JY. Renal liposarcoma. Am J Surg Pathol. 1990;14(3):268–73.
72. Israel GM, Bosniak MA, Slywotzky CM, Rosen RJ. CT differentiation of large exophytic renal angiomyolipomas and perirenal liposarcomas. AJR Am J Roentgenol. 2002;179(3):769–73.
73. Amin MB, Grignon DJ, Srigley JR. Urological pathology. 1st ed. Philadelphia: Wolters Kluwer Health, Lippincott Williams & Wilkins; 2014.
74. Binder SC, Katz B, Sheridan B. Retroperitoneal liposarcoma. Ann Surg. 1978;187(3):257–61.
75. Shastri C, Kumar J, Jaiswal S, Mandhani A. Renal dedifferentiated liposarcoma with intracaval tumor thrombus: a rare case. Indian J Urol. 2012;28(2):208–10.
76. Antman K, Crowley J, Balcerzak SP, et al. An intergroup phase III randomized study of doxorubicin and dacarbazine with or without ifosfamide and mesna in advanced soft tissue and bone sarcomas. J Clin Oncol Off J Am Soc Clin Oncol. 1993;11(7):1276–85.
77. Williams JP, Savage PT. Liposarcoma of kidney. Br J Surg. 1958;46(197):225–31.
78. Matsushita M, Ito A, Ishidoya S, Endoh M, Moriya T, Arai Y. Intravenous extended liposarcoma arising from renal sinus. Int J Urol. 2007;14(8):769–70.
79. Brescia A, Pinto F, Gardi M, Maria Vecchio F, Bassi PF. Renal hemangiopericytoma: case report and review of the literature. Urology. 2008;71(4):755 e759–712.
80. Stout AP, Murray MR. Hemangiopericytoma: a vascular tumor featuring Zimmermann's pericytes. Ann Surg. 1942;116(1):26–33.
81. Chaudhary A, Seenu V, Sedain G, et al. Hemangiopericytoma of renal pelvis – an unusual tumor in an adolescent. Urology. 2007;70(4):811.e813–4.
82. Black HR, Heinemann S. Hemangiopericytoma: report of a case involving the kidney. J Urol. 1955;74(1):42–6.
83. Argyropoulos A, Liakatas I, Lykourinas M. Renal haemangiopericytoma: the characteristics of a rare tumour. BJU Int. 2005;95(7):943–7.
84. Hu Q, Fang Z, Zhou Z, Zheng J. Renal hemangiopericytoma secondary to refractory hypertension in a child: a case report. Oncol Lett. 2014;8(6):2493–5.
85. Simon R, Greene RC. Perirenal hemangiopericytoma: a case associated with hypoglycemia. JAMA. 1964;189(2):155–6.
86. Lee SJ, Kim ST, Park SH, et al. Successful use of pazopanib for treatment of refractory metastatic hemangiopericytoma. Clin Sarcoma Res. 2014;4:13.

87. Hayasaka K, Nihashi T, Nojiri Y, Okamuara K. Computed tomography manifestations of renal hemangiopericytoma. Acta Radiol (Stockh Sweden: 1987). 2007;48(8):934–7.
88. Yaghmai I. Angiographic manifestations of soft-tissue and osseous hemangiopericytomas. Radiology. 1978;126(3):653–9.
89. Enzinger FM, Smith BH. Hemangiopericytoma. An analysis of 106 cases. Hum Pathol. 1976;7(1):61–82.
90. Lee HC, Kay S. Hemangiopericytoma: report of a case involving the kidney with an 11-year follow up. Ann Surg. 1962;156(1):125–8.
91. Ares Valdes Y, Ares Valdes N, Contreras Duvelgel DM. Renal fibrosarcoma. Report of a case. Arch Esp Urol. 2003;56(9):1041–3.
92. Kansara V, Powell I. Fibrosarcoma of kidney. Urology. 1980;16(4):419–21.
93. Katabathina VS, Vikram R, Nagar AM, Tamboli P, Menias CO, Prasad SR. Mesenchymal neoplasms of the kidney in adults: imaging spectrum with radiologic-pathologic correlation. Radiographics. 2010;30(6):1525–40.
94. Gupta M, Bahri NU, Watal P, Chudasama SL, Brahmbhatt SG, Yant H. Malignant mesenchymal renal tumor: a rare case of primary renal fibrosarcoma. J Clin Imag Sci. 2013;3:52.
95. Agarwal K, Singh S, Pathania OP. Primary renal fibrosarcoma: a rare case report and review of literature. Indian J Pathol Microbiol. 2008;51(3):409–10.
96. Chaudhari S, Hatwal D, Suri V. A rare case of primary fibrosarcoma of kidney. Iran J Kidney Dis. 2013;7(1):67–9.
97. Cavaliere A, Fratini D, Legittimo C, Tosi F, Lolli E. Renal fibrosarcoma. Single case in a ten-year survey. Pathologica. 1984;76(1045):615–21.
98. Srinivas V, Sogani PC, Hajdu SI, Whitmore Jr WF. Sarcomas of the kidney. J Urol. 1984;132(1):13–6.
99. Pettirssen R. Mesenchymal neoplasms of kidney. In: Petersen RO, editor. Urologic pathology. Philadelphia: JB Lippincott; 1986. p. 113.
100. Fletcher CD. The evolving classification of soft tissue tumours – an update based on the new 2013 WHO classification. Histopathology. 2014;64(1):2–11.
101. Altunkol A, Savas M, Ciftci H, Gulum M, Yagmur I, Bitiren M. Primary giant cell malignant fibrous histiocytoma-associated with renal calculus. Can Urol Assoc J J Assoc Urologues Can. 2014;8(3–4):E193–5.
102. Eble JN SG, Epstein JI, Sesterhenn IA. World Health Organization classification of tumours: pathology and genetics of tumours of the urinary system and male genital organs. Lyon: IARC; 2004.
103. Pathrose G, John NT, Manojkumar R. A rare case of malignant fibrous histiocytoma/pleomorphic undifferentiated sarcoma of the kidney. J Clin Diagn Res. 2015;9(1):D27–9.
104. Kim KH, Lee SH, Cha SH, Kim YS, Sung DJ. Malignant fibrous histiocytoma arising from a hydronephrotic kidney: a case report and review of the literature. Clin Imaging. 2012;36(3):239–42.
105. Kitajima K, Kaji Y, Morita M, Okuda Y, Sugimura K. Malignant fibrous histiocytoma arising from the renal capsule. Magn Reson Med Sci. 2003;2(4):199–202.
106. Singh SK, Mandal AK, Agarwal MM, Das A. Primary renal inflammatory malignant fibrous histiocytoma: a diagnostic challenge. Int J Urol. 2006;13(7):1000–2.
107. Eroglu M, Bakirtas H, Cimentepe E, Unsal A, Ataoglu O, Balbay MD. Malignant fibrous histiocytoma arising from the renal capsule. Urol Int. 2005;75(4):368–70.
108. Gil-Julio H, Vazquez-Alonso F, Puche-Sanz I, Fernandez-Sanchez AJ, Cozar-Olmo JM. Conservative treatment of malignant fibrous histiocytoma of the kidney: a case report. Curr Urol. 2012;6(1):46–9.
109. Chen Y, Rao D, Zhu H, Yu H, Yang S. Primary malignant fibrous histiocytoma of the renal pelvis: a 78-month follow-up case report. Oncol Targets Ther. 2013;7:1–3.
110. Bayindir P, Guillerman RP, Hicks MJ, Chintagumpala MM. Cellular mesoblastic nephroma (infantile renal fibrosarcoma): institutional review of the clinical, diagnostic imaging, and pathologic features of a distinctive neoplasm of infancy. Pediatr Radiol. 2009;39(10): 1066–74.

111. Fanous RN, Mayer EK, Vale J, Lloyd J, Walker MM. Primary renal embryonal rhabdomyosarcoma in adults: a case report and review of the literature. Case Rep Oncol Med. 2012;2012:460749.
112. Raney B, Anderson J, Arndt C, et al. Primary renal sarcomas in the Intergroup Rhabdomyosarcoma Study Group (IRSG) experience, 1972–2005: a report from the Children's Oncology Group. Pediatr Blood Cancer. 2008;51(3):339–43.
113. Sola JE, Cova D, Casillas J, Alvarez OA, Qualman S, Rodriguez MM. Primary renal botryoid rhabdomyosarcoma: diagnosis and outcome. J Pediatr Surg. 2007;42(12):e17–20.
114. Linardic CM. PAX3-FOXO1 fusion gene in rhabdomyosarcoma. Cancer Lett. 2008;270(1):10–8.
115. Dalfior D, Eccher A, Gobbo S, et al. Primary pleomorphic rhabdomyosarcoma of the kidney in an adult. Ann Diagn Pathol. 2008;12(4):301–3.
116. Grignon DJ, McIsaac GP, Armstrong RF, Wyatt JK. Primary rhabdomyosarcoma of the kidney. A light microscopic, immunohistochemical, and electron microscopic study. Cancer. 1988;62(9):2027–32.
117. Walther A, Cost NG, Garrison AP, Geller JI, Alam S, Tiao GM. Renal rhabdomyosarcoma in a pancake kidney. Urology. 2013;82(2):458–60.
118. Argani P, Faria PA, Epstein JI, et al. Primary renal synovial sarcoma: molecular and morphologic delineation of an entity previously included among embryonal sarcomas of the kidney. Am J Surg Pathol. 2000;24(8):1087–96.
119. Lv XF, Qiu YW, Han LJ, et al. Primary renal synovial sarcoma: computed tomography imaging findings. Acta Radiol. 2015;56(4):493–9.
120. Nishida T, Inamoto T, Uehara H, et al. Monophasic primary renal synovial sarcoma accompanied with a hemorrhagic cyst. Urol J. 2011;8(3):244–7.
121. Iacovelli R, Altavilla A, Ciardi A, et al. Clinical and pathological features of primary renal synovial sarcoma: analysis of 64 cases from 11 years of medical literature. BJU Int. 2012;110(10):1449–54.
122. Chen S, Bhuiya T, Liatsikos EN, Alexianu MD, Weiss GH, Kahn LB. Primary synovial sarcoma of the kidney: a case report with literature review. Int J Surg Pathol. 2001;9(4):335–9.
123. Lopes H, Pereira CA, Zucca LE, et al. Primary monophasic synovial sarcoma of the kidney: a case report and review of literature. Clin Med Insights Oncol. 2013;7:257–62.
124. Bella AJ, Winquist EW, Perlman EJ. Primary synovial sarcoma of the kidney diagnosed by molecular detection of SYT-SSX fusion transcripts. J Urol. 2002;168(3):1092–3.
125. Abbas M, Dammrich ME, Braubach P, et al. Synovial sarcoma of the kidney in a young patient with a review of the literature. Rare Tumor. 2014;6(2):5393.
126. Lalwani N, Prasad SR, Vikram R, Katabathina V, Shanbhogue A, Restrepo C. Pediatric and adult primary sarcomas of the kidney: a cross-sectional imaging review. Acta Radiol (Stockhol Sweden: 1987). 2011;52(4):448–57.
127. Erturhan S, Seckiner I, Zincirkeser S, et al. Primary synovial sarcoma of the kidney: use of PET/CT in diagnosis and follow-up. Ann Nucl Med. 2008;22(3):225–9.
128. Majumder A, Dey S, Khandakar B, Medda S, Chandra PP. Primary renal synovial sarcoma: a rare tumor with an atypical presentation. Arch Iran Med. 2014;17(10):726–8.
129. Park SJ, Kim HK, Kim CK, et al. A case of renal synovial sarcoma: complete remission was induced by chemotherapy with doxorubicin and ifosfamide. Korean J Intern Med. 2004;19(1):62–5.
130. Rosen G, Forscher C, Lowenbraun S, et al. Synovial sarcoma. Uniform response of metastases to high dose ifosfamide. Cancer. 1994;73(10):2506–11.

Adult Wilms' Tumor

5

Ankit Madan and Guru Sonpavde

Introduction

Wilms' tumor or nephroblastoma, named after nineteenth-century German surgeon Carl Max Wilhelm Wilms, is an embryonal kidney tumor that occurs primarily in children. It is a rare tumor and represents 5–6 % of all childhood cancer cases in Europe and United States and is the most common pediatric primary malignant tumor of the kidneys [1]. The median age at diagnosis for children is 3–4 years, and 90 % of children are diagnosed before the age of 7 years [2]. In Europe and the United States, the incidence rate of Wilms' tumor in children (0–14 years) is about ten per million [3]. Approximately 510 children are diagnosed every year in the United States [4].

Wilms' tumor is extremely rare among the adolescent and adult population. Until 2004, only 300 cases had been reported in adults worldwide [5]. According to a population-based European epidemiological study from European cancer registries' study on cancer patients' survival and care (EUROCARE) project, which included data from years 1983 to 1994 from 67 cancer registries that covered a combined population of 100 million in 22 European countries, the overall crude incidence rate was 0.19 per million adults. The proportion of adult Wilms' tumor among all kidney cancers was 0.33 % or less in most registries. Recent data indicates that approximately 70 new cases arise in adults in Europe each year [2].

A. Madan, MD
Department of Medicine, Section of Hematology-Oncology, University of Alabama at Birmingham (UAB), Birmingham, AL, USA

G. Sonpavde, MD (✉)
Department of Medicine, Section of Hematology-Oncology, University of Alabama at Birmingham (UAB), Birmingham, AL, USA
e-mail: gsonpavde@uabmc.edu

L. Pagliaro (ed.), *Rare Genitourinary Tumors*,
DOI 10.1007/978-3-319-30046-7_5

Pathogenesis

Histopathology

The histology and cytology of Wilms' tumor in adults are similar to that of pediatric patients [6]. During embryonic development, the fetal kidney and collecting ducts from the ureteric bud and the metanephric mesenchyme or blastema form the stroma and proximal tubular structures, glomeruli, proximal and distal tubules, and loop of Henle (which requires mesenchymal to epithelial transition) [7]. The blastema usually disappears by 36 weeks of gestation. However, at birth approximately 1 % of infants retain residual blastema within their kidney [8, 9]. These abnormally persistent cells were defined by Beckwith as nephrogenic rests [8]. Interestingly, in 40 % of Wilms' tumor patients, nephrogenic rests can be identified. Nephrogenic rests are thought to be the precursor lesions of Wilms' tumors [10]. Although nephrogenic rests may regress or lie dormant, a proportion will proliferate and may undergo neoplastic transformation into Wilms' tumor.

Progression of disease is thought to result from the acquisition of stable somatic changes, either in the form of genetic mutations or epimutations [8, 10]. Morphologically, three major components are present in most tumors – undifferentiated blastema, mesenchymal stroma, and epithelial cells (Fig. 5.1). The blastema is extremely cellular and composed of small round to oval primitive cells or spindle

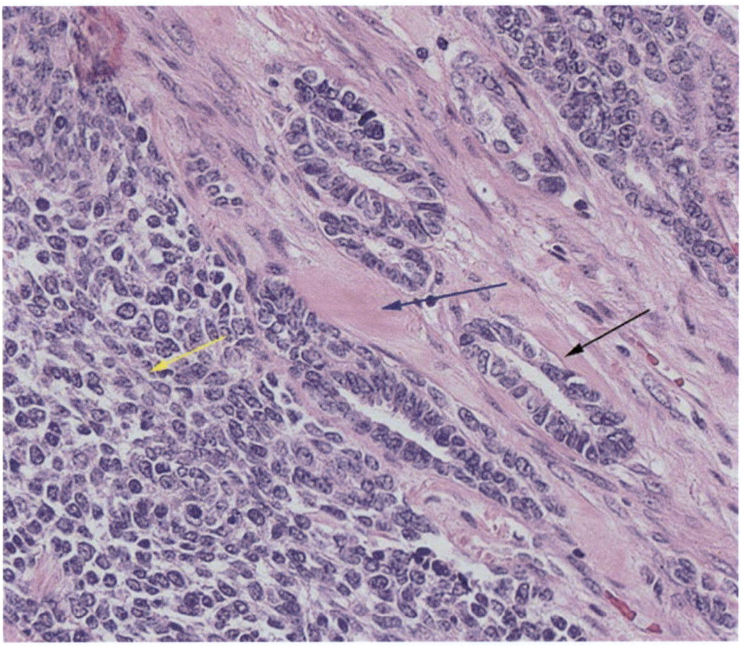

Fig. 5.1 Histopathology of Wilms' tumor. This image shows all the three components of Wilms' tumor – epithelial component (*black arrow*), blastemal component (*yellow arrow*), and mesenchymal component (*Blue arrow*) (Courtesy of Jennifer Beth Gordetsky, MD, Dept. of Pathology, UAB Birmingham, AL)

cells with scanty cytoplasm. The pattern of growth may be diffuse, nodular, cord-like, or basaloid. The mesenchymal elements usually have a spindle-cell fibroblastic configuration but may exhibit a varied differentiation, including smooth and striated muscle cells and neurons. The epithelial component is characterized by the formation of embryonic tubular or glomerular structures, which closely recapitulates the appearance of normal developing metanephric tubules and glomeruli. The key to recognizing Wilms' tumor in a biopsy is to identify these three components of the tumor in the renal mass; the most conspicuous being the blastemal component [11].

Immunohistochemistry (IHC) can provide supportive evidence with the presence of WT1 in the malignant blastemic and epithelial components. Additionally, IHC for cytokeratin, vimentin, desmin, and actin helps to distinguish Wilms' tumor from other malignancies such as renal sarcoma and clear cell sarcoma as well. Kilton and colleagues established diagnostic criteria for adult Wilms' tumor which include: [12]

- Primary renal neoplasm
- Presence of primitive blastemic spindle- or round-cell component
- Formation of abortive or embryonal tubules or glomerular structures
- No areas of tumor diagnostic of renal cell carcinoma
- Pictorial confirmation of histology
- Age >15 years

Blastemal-predominant Wilms' tumor is more aggressive than other types and confers poor outcomes. In contrast, epithelial and stromal component predominant tumors confer intermediate risk. Anaplastic features, i.e., the presence of substantial nuclear and mitotic atypia, have also been associated with a poorer outcome and resistance to chemotherapy [13].

Histologic Classification

The International Society of Pediatric Oncology (SIOP) approach classifies tumor into three prognostic risk groups (low, intermediate, and high) based on histology which captures chemotherapy-induced regressive changes and has allowed the use of tailored therapy (Table 5.1) [14]. In contrast, the National Wilms' Tumor Study Group (NWTSG) approach which is used by the Children's Oncology Group (COG) classifies Wilms' tumor into two groups based on presence or absence of anaplasia.

Genetics

Wilms' tumor is known to be genetically heterogeneous in the pediatric. Thus far, the paucity of data available in adults makes it difficult to determine whether Wilms' tumor in adults and children is biologically comparable and similar tumor entities occurring in a different age group as suggested by their morphological similarities. More research needs to be done to elicit the genetic landscape of adult Wilms'

Table 5.1 Histological subtyping and risk grouping of renal tumors in children according to SIOP initial treatment approach [14]

Low risk tumor	Intermediate risk tumor	High risk tumor
Mesoblastic nephroma	Epithelial type	Blastema type
Necrotic nephroblastoma	Stromal type	Diffuse anaplasia
Cystic partially differentiated nephroblastoma	Regressive type	Clear cell sarcoma of kidney
	Mixed type	Rhabdoid tumor of kidney
	Focal anaplasia	

Adapted from Vujanić et al. [14]

tumor. Wilms' tumor is generally a sporadic disease. Nevertheless, congenital disorders due to germline WT1 gene alterations that predispose to pediatric Wilms' tumor, like the WAGR (Wilms' tumor, aniridia, genitourinary anomalies, and mental retardation) syndrome, Denys-Drash syndrome (renal disease, male pseudohermaphroditism, and Wilms' tumor), and the Beckwith-Wiedemann syndrome (associated with microduplication mutations in the 11p11.5 regions of imprinting genes), do not seem to be associated with adult Wilms' tumor [15].

Somatic mutations in Wilms' tumor 1 (WT1) gene located on the short arm of chromosome 11 at position 13 (11p13), Wilms' tumor gene on the X chromosome (WTX; also known as AMER1), β-catenin (CTNNB1), and TP53 occur either singly or in combination in a third of cases (Fig. 5.2) [16–18]. Cytogenetic analysis of germline DNA from patients with the rare congenital WAGR syndrome detected deletion of band 13 of the short arm of chromosome 11, which led to the identification and isolation of WT1 tumor suppressor gene from that region [19, 20]. Data suggest that WT1 expression plays a role in metanephric stem cell differentiation [21]. Consistent with its vital role in the development of the kidney and gonad, in addition to predisposition to Wilms' tumor, WT1 germline mutations can engender genitourinary tract anomalies and glomerulosclerosis, leading to renal failure [22, 23]. The CTNNB1 or catenin (cadherin-associated protein) beta 1 gene encodes β-catenin and upregulates the WNT pathway leading to tumorigenesis. A positive correlation exists between CTNNB1 mutation and WT1 gene mutation with many WT1-mutated Wilms' tumors also harboring CTNNB1 mutations [24]. The WTX (Wilms' tumor on the X, Xq11.1) tumor suppressor gene is altered in 7–29 % of Wilms' tumors, with two-thirds of these tumor's carrying deletions of the entire WTX gene [16, 25–28]. The remaining one-third of WTX-mutated Wilms' tumors carry mutations such as nonsense mutations and insertions and deletions that cause frameshifts that can result in termination codons or missense mutations [24]. The WTX gene encodes a protein that negatively regulates the WNT pathway. WTX mutations appear to be equally frequent in tumors with and without mutations in WT1 [16, 28]. Although p53 tumor suppressor gene alterations are the most common genetic abnormality detected in adult tumors, they are rare in pediatric malignancies, including Wilms' tumor with the exception of the anaplastic histologic subtype of Wilms' tumor. This finding provides a biologic rationale for the poor outcomes in anaplastic tumors with current chemotherapy. Their p53-dependent apoptotic pathway may have become inactivated [29].

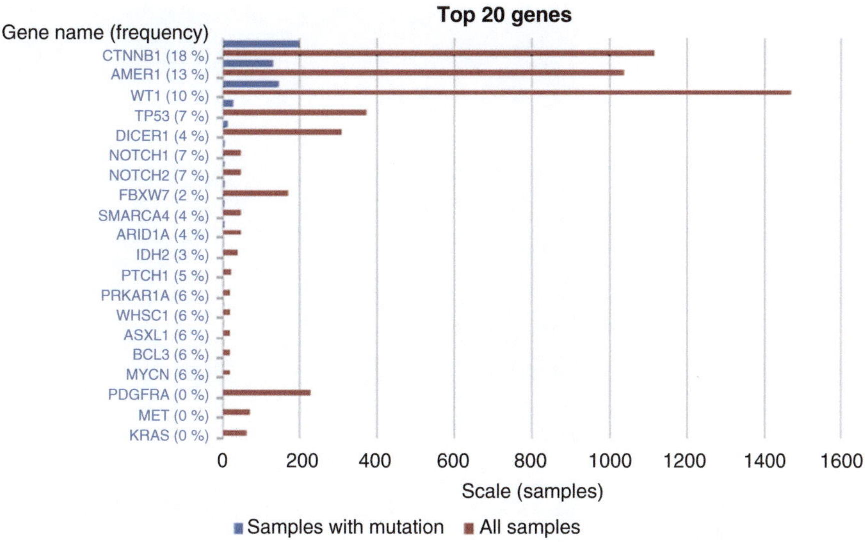

Fig. 5.2 Common somatic mutations in Wilms' tumor. CTNNB1, AMER1, WT1, and TP53 appear to be the most commonly mutated genes in Wilms' tumors (Courtesy of cancer.sanger.ac.uk and Forbes et al. COSMIC: exploring the world's knowledge of somatic mutations in human cancer 2014 [16–18])

Other loci, including 11p15, 1p, 2q, 7p, 9q, 14q, 16q, and 22, have also been implicated in the etiology of Wilms' tumor. Patients with LOH for chromosome 16q had relapse rates three times higher and a significantly higher mortality, i.e., more than ten times higher than patients without this alteration, suggesting that a gene within this site may be responsible for more aggressive biology [30]. National Wilms' Tumor Study (NWTS) Group-5 trial also identified that in favorable histology Wilms' tumors, the presence of both LOH of chromosome 16p and 1p was associated with an increased risk of relapse and death [31]. Genome loss at 4q and 14q has been identified for anaplastic tumors as well [32]. Additionally, gain of chromosome 1q observed in approximately 25 % of cases appears to be associated with poor survival as demonstrated in the NWTS-4 favorable histology cohort [33, 34].

Clinical Features

Clinical Presentation

Adult Wilms' tumor presents with flank or abdominal pain in approximately 80 % of patients. This is accompanied by nonspecific symptoms including weight loss, anorexia, gross or microscopic hematuria, and decline in performance status. Rarely, it can present as a palpable abdominal mass. The median age of diagnosis reported in adults with Wilms' tumor has varied between 18 and 34 years in different case

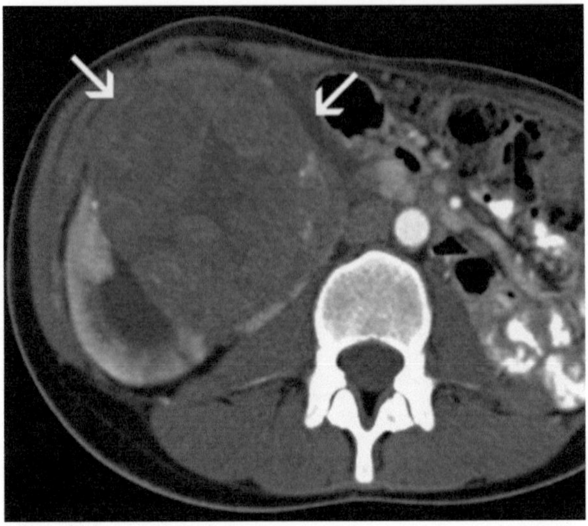

Fig. 5.3 The Wilms' tumor is shown by the *white arrows* (Courtesy of Mark Lockhart, MD Dept. of Radiology UAB Birmingham, AL)

series [35, 36]. In contrast, children typically present with an asymptomatic abdominal mass, malaise, pain, and either microscopic or gross hematuria. Approximately 25 % of children with Wilms' tumor have hypertension presumably due to increased renin activity [20].

Imaging

Imaging plays an important role in the early diagnosis of Wilms' tumor. Ultrasound is the most common method for initial diagnosis of Wilms' tumor. It is noninvasive and affordable [37]. However, it provides poor cross-sectional anatomical information and is less accurate than computerized tomography (CT) scan in tumor staging. Intravenous urography (IVU) can assess physiological or functional ability of the kidney(s) and is also helpful in preoperative differentiation between neuroblastoma and Wilms' tumor [38]. However, IVU is suboptimal to differentiate between solid tumors and benign lesions. CT and magnetic resonance imaging (MRI) are superior to conventional ultrasound and IVU in the preoperative evaluation of patients with Wilms' tumor, owing to their better accuracy and detail [37, 39]. CT chest may be performed to detect pulmonary metastases. CT scan provides excellent visualization of the renal mass, intravascular extension of tumor, and contiguous structures like vessels and lymph nodes along with status and function of the contralateral kidney. On CT, Wilms' tumor usually appears as a bulky, spherical intra-renal mass, usually with a well-defined rim of compressed renal parenchyma or surrounding pseudo capsule (Fig. 5.3) [39]. Some tumors may arise from the periphery of the cortex and grow in an exophytic manner. A heterogeneous mass replacing the kidney and displacing adjacent organs can also be observed. The tumor is hypodense as compared to the surrounding normal renal parenchyma on contrast-enhanced CT scans with the areas of low attenuation coinciding with tumor necrosis, fat deposition, or both [40]. MRI may be superior to CT for determining the extent of intravascular involvement [41]. Wilms' tumor in adults can be indistinguishable from the more common adult renal neoplasm renal cell carcinoma [42].

Management

Staging

Available adult series report a higher incidence of advanced stage 3 or 4 disease in greater than 50 % of patients compared with the pediatric series where approximately one-third of children are classified as stage 3 or 4 disease [5, 43]. Staging investigations should include a CT scan of the chest and abdomen to detect pulmonary and hepatic metastases and to assess tumor extension, involvement of inferior vena cava, and function of the contralateral kidney. There are two main staging systems: a pre-chemotherapy, surgery-based system developed by the NWTS group and a post-chemotherapy-based system developed by the SIOP [14, 44]. Both staging systems are described in detail in Tables 5.2 and 5.3.

Table 5.2 Wilms' tumor pre-chemotherapy staging by the National Wilms' Tumor Study Group (NWTSG) [44]

NWTSG staging system (pre-chemotherapy)
Stage 1
Tumor is limited to the kidney and completely resected
Tumor was not ruptured before or during removal
Vessels of the renal sinus are not involved beyond 2 mm
There is no residual tumor apparent beyond the margins of excision
Stage 2
Tumor extends beyond the kidney but is completely excised
No residual tumor is apparent at or beyond the margins of excision
Tumor thrombus in vessels outside the kidney is stage 2 if the thrombus is removed en bloc with the tumor
Stage 3
Residual tumor confined to the abdomen
Lymph nodes in the renal hilum or the periaortic chains or beyond are found to contain the tumor
Diffuse peritoneal contamination by the tumor
Tumor extends beyond the surgical margins either microscopically or glossy
Tumor is not completely resectable because of local infiltration into vital structures
Stage 4
Presence of hematogenous metastases or metastases to distal lymph nodes
Stage 5
Bilateral renal involvement at the time of initial diagnosis

Table 5.3 Wilms' tumor post-chemotherapy staging by the International Society of Pediatric Oncology (SIOP) [14]

SIOP staging system (post-chemotherapy)
Stage 1
Tumor is limited to kidney or surrounded with fibrous pseudocapsule. If outside the normal contours of the kidney, the renal capsule or pseudocapsule may be infiltrated with the tumor, but it does not reach the outer surface and is completely resected (resection margins "clear")
The tumor may be protruding into the pelvic system and "dipping" into the ureter (but it is not infiltrating their walls)
The vessels of the renal sinus are not involved
Intra-renal vessel involvement may be present
Stage 2
The tumor extends beyond kidney or penetrates through the renal capsule and/or fibrous pseudocapsule into peri-renal fat but is completely resected (resection margins "clear")
The tumor infiltrates the renal sinus and/or invades blood and lymphatic vessels outside the renal parenchyma but is completely resected
The tumor infiltrates adjacent organs or vena cava but is completely resected
Stage 3
Incomplete excision of the tumor, which extends beyond resection margins (gross or microscopic tumor remains postoperatively)
Any abdominal lymph nodes are involved
Tumor rupture before or intraoperatively (irrespective of other criteria for staging)
The tumor has penetrated through the peritoneal surface
Tumor thrombi present at resection margins of vessels or ureter transected or removed piecemeal by surgeon
The tumor has been surgically biopsied (wedge biopsy) prior to preoperative chemotherapy or surgery
Stage 4
Hematogenous metastases (lung, liver, bone, brain, etc.) or lymph node metastases outside the abdominopelvic region
Stage 5
Bilateral renal tumors at diagnosis

Treatment

To achieve the best outcomes in adults, a multimodality approach using pediatric protocols which includes surgery (nephrectomy), chemotherapy, and radiation treatment is advocated.

Surgery: In children, there are two protocols (SIOP and COG) for the treatment of Wilms' tumor. The protocols differ on the timing of surgery (nephrectomy). The COG which took forward clinical trials run by NWTS in 1969 recommends resection of the primary tumor (nephrectomy) for precise pathologic assessment of tumor extent (stage) and histology before adjuvant chemotherapy is instituted. In contrast, the SIOP nephroblastoma group, which commenced its trials in 1971, favors preoperative (neoadjuvant) chemotherapy to reduce the complications of surgery and tumor spillage, at the time of delayed nephrectomy which takes place 4–6 weeks after chemotherapy [22].

Most adult patients are treated with initial nephrectomy because in majority of patients the diagnosis is made unexpectedly after nephrectomy is performed for presumed RCC. Even when Wilms' tumor is diagnosed before nephrectomy, total nephrectomy is still recommended according to adult nephrectomy guidelines for any renal cancer. The surgery of choice is open total nephrectomy with lymph node sampling and immediate review by pathology [45]. A review of lymph node sampling has demonstrated a false-negative rate of more than 30 % [46]. Hence although formal lymph node dissection is not considered necessary, lymph node sampling is critically important during the surgical procedure regardless of benign appearing nodes on preoperative imaging or during surgery. Conversely, enlarged lymph nodes seen on preoperative imaging may be "reactive," and there is no definitive evidence that routine lymphadenectomy improves survival. The absence of node sampling may result in under-staging and undertreatment of the tumor as reported by NWTS group in 2005, which could result in an increase of relative risk of local recurrence [46–48]. The surrounding structures are infrequently invaded by Wilms' tumors. The en bloc excision of the tumor with closely adherent structures is necessary when they cannot be cleanly separated, e.g., hepatic invasion [46].

In the pediatric population, there was no difference in event-free or overall survival with immediate nephrectomy versus preoperative chemotherapy followed by nephrectomy in the United Kingdom Children's Cancer Study Group (UKCCS group) trial [49, 50]. In this trial, 205 pediatric patients (186 had confirmed Wilms' tumor) with newly diagnosed potentially resectable renal tumors were randomly selected to undergo immediate nephrectomy, or percutaneous renal biopsy, followed by 6 weeks of neoadjuvant vincristine and actinomycin-D chemotherapy followed by nephrectomy. There was no difference between the two groups in 5-year event-free survival (~80 %), although clinical downstaging was observed with neoadjuvant chemotherapy. In a subsequent report of 520 pediatric patients from the UKCCS group including the aforementioned trial and other off-protocol patients, delayed nephrectomy preceded by preoperative chemotherapy was reported to be associated with fewer surgical complications including tumor rupture and spillage compared with immediate nephrectomy (1 % versus 20.4 %) [15]. For patients with bilateral Wilms' tumor, surgical management is complicated and the risk of renal failure is a concern [46]. The treatment strategy relies on nephron sparing surgery after preoperative chemotherapy which often results in significant reduction of tumor size [51]. The incidence of end-stage renal disease is approximately 15 % at 15 years post-surgery [52].

Chemotherapy: Over the years, adopting pediatric regimens of chemotherapy for treating adults has proven to be effective in improving outcomes. Wilms' tumor is quite sensitive to chemotherapy with partial or complete responses seen in 40–60 % of metastatic tumors. The backbone of chemotherapy regimens for Wilms' tumor comprises vincristine and actinomycin-D, which is administered as perioperative therapy for stage 1 and favorable stage 2 disease. Doxorubicin is added to this backbone, in high-risk stage 2, 3, and 4 disease. Ifosfamide, carboplatin, and etoposide (ICE) are generally reserved for recurrent advanced disease [45]. The duration of therapy requires further study. Currently, protocols are using 4–6 weeks of neoadjuvant chemotherapy followed by 4–6 months of adjuvant chemotherapy for operable localized disease. For recurrent metastatic disease, the ICE regimen and clinical trials may be considered.

The COG protocol recommends metastatic or "inoperable" cases be diagnosed by preoperative biopsy to receive preoperative chemotherapy based on histology. In their current protocol, children with stage 2 favorable histology Wilms' tumor are treated without doxorubicin. The recommendation for adults is to include doxorubicin in patients who harbor LOH at 1p and 16q, since this molecular subset of patients exhibit poor outcomes with the two-drug regimen. Vincristine intensity is also decreased in these guidelines as compared with current childhood protocols, as adults frequently develop severe neurological toxicities. Sperm banking in males or ovarian preservation in females could be considered immediately before instituting chemotherapy, especially when delivering regimens containing cyclophosphamide or carboplatin [53].

Radiation: Nephroblastoma is a radiotherapy-sensitive cancer as well. In general, radiation therapy is a component of treatment for more advanced stages of Wilms' tumor (stage 3–5). Minor differences in recommendations exist between the SIOP and COG protocol. According to SIOP, radiation therapy is also indicated as adjuvant therapy for node-positive and stage >2 with high risk disease. For the intermediate-risk group, the dose recommended is 15 Gray (Gy) with 15 Gy boost and for the high-risk group, 30 Gy with 5 Gy boost [36]. In the COG protocol, in addition to stage >3, radiation therapy is also recommended for stage 1–2 with unfavorable histology. Radiotherapy is usually instituted by day 14 post-nephrectomy although starting by day 30 is also considered acceptable [45]. Pulmonary radiotherapy is reserved for patients with evidence of pulmonary metastases on chest imaging.

Outcomes

Adults with Wilms' tumor were reported to have worse outcomes in the past as compared with pediatric patients, with historically recorded long-term survival rates of 18–27 % [54, 55]. These results are attributable in part to the fact that the disease usually presented at an advanced stage in adults. Patients with stage 3 and stage 4 diseases were reported to account for more than 50 % of most adult series. Byrd et al. demonstrated that the prognosis was worse in adults than in children even stage for stage. Uncorrected for histology, the recorded 3-year actuarial survival rates in adults were 48 % for stages 1–2 aggregated and 11 % for stage 4, with an

Table 5.4 Outcomes in adult patients with Wilms' tumor reported by different studies

Study (year)	Year	*n* (F/M)	Median age (years)	EFS (%)	OS,% 5 years	Ref. no.
Mitry et al. (2006)	1983–1994	133 (69/64)	34 (15–60)	N/A	47.3	[2]
Izawa et al. (2008)	1973–2006	128	26 (15–73)	N/A	68	[57]
Terenziani et al. (2004)	1983–2001	17 (11/6)	17.5 (16–29)	45	62.4	[5]
Kattan et al. (1994)	1973–1992	22 (14/8)	24 (16–40)	41	55	[35]
Reinhard et al. (2004)	1994–2001	30 (13/17)	25.4 (15–62)	57	83	[36]
Kalapurakal et al. (2004)	1988–2001	23 (13/10)	21.9 (16–51)	77.3	82.6	[58]
Arrigo et al. (1990)	1979–1987	27 (N/A)	24 (16–74)	NA	67	[56]

overall survival of 24 %. In contrast, children of that era had corresponding survival rates of 87 %, 53 %, and 74 %, respectively, also uncorrected for histology [43]. This prompted treating adults with protocols that were designed for and used in pediatric patients involving different modalities of treatment. Using pediatric protocol, the experience of Arrigo and associates with 27 patients between 1979 and 1987 yielded 3-year survival rates of 67 % when anaplastic tumors were included and 79 % when they were excluded (Table 5.4) [56–60]. This data represented an important improvement over prior results and led to the following recommendations: perioperative two-drug chemotherapy for patients with stage 1 disease and perioperative three-drug chemotherapy and adjuvant radiotherapy to the tumor bed (2,000 cGy) for patients with stage ≥2 disease [56]. Subsequently, other retrospective case series of patients reported similar long-term outcomes with multimodality therapy (Table 5.4) [2, 5, 35, 36, 56–58].

In one noteworthy study, a German group using the SIOP perioperative treatment protocol focused on 30 adult patients who were treated according to the SIOP 93-01 study. All of the patients had a central pathology review, and six tumors (13 %) were classified as having high-risk histology. Ten patients (33 %) were found to have distant metastases at the time of diagnosis. All patients underwent primary surgery, all received chemotherapy, and 14 of the 30 patients received radiation as well. At a median follow-up of 4 years, the event-free survival and the OS rates were 57 % and 83 %, respectively [36].

Treatment Toxicity and Monitoring

Neurotoxicity secondary to vincristine and hepatotoxicity or veno-occlusive disease (VOD) due to actinomycin-D is also reported in adults similar to children [36, 58]. The SIOP 9301 study done by the German group reported that 13 out of 27 (48 %) adults suffered from severe (grade 3–4) neurotoxicity, resulting in treatment delay, dose reduction, or even discontinuation of treatment (40.7 %) [36]. In children, the incidence of VOD varies from 5 to 8 % [59–61]. If supportive management is initiated adequately and timely, it is mostly reversible. The SIOP 9301 also reported severe VOD in 1 out of 30 (3 %) adult renal tumor patients (27 Wilms' tumor and 3 clear cell sarcoma of the kidney) that resolved without residual effects [36]. Kalapurakal and his associates reported 23 adult Wilms' tumor patients of whom 3 (13 %) died after treatment-related liver toxicity, 3–6 months after treatment with actinomycin-D [58].

A late adverse effect associated with a cumulative dose of anthracyclines exceeding 300 mg/m^2 is cardiotoxicity. Anthracycline-mediated cardiotoxicity may be severe if pulmonary irradiation has been administered. Pulmonary irradiation can itself result in restrictive lung disease, whereas abdominal radiotherapy can cause fertility problems and impaired renal function. Renal dysfunction has been described after cyclophosphamide and carboplatin as well in adults [62–66]. Long-term survivors of Wilms' tumor have an increased risk of developing subsequent secondary malignant neoplasms (6.7 % at 40 years from diagnosis) [67]. Secondary malignancies can include bone and soft-tissue sarcomas, breast cancer, lymphoma, leukemia, and melanoma [51].

Toxicity monitoring should comprise of complete blood count and a complete metabolic panel before administration of each dose of chemotherapy. Disproportionate thrombocytopenia and signs of hepatotoxicity will alert the physician to the possibility of VOD. Monitoring for impaired renal function (both glomerular and tubular) as well as possible cardiac function by an echocardiogram (especially in cases with lung irradiation in combination with doxorubicin) or impaired lung function is recommended in patients bearing this risk. During and after therapy, tumor monitoring by chest and abdominal imaging is recommended periodically for 2 years, since most of the relapses occur within first 2 years of completion of therapy [5, 15, 35, 36, 56].

Conclusion

Over the years, the outcomes in the adult Wilms' tumor population have been steadily improving with the adoption of aggressive multimodality pediatric protocols. Further appropriate application of diagnostic and treatment strategies as applied to childhood Wilms' tumor patients and more effective cooperation with pediatric oncologists and pediatric surgeons are important steps in achieving even more improved outcomes. Better understanding of the molecular biology of the disease is critical to make further advances.

Acknowledgment We thank Jennifer Beth Gordetsky, MD, and Mark Lockhart, MD, for providing histology and radiology images, respectively. We also acknowledge cancer.sanger.ac.uk and Forbes et al. (2014) COSMIC: exploring the world's knowledge of somatic mutations in human cancer for providing mutation information.

Potential Conflicts

Ankit Madan: None

Guru Sonpavde: Research support from Onyx, Bayer; Consultant/advisory board of Sanofi, Merck, Genentech, Bayer

References

1. Zugor V, Schott GE, Lausen B, et al. Clinical and surgical experience with Wilms tumor. Long-term results of a single institution. Anticancer Res. 2010;30:1735–9.
2. Mitry E, Ciccolallo L, Coleman MP, et al. Incidence of and survival from Wilms' tumor in adults in Europe: data from the EUROCARE study. Eur J Cancer. 2006;42:2363–8.
3. Parkin D, Kramarova E, Draper G, et al. International incidence of childhood cancer, vol. 2. Lyon: International Agency for Research on Cancer; 1998.
4. Surveillance, Epidemiology and End Results (SEER) Program (www.seer.cancer.gov) SEER*Stat Database: NAACCR Incidence–CiNA Analytic File, 1995–2010, for NHIAv2 Origin, Custom File With County, ACS Facts and Figures Projection Project, North American Association of Central Cancer Registries.
5. Terenziani M, Spreafico F, Collini P, et al. Adult Wilms' tumor: a mono-institutional experience and a review of the literature. Cancer. 2004;101(2):289–93.
6. Huszno J, Starzyczny–Słota D, Jaworska M, Nowara E. Adult Wilms tumor-diagnosis and current therapy. Cent Eur J Urol. 2013;66(1):39–44.
7. Rivera MN, Haber DA. Wilms' tumor: connecting tumorigenesis and organ development in the kidney. Nat Rev Cancer. 2005;5:699–712.
8. Beckwith JB, Kiviat NB, Bonadio JF. Nephrogenic rests, nephroblastomatosis, and the pathogenesis of Wilms' tumor. Pediatr Pathol. 1990;10:1–36.
9. Breslow N, Olshan A, Beckwith JB, et al. Epidemiology of Wilms-tumor. Med Pediatr Oncol. 1993;21:172–81.
10. Breslow NE, Beckwith JB, Perlman EJ, et al. Age distributions, birth weights, nephrogenic rests, and heterogeneity in the pathogenesis of Wilms tumor. Pediatr Blood Cancer. 2006; 47:260–7.
11. Peng L, Perle MA, Scholes JV, Yang GCH. Wilms tumor is adults: aspiration cytology and cytogenetics. Diagn Cytopathol. 2002;26:99–103.
12. Kilton L, Matthews MJ, Cohen MH. Adult Wilms tumor: a report of prolonged survival and review of literature. J Urol. 1980;124:1–5.
13. M.D. Faria P, M.D. Beckwith JB, M.D. Kiran M. Focal versus diffuse anaplasia in Wilms tumor—new definitions with prognostic significance: a report from the National Wilms Tumor Study Group. Am J Surg Pathol. 1996;20(8):909–20.
14. Vujanić GM, Sandstedt B, Harms D, et al. Revised International Society of Paediatric Oncology (SIOP) working classification of renal tumors of childhood. Med Pediatr Oncol. 2002;38:79–82.
15. Spreafico F, Bellani FF. Wilms' tumor: past, present and (possibly) future. Expert Rev Anticancer Ther. 2006;6:249–58.
16. Ruteshouser EC, Robinson SM, Huff V. Wilms tumor genetics: mutations in WT1, WTX, and CTNNB1 account for only about one-third of tumors. Genes Chromosomes Cancer. 2008; 47(6):461–70.
17. Forbes SA, Beare D, et al. COSMIC: exploring the world's knowledge of somatic mutations in human cancer. Nucl Acids Res. 2015;43(D1):D805–11.
18. Cancer.sanger.ac.uk.
19. Call KM, Glaser T, Ito CY, et al. Isolation and characterization of a zinc finger polypeptide gene at the human chromosome 11 Wilms' tumor locus. Cell. 1990;60:509–20.
20. Andrew M. Davidoff Wilms tumor. Adv Pediatr. 2012;59(1):247–67.
21. Grubb GR, Yun K, Williams BR, et al. Expression of WT1 protein in fetal kidneys and Wilms tumors. Lab Invest. 1994;71:472–9.
22. Szychot E, Apps J, Pritchard-Jones K. Wilms' tumor: biology, diagnosis and treatment. Transl Pediatr. 2014;3(1):12–24.
23. Pelletier J, et al. Germline mutations in the Wilms' tumor suppressor gene are associated with abnormal urogenital development in Denys-Drash syndrome. Cell. 1991;67:437–47.
24. Huff V. Wilms' tumours: about tumour suppressor genes, an oncogene and a chameleon gene. Nat Rev Cancer. 2011;11(2):111–21. doi:10.1038/nrc3002.

25. Rivera MN, et al. An X chromosome gene, WTX, is commonly inactivated in Wilms tumor. Science. 2007;315:642–5.
26. Perotti D, et al. Functional inactivation of the WTX gene is not a frequent event in Wilms' tumors. Oncogene. 2008;27:4625–32.
27. Wegert J, et al. WTX inactivation is a frequent, but late event in Wilms tumors without apparent clinical impact. Genes Chromosomes Cancer. 2009;48:1102–11.
28. Fukuzawa R, Anaka MR, Weeks RJ, Morison IM, Reeve AE. Canonical WNT signaling determines lineage specificity in Wilms tumour. Oncogene. 2009;28:1063–75.
29. Bardeesy N, Falkoff D, Petruzzi MJ, et al. Anaplastic Wilms' tumour, a subtype displaying poor prognosis, harbours p53 gene mutations. Nat Genet. 1994;7:91–7.
30. Grundy PE, Telzerow PE, Breslow N, et al. Loss of heterozygosity for chromosomes 16q and 1p in Wilms' tumors predicts an adverse outcome. Cancer Res. 1994;54:2331–3.
31. Grundy PE, Breslow NE, Li S, National Wilms Tumor Study Group, et al. Loss of heterozygosity for chromosomes 1p and 16q is an adverse prognostic factor in favorable-histology Wilms tumor: a report from the National Wilms Tumor Study Group. J Clin Oncol. 2005;23:7312–21.
32. Williams RD, Al-Saadi R, Natrajan R, et al. Molecular profiling reveals frequent gain of MYCN and anaplasia-specific loss of 4q and 14q in Wilms tumor. Genes Chromosomes Cancer. 2011;50:982–95.
33. Gratias EJ, Jennings LJ, Anderson JR, et al. Gain of 1q is associated with inferior event-free and overall survival in patients with favorable histology Wilms tumor: a report from the Children's Oncology Group. Cancer. 2013;119:3887–94.
34. Perotti D, Spreafico F, Torri F, et al. Genomic profiling by whole-genome single nucleotide polymorphism arrays in Wilms tumor and association with relapse. Genes Chromosomes Cancer. 2012;51:644–53.
35. Kattan J, Tournade MF, Culine S, Terrier-Lacombe MJ, Droz JP. Adult Wilms tumour: review of 22 cases. Eur J Cancer. 1994;30A:1778–82.
36. Reinhard H, Aliani S, Ruebe C, Stöckle M, Leuschner I, Graf N. Wilms' tumor in adults: results of the Society of Pediatric Oncology (SIOP) 93-01/Society for Pediatric Oncology and Hematology (GPOH) Study. J Clin Oncol. 2004;22(22):4500–6.
37. Cushing B, Slovis TL. Imaging of Wilms' tumor: what is important! Urol Radiol. 1992;14:241–51.
38. Damgaard-Pedersen K. CT and IVU in the diagnosis of Wilms' tumour. A comparative study. Pediatr Radiol. 1980;9:207–11.
39. Fishman EK, Hartman DS, Goldman SM, Siegelman SS. The CT appearance of Wilms tumor. J Comput Assist Tomogr. 1983;7:659–65.
40. Geller E, Smergel EM, Lowry PA. Renal neoplasms of childhood. Radiol Clin North Am. 1997;35:1391–413.
41. Adegboyega Olukayode, Osuoji Richard I, Akinola Rachael O, Balogun Babajide O, Faturoti Ireti O, Awosanya Gbolahan O. Pattern of computed tomography scan findings in children with Wilms' tumor in a tertiary hospital in Lagos, Nigeria. Indian J Med Paediatr Oncol. 2014;35(1):31–5.
42. Lowe LH, Isuani BH, Heller RM, et al. Pediatric renal masses: Wilms' tumor and beyond. Radiographics. 2000;20(6):1585–603.
43. Byrd RL, Evans AE, D'Angio GJ. Adult Wilms' tumor: effect of combined therapy on survival. J Urol. 1982;127:648–65.
44. Kalapurakal JA, Dome JS, Perlman EJ, et al. Management of Wilms' tumour: current practice and future goals. Lancet Oncol. 2004;5:37–46.
45. Segers H, van den Heuvel-Eibrink MM, Pritchard-Jones K, SIOP-RTSG and the COG-Renal Tumor Committee, et al. Management of adults with Wilms' tumor: recommendations based on international consensus. Expert Rev Anticancer Ther. 2011;11:1105–13.
46. Davidoff AM. Wilms' tumor. Curr Opin Pediatr. 2009;21:357–64.
47. Scott RH, Walker L, Olsen ØE, et al. Surveillance for Wilms tumor in at-risk children: pragmatic recommendations for best practice. Arch Dis Child. 2006;91:995–9.

48. Stiller CA, Allen MB, Eatock EM. Childhood cancer in Britain: the National Registry of Childhood Tumors and incidence rates 1978–1987. Eur J Cancer. 1995;31A:2028–34.
49. Mitchell C, Pritchard-Jones K, Shannon R, et al. United Kingdom Cancer Study Group. Immediate nephrectomy versus pre-operative chemotherapy in the management of non-metastatic Wilms' tumor: results of a randomized trial (UKW3) by the UK Children's Cancer Study Group. Eur J Cancer. 2006;42:2554–62.
50. Pritchard-Jones K, Moroz V, Vujanic G, Children's Cancer and Leukaemia Group (CCLG) Renal Tumors Group, et al. Treatment and outcome of Wilms' tumor patients: an analysis of all cases registered in the UKW3 trial. Ann Oncol. 2012;23:2457–63.
51. Ko EY, Ritchey ML. Current management of Wilms' tumor in children. J Pediatr Urol. 2009;5:56–65.
52. Ritchey ML, Green DM, Thomas PR, et al. Renal failure in Wilms' tumor patients: a report from the National Wilms' Tumor Study Group. Med Pediatr Oncol. 1996;26:75–80.
53. Van Casteren NJ, Dohle GR, Romijn JC, de Muinck Keizer-Schrama SM, Weber RF, van den Heuvel-Eibrink MM. Semen cryopreservation in pubertal boys before gonadotoxic treatment and the role of endocrinologic evaluation in predicting sperm yield. Fertil Steril. 2008;90(4):1119–25.
54. Culp O, Hartman FW. Mesoblastic nephroma in adults: a clinicopathologic study of Wilms and related renal neoplasms. J Urol. 1948;60:552.
55. Foot NC, Humphreys GA, Whitmore WF. Renal tumors: pathology and prognosis in 295 cases. J Urol. 1951;66:190–7.
56. Arrigo S, Beckwith J, Sharples K, D'Angio G, Haase G. Better survival after combined modality care for adults with Wilms' tumor. A report from the National Wilms' Tumor Study. Cancer. 1990;66:827–30.
57. Izawa JI, Al-Omar M, Winquist E, et al. Prognostic variables in adult Wilms' tumour. Can J Surg. 2008;51(4):252–6.
58. Kalapurakal JA, Nan B, Norkool P, et al. Treatment outcomes in adults with favorable histologic type Wilms' tumor-an update from the National Wilms' Tumor Study Group. Int J Radiat Oncol Biol Phys. 2004;60(5):1379–84.
59. Bisogno G, de Kraker J, Weirich A, et al. Veno-occlusive disease of the liver in children treated for Wilms' tumor. Med Pediatr Oncol. 1997;29(4):245–51.
60. Czauderna P, Katski K, Kowalczyk J, et al. Venoocclusive liver disease (VOD) as a complication of Wilms' tumour management in the series of consecutive 206 patients. Eur J Pediatr Surg. 2000;10(5):300–3.
61. Ludwig R, Weirich A, Abel U, Hofmann W, Graf N, Tournade MF. Hepatotoxicity in patients treated according to the nephroblastoma trial and study SIOP-9/GPOH. Med Pediatr Oncol. 1999;33(5):462–9.
62. Beyer J, Rick O, Weinknecht S, Kingreen D, Lenz K, Siegert W. Nephrotoxicity after high-dose carboplatin, etoposide and ifosfamide in germ-cell tumors: incidence and implications for hematologic recovery and clinical outcome. Bone Marrow Transplant. 1997;20(10):813–9.
63. Chauvergne J, Chinet-Charrot P, Stockle E, Thomas L, Toulouse C. Carboplatin and etoposide combination for the treatment of recurrent epithelial ovarian cancer. Bull Cancer. 1996;83(4):315–23.
64. Thatcher N, Qian W, Clark PI, et al. Ifosfamide, carboplatin, and etoposide with midcycle vincristine versus standard chemotherapy in patients with small-cell lung cancer and good performance status: clinical and quality-of-life results of the British Medical Research Council multicenter randomized LU21 trial. J Clin Oncol. 2005;23(33):8371–9.
65. White SC, Lorigan P, Middleton MR, et al. Randomized phase II study of cyclophosphamide, doxorubicin, and vincristine compared with single-agent carboplatin in patients with poor prognosis small cell lung carcinoma. Cancer. 2001;92(3):601–8.
66. De Kraker J, Graf N, van Tinteren H, et al. Reduction of postoperative chemotherapy in children with stage I intermediate-risk and anaplastic Wilms' tumour (SIOP 93-01 trial): a randomised controlled trial. Lancet. 2004;364(9441):1229–35.
67. Breslow NE, Lange JM, Friedman DL, et al. Secondary malignant neoplasms after Wilms tumor: an international collaborative study. Int J Cancer. 2010;127:657–66.

6 Urothelial Carcinoma with Variant Histology: Sarcomatoid, Plasmacytoid, and Micropapillary

Stephen B. Williams and Ashish M. Kamat

Introduction

Approximately 80 % of bladder cancer is diagnosed as "conventional" urothelial carcinoma (UC) with 10–25 % nonurothelial and "variants" of urothelial carcinoma (UC) [1, 2]. For the current discussion, variant histology will refer to any bladder malignancy other than pure UC. Furthermore, we have limited our review to the specific histologic variants sarcomatoid, plasmacytoid, and micropapillary bladder cancer. Before we discuss each of these variants in detail, we should mention that each of these histologic descriptions is based on morphologic features from H&E pathologic sections with little insight into their biology. Moreover, mixed histologies are often present (including so-called urothelial and nonurothelial carcinomas), for which the term variant histology is generally used. Table 6.1 describes the histological classification of tumors arising from the urinary tract and was adapted from the 2004 World Health Organization classification of tumors.

Challenges in the Study of Variant Histology

Sampling error and tumor heterogeneity at transurethral resection (TUR) have been reported to detect only 39 % of variant cancers [3, 4]. It has been estimated that up to 44 % of cases of histologic variants are not recognized or documented by community pathologists which further leads to underreporting and potential mismanagement. Initial reports have suggested variant tumors were uniformly present at a high stage with invasion into muscularis propria [1]. However, more recent studies have shown variant histology present within non-muscle-invasive (NMI) tumors

S.B. Williams, MD • A.M. Kamat, MD, MBBS, FACS (✉)
Department of Urology, The University of Texas MD Anderson Cancer Center, 1515 Holcombe Blvd., Unit 1373, Houston, TX 77030, USA
e-mail: akamat@mdanderson.org

L. Pagliaro (ed.), *Rare Genitourinary Tumors*,
DOI 10.1007/978-3-319-30046-7_6

Table 6.1 Histological classification of tumors arising from the urinary tract and was adapted from the 2004 World Health Organization classification of tumors

Urothelial tumors
Infiltrating urothelial carcinoma
With squamous differentiation
With glandular differentiation
With trophoblastic differentiation
Nested
Microcystic
Micropapillary
Lymphoepithelioma-like
Lymphoma-like
Plasmacytoid
Sarcomatoid
Giant cell
Undifferentiated
Noninvasive urothelial neoplasias
Urothelial carcinoma in situ
Noninvasive papillary urothelial carcinoma, high grade
Noninvasive papillary urothelial carcinoma, low grade
Noninvasive papillary urothelial neoplasm of low malignant potential
Urothelial papilloma
Inverted urothelial papilloma
Squamous neoplasms
Squamous cell carcinoma
Verrucous carcinoma
Squamous cell papilloma
Glandular neoplasms
Adenocarcinoma
Enteric
Mucinous
Signet-ring cell
Clear cell
Villous adenoma
Neuroendocrine tumors
Small cell carcinoma
Carcinoid
Paraganglioma
Melanocytic tumors
Malignant melanoma
Nevus
Mesenchymal tumors
Rhabdomyosarcoma
Leiomyosarcoma
Angiosarcoma

Table 6.1 (continued)

Osteosarcoma
Malignant fibrous histiocytoma
Leiomyoma
Hemangioma
Other
Hematopoietic and lymphoid tumors
Lymphoma
Plasmacytoma
Miscellaneous tumors
Carcinoma of Skene, Cowper, and Littre glands
Metastatic tumors and tumors extending from other organs

Reference: Eble et al. [50]

[5–10]. In a large bladder cancer patient registry from the Netherlands, 23 % of all variant tumors identified within the registry presented with NMI disease [11].

While this is likely a reflection of increased awareness and recognition within the scientific community, variant histology often carries an aggressive and lethal diagnosis. One early study proposed that up to 20 % variant histology within a bladder specimen was associated with worse survival outcomes [12]. However, no consistency has been shown among subsequent studies, and it has become quite apparent that each bladder cancer variant behaves differently and needs to be addressed individually to assess its impact on the overall biology of the disease. In a recent retrospective study evaluating pathologic and survival outcomes among patients with variant histology, micropapillary and plasmacytoid variants were independently associated with twice the risk of all-cause mortality compared with nonvariant UC [13]. The significance of the extent of each specific variant remains an area of significant interest.

Diagnosing variant histology has been the rate-limiting step at understanding the biology and development of appropriate treatment algorithms. Figure 6.1 illustrates the most common histologic appearances of sarcomatoid, plasmacytoid, and micropapillary bladder cancer. In an effort to combat these challenges, many groups are collaborating to outline standards and guidelines in the identification and reporting of variant histology [4]. With the incorporation of collaborative efforts and centralized pathologic review, further improvements in the identification and treatment of variant bladder cancer will result. Figure 6.2 provides a decision tree utilized for the diagnosis and treatment of non-muscle-invasive variant histology bladder cancer. When feasible in muscle invasive disease, we believe that up-front radical cystectomy is the treatment of choice for reasons we will explain further in this chapter.

Significance of Variant Histology

Variant histology often portends to worse oncologic outcomes when compared to conventional urothelial carcinoma. Several retrospective studies suggest to be the result of a higher propensity of locally aggressive disease, higher rates of distant

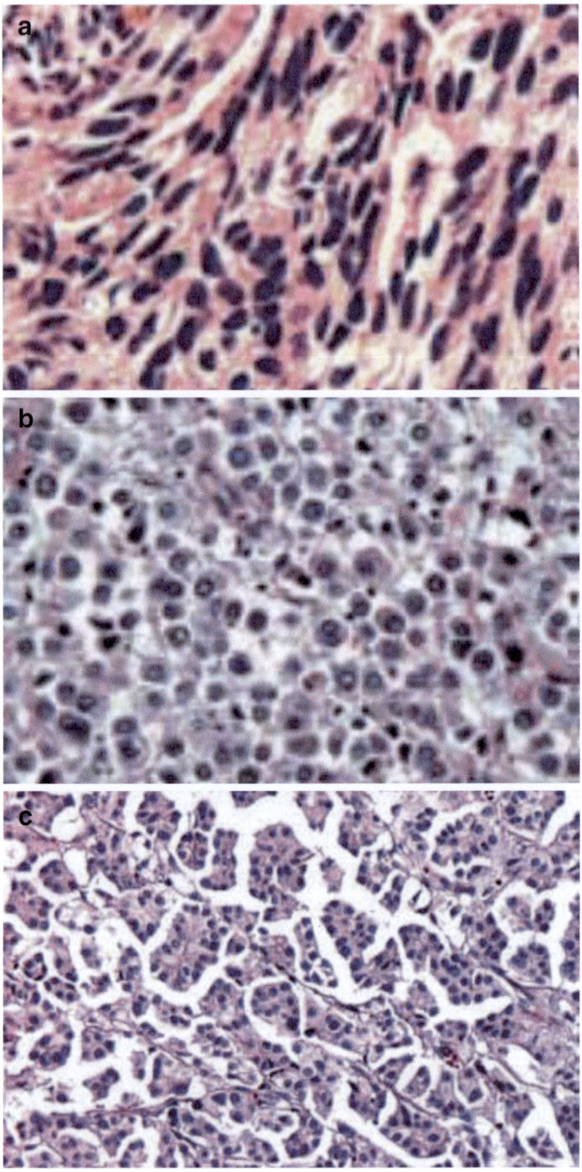

Fig. 6.1 Histologic variants: sarcomatoid, plasmacytoid, and micropapillary. (**a**) Infiltrative urothelial carcinoma. Sarcomatoid variant without heterologous elements showing spindle cell morphology. (**b**) Infiltrating urothelial carcinoma of the bladder, plasmacytoid variant. (**c**) Micropapillary urothelial carcinoma (Reference: Eble et al. [50])

metastasis, and a different response to chemotherapy or radiotherapy as compared to conventional UC. In a study of 448 consecutive TURBT cases with 295 subsequent cystectomies, mixed histology was present in 25 %, and the presence of variant architecture almost uniformly predicted the presence of locally advanced disease at cystectomy [1]. Another study observed that among 600 cystectomy patients,

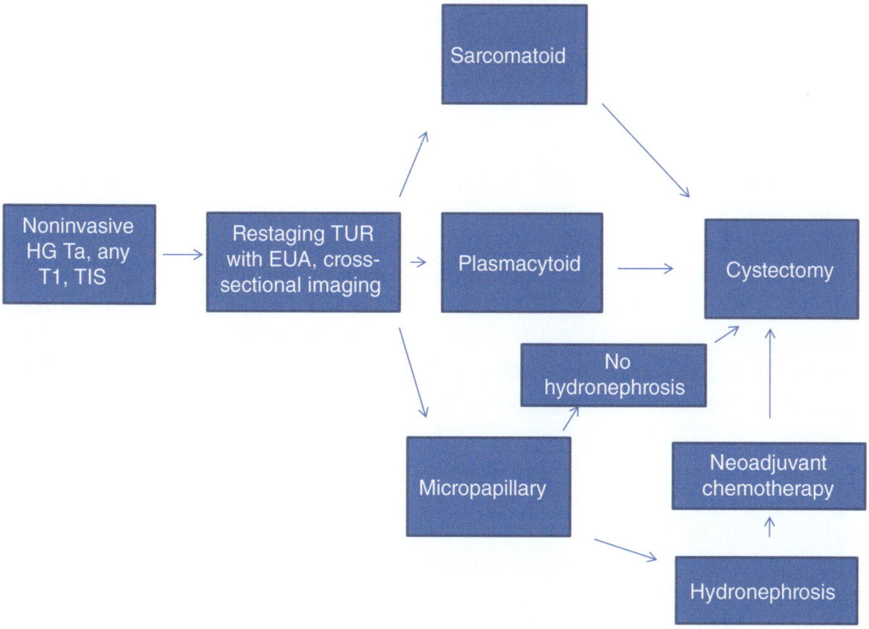

Fig. 6.2 Decision tree for the clinical management of variant NMIBC

variant histology predicted upstaging at the time of cystectomy with an odds ratio of 2.77 [14]. The presence of variant histology has also been found to be associated with increased rates of pathologic lymph node metastasis leading to worse survival outcomes [15, 16]. In one of the largest multi-institutional studies pertaining to variant histology, identified patients with adenocarcinoma, small cell carcinoma, or other histologic subtypes had worse disease-specific survival compared to conventional UC even adjusting for stage, adjunctive treatment, and lymphovascular invasion on multivariate analyses [17].

However, other studies have presented conflicting evidence that these trends may not be true for all variant types of bladder cancer. The Southwest Oncology Group (SWOG)-randomized trial S8710 showed increased survival for neoadjuvant MVAC (methotrexate, vinblastine, Adriamycin, cisplatin) plus cystectomy over cystectomy alone in patients with locally advanced (cT2-T4a) bladder cancer [18]. In a secondary analysis they demonstrated that patients with mixed histology (squamous and glandular differentiation) had improved survival rates after neoadjuvant MVAC chemotherapy as well as a higher rate of pT0 downstaging (34 %) versus cystectomy alone (4 %). This translated to improved survival rates for patients with mixed histology after neoadjuvant chemotherapy, though statistical significance was not achieved. This secondary analysis challenges the notion that all variant histology leads to a worse overall prognosis and outcome.

Non-muscle-Invasive Variant Bladder Cancer

There is intense controversy regarding non-muscle-invasive bladder cancer with variant histology, both in terms of diagnosis, role of intravesical therapy, and aggressive up-front radical cystectomy. Clinical staging for NMI variant bladder cancer is critical. While this is important for conventional UC, some argue that since variant tumors notoriously are associated with advanced disease, there may be a potentially higher risk of understaging for variant tumors. Thus, intravesical therapy would be less effective and potentially lead to missed opportunity for cancer cure. Several studies for cT1 NMI variant bladder cancer have reported local understaging rates ranging from 27 to 57 % [1, 4, 19]. Rates of occult metastatic disease have also been reported as high as 27–44 % among NMI variant tumors [5] with divergent histology being associated with the presence of lymph node metastasis and decreased survival [20]. Thus, in the setting of NMI variant bladder cancer, a more aggressive treatment strategy might be warranted. However, other studies have reported progression rates of approximately 40 % which is similar to conventional UC with high-risk features [5, 10, 19, 21]. Caution must be made when extrapolating results from these studies as they included tumors with squamous or glandular differentiation, nested variant, and micropapillary disease. The role of intravesical treatment for variant NMIBC should be considered based on the unique subtype and should be weighed against the risk of understaging in order to optimize oncologic outcomes.

Sarcomatoid

Carcinosarcomas (CS) are biphasic malignant neoplasms with morphological evidence of both epithelial (carcinomatous) and mesenchymal (sarcomatous) differentiation. It is different from sarcomatoid carcinoma (SaC) of the bladder, which is a malignant spindle cell neoplasm, in which epithelial differentiation may be demonstrated by immunohistochemical or ultrastructural studies. However, World Health Organization classification system acknowledges the controversy surrounding the terminology and histogenesis of these tumors of the bladder and now includes what used to be called carcinosarcoma together with sarcomatoid UC.

Sarcomatoid variant is a rare variant of UC, which accounts for approximately 0.3 % of all urothelial tumors [22]. A history of radiation and intravesical cyclophosphamide chemotherapy has been associated. Macroscopically, tumors are often polypoid with often advanced large intraluminal masses.

Microscopically, the sarcomatous component is usually a high-grade spindle cell neoplasm, whereas the epithelial component can be in the form of conventional UC, squamous cell carcinoma, adenocarcinoma, small cell carcinoma, or overlying carcinoma in situ. The immunohistochemical profile of the sarcomatoid variant of UC includes positivity for epithelial markers, at least focally, including cytokeratin and epithelial membrane antigen. This immunohistochemical profile distinguishes this entity from pure sarcomas [23].

Similar to other variants, sarcomatoid carcinoma also tends to present with advanced stage, distant metastasis, and local progression [10, 19]. The mean age of presentation is 66 years (50–77) with presentation similar to conventional UC with hematuria as the usual presenting symptom. These tumors are typically diagnosed at advanced local stage, and they often exhibit nodal or distant metastases. The significance of this variant lies in its association with a poor prognosis [24]. After controlling for stage, patients with sarcomatoid disease have a worse survival and higher disease-specific mortality (almost twofold greater) than those with conventional UC [10, 25]. Pathological stage is the best predictor of survival in sarcomatoid variants [24]. Good prognostic factors include negative surgical margins and absence of metastatic disease at the initial presentation; however, even with these favorable prognostic factors taken into account, 2-year mortality is almost 70 %.

Few case reports/series have been reported with few population-based analyses providing further information on this rare variant. Wright et al. presented a SEER database of patients with SaC, CS, and urothelial carcinoma (UC) treated between 1988 and 2003 [10]. It was found that patients with both SaC and CS presented more frequently with locally advanced or metastatic disease. Survival was worse for sarcomatoid variants compared with UC in organ-confined and metastatic disease. Five-year survival was 17 % and 37 % in SaC and CS, respectively, compared with 47 % in UCs.

Appropriate modalities and sequence of administration remain to be defined. However, given the aggressive behavior of the tumor precludes radical therapy whenever possible. A variety of treatment modalities have been described, but optimal treatment requires rather a multimodality approach. The effectiveness of different modalities is not known because of varying rates of usage of adjuvant radiation (15–45 %) and chemotherapy (5–60 %) and varying results of each case [26]. Transurethral resection and partial cystectomy carry the risk of incomplete tumor resection. Radical cystectomy with pelvic lymphadenectomy is the mainstay of treatment, although patients tend to develop local recurrence after surgery [10].

Wang et al. presented SEER databases, which included 221 patients, between 1973 and 2004. Median age of the patients was 75 years (range 41–96) [25]. 72.5 % had a locally advanced or distant stage. 53.9 % of patients underwent transurethral resection only, 35.8 % of patients had radical or partial cystectomy, and 15.8 % of patients received surgery followed by radiation therapy. The median overall survival was 14 months (95 % confidence interval 7–21 months). The overall 1-, 5-, and 10-year survival rates were 53.9 %, 28.4 %, and 25.8 %. The overall 5-year survival rate after cystectomy was only 20.3 %, suggesting a high risk of early dissemination. Cancer-specific survival was significantly better for those who underwent cystectomy instead of transurethral resection.

The rationale for the use of adjuvant chemotherapy in this variant is the aggressive nature of the disease. Probability of metastasis is high (50–70 %). The combination of gemcitabine and cisplatin is an effective and well-tolerated chemotherapy regimen for the treatment of advanced UC. However, no data are available regarding its use in bladder sarcomatoid UC. The use of this chemotherapy regimen in sarcomatoid variants was first reported by Froehner in a single case of metastatic (pulmonary) SC showing durable, complete local, and pulmonary remission, but, the pathological stage, was not reported (pTxNxM1) in this study, and hence no conclusion can therefore be drawn [27]. Other platinum-based regimens have been utilized with varying responses and include methotrexate, vinblastine, doxorubicin, and cisplatin as well as gemcitabine and cisplatin when concerned for nephrotoxicity. As mentioned in most of the studies, favorable outcomes may be explained by good performance status, absence of nodal and metastatic involvement, and delivery of chemotherapeutic agents at the full dose.

The role of adjuvant radiation in SC can be justified on the basis of high chances of local invasion and pelvic lymph node metastasis, known with this variant. Adjuvant radiotherapy to the dose of 50–60 Gy, along with the various combinations of chemotherapy has been used in certain case reports, but has yielded inconsistent results. No definite effect of adjuvant radiation on local control can be concluded in view of limited case studies and high disease-specific mortality.

Plasmacytoid

Plasmacytoid urothelial carcinoma (PUC) is uncommon; however, as with other variant bladder cancers, it exhibits a unique clinical behavior. As is the case with the prior variants, PUC is associated with advanced local and distant disease at presentation in an often younger subset of patients than conventional UC [28]. Morphologically, PUC presents with a discohesive, single cell growth pattern, with eccentrically located nuclei and an abundant eosinophilic cytoplasm [28]. PUC is usually diagnosed at an advanced pathological stage, and survival appears to be more unfavorable to what has been described for conventional UC [3]. PUC often expresses unfavorable molecular features, such as the loss of CK20, high proliferation index, p53 accumulation, and complete loss of membranous E-cadherin expression [29]. Loss of E-cadherin is a sign of epithelial-mesenchymal transition (EMT), and upregulation of transcriptional repressors of E-cadherin may contribute to the aggressiveness of these tumors which may portend to reduced sensitivity to chemotherapeutic agents [29, 30]. Interestingly, even in the setting of negative surgical margins, the peritoneum remains a site of major recurrence. Because of this predisposition for peritoneal metastasis, CEA, CA125, and CA19-9 have been incorporated as potential tumor markers for PUC [31, 32].

While few studies on PUC exist, a 31-patient case series has been published in patients with >50 % PUC at the time of TUR to determine the utility of neoadjuvant chemotherapy [32]. Median overall survival was 17.7 months (stage I–III vs IV; 45.8 vs 13.3). In patients who presented with metastatic disease and were treated with chemotherapy, median survival was 12.6 months. Moreover, no survival difference was noted between those receiving neoadjuvant chemotherapy and those proceeding to up-front cystectomy, though some chemotherapeutic responses were observed. A recent study found therapeutic strategies with radical cystectomy, and cisplatin-based chemotherapy was not as effective for PUC as it was described for locally advanced UC or micropapillary bladder cancer, however, a complete response to adjuvant chemotherapy administering MVAC and neoadjuvant chemotherapy using gemcitabine and cisplatin may occur in a subgroup of PUC patients [33]. Therefore, chemotherapy in a neoadjuvant or adjuvant setting should be included in the treatment paradigm. PUC tumor biology represents a negative prognostic factor for patients suffering from this histologic variant. Because of the aggressive nature of PUC and the high rates of peritoneal metastasis, aggressive therapy incorporating radical cystectomy is likely required for both invasive and NMI forms of PUC.

Micropapillary

Micropapillary bladder carcinoma (MPBC) has been a recent interest of many groups with a majority of variant studies published on this particular variant. MPBC is a distinct variant of conventional UC and resembles papillary serous carcinoma of the ovary. MPBC is typically found in the background of conventional UC to varying degrees of involvement but can also be associated with squamous cell carcinoma of the bladder [34], adenocarcinoma [35], small cell carcinoma [36], and sarcomatoid carcinoma [37]. Studies of MPBC have helped elucidate the void in our understanding variant bladder cancer. Published literature has demonstrated not only that MPBC has a relatively poor recognition in community practices but great heterogeneity even among academic pathologists regarding the histologic diagnosis of micropapillary architecture with only classical cases of MPBC showing consensus [38].

A majority of MPBC studies have consistently shown that muscle invasive MPBC is associated with high rates of locally advanced, metastatic disease associated with limited overall survival [6, 8, 35, 37, 39]. As previously mentioned, MPBC often exists within the background of conventional UC with small amounts of MPBC within the tumor being clinically significant with >10 % MPBC associated with worse clinical outcomes [39, 40]. The largest single institution series to date from MD Anderson Cancer Center demonstrated that the overall prognosis of MPBC was poor with 5- and 10-year OS rates of 54 % and 27 %, respectively [21], despite a relatively high proportion of patients with NMI-MPBC at presentation (44 %). Moreover, there were high rates of upstaging at the time of radical cystectomy (52.7 %) and occult lymph node metastases identified in 27.3 % of patients. Others studies have reported rates of occult metastatic disease as high as 35 and 86 % [6]. In the MD Anderson cohort, the lymph node metastases were often reported to contain micropapillary features, independent of percentage of involvement of MPBC in the primary tumor, suggesting a predisposition of MPBC to spread by lymphatic invasion. Interestingly, case-matched studies with conventional UC have demonstrated that stage for stage, there is no survival difference in MPBC and conventional UC [41, 42].

There remains limited consensus regarding the clinical management of MPBC [43]. The utilization of multimodality treatments including neoadjuvant chemotherapy varies, and the definition of risk stratification groups within the arena of MPBC remains to be elucidated. The MD Anderson experience suggested MPBC might not respond to chemotherapy with worse survival identified among those receiving neoadjuvant chemotherapy after controlling for stage [21]. However, others have argued due to high rates of upstaging at surgery and high rates of lymph node metastasis, systemic chemotherapy should be incorporated [6]. A retrospective cohort reported a 45 % pathologic pT0 downstaging rate among MPBC patients after neoadjuvant chemotherapy compared to 13 % downstaging in those patients who underwent up-front cystectomy. They also noted a survival advantage with neoadjuvant chemotherapy for patients that were downstaged [44]. While there are limitations to all of these studies including retrospective nature, small sample size, relatively short follow-up, and few quality controls for chemotherapy regimens, the role of neoadjuvant chemotherapy for organ-confined MPBC remains controversial.

The initial MD Anderson study was one of the first to help develop an awareness of variant histology among NMI-MPBC as well as diagnostic and therapeutic strategies needed to optimize oncologic outcomes. In one study, 44 patients with NMI-MPBC were treated with intravesical bacillus Calmette-Guérin (BCG) versus up-front radical cystectomy [5]. Cancer progression was 67 % in the BCG group with progression to metastatic disease in 22 %. Patients who underwent delayed cystectomy after BCG failure were found to have worse disease-specific survival rates compared to up-front radical cystectomy. In a follow-up study, patients who received BCG had recurrence, progression, and lymph node metastasis in 75 %, 45 %, and 35 %, respectively [45]. Patients treated with up-front cystectomy had improved survival compared to patients treated with primary BCG (5-year disease-specific survival 100 % vs 60 %, $p=0.006$) and patients who underwent delayed cystectomy after recurrence (5-year disease-specific survival 62 %, $p=0.015$). Prognosis was especially poor in patients who waited for progression before undergoing radical cystectomy with an estimated 5-year disease-specific survival of only 24 % and a median survival of 35 months. In patients treated with up-front cystectomy, pathological upstaging was done in 27 %, including 20 % with lymph node metastasis. In these studies, the authors concluded that because of the high rates of occult metastatic disease and the poor prognosis associated with BCG failure, up-front radical cystectomy was the treatment of choice for cT1 MPBC. These findings coincide with a recent population-based study which identified 120 patients with MPBC. After controlling for stage, there was no difference in survival between MPBC and conventional UC except among patients with NMI-MPBC where worse survival outcomes was noted [8].

Other authors have suggested intravesical BCG might be an appropriate therapy for NMI-MPBC. In a publication from Memorial Sloan Kettering Cancer Center, they noted equivalent survival outcomes between intravesical BCG and up-front radical cystectomy. While no survival difference was noted, there was a 21 % incidence of metastasis in the BCG cohort with a 27 % rate of occult metastatic disease in those patients who underwent up-front cystectomy [46]. Other reports have made similar conclusions regarding intravesical BCG which have also suggested that BCG might be appropriate in patients with a small percentage of micropapillary component in the tumor [9].

While no universal guidelines exist for the management of MPBC, radical cystectomy is encouraged for invasive disease. Conflicting evidence exists regarding the optimal management for NMI-MPBC; however, many experts still favor up-front radical cystectomy over BCG due to high rates of distant metastasis and the poor survival after BCG failure [45, 47].

Future Therapy

In order to direct appropriate therapy for variant histologies including sarcomatoid, plasmacytoid, and micropapillary bladder cancer, we need precise diagnosis at the onset. Moreover, due to the limited diagnoses made relative to conventional UC, the likelihood of developing randomized controlled trials is dismal, and we must rely on data combined from large centers in order to direct future therapies. It appears aggressive local therapy with radical cystectomy when diagnosis is made and surgically feasible remains the mainstay of treatment. Tissue from these patients can then be studied in order to direct targeted therapies desperately needed among these aggressive histologic variants. Subtyping of bladder cancer has been performed by several groups, including our own [48], suggesting that several distinct classes of bladder cancer exist based on gene expression platform data. It is important that this is performed with tumors showing variant histologies, which would enhance our understanding of the innate biology of these subtypes and establish treatment paradigms based on putative cell pathways and target identification. Unfortunately, there are no targeted therapies to date as in the case of conventional UC; however, we are optimistic that further collaborative efforts among UC studies may help direct treatment options for these aggressive histologic variants as well [49].

Conclusion

Precise identification and staging of variants including sarcomatoid, plasmacytoid, and micropapillary bladder cancer is cornerstone to making appropriate treatment decisions. Radical cystectomy is the mainstay of treatment with multimodal chemotherapy treatments also considered when feasible. Further research directed at risk stratification within each of the variant histologies is needed in order to identify appropriate treatments to ameliorate the often poor survival outcomes among these patients. As with the case of conventional UC, targeted therapies are needed, and further research among these variants as well as conventional UC may elucidate targeted agents for these variant histologies.

References

1. Wasco MJ, Daignault S, Zhang Y, et al. Urothelial carcinoma with divergent histologic differentiation (mixed histologic features) predicts the presence of locally advanced bladder cancer when detected at transurethral resection. Urology. 2007;70(1):69–74.
2. Kantor AF, Hartge P, Hoover RN, Fraumeni Jr JF. Epidemiological characteristics of squamous cell carcinoma and adenocarcinoma of the bladder. Cancer Res. 1988;48(13):3853–5.
3. Abd El-Latif A, Watts KE, Elson P, Fergany A, Hansel DE. The sensitivity of initial transurethral resection or biopsy of bladder tumor(s) for detecting bladder cancer variants on radical cystectomy. J Urol. 2013;189(4):1263–7.

4. Hansel DE, Amin MB, Comperat E, et al. A contemporary update on pathology standards for bladder cancer: transurethral resection and radical cystectomy specimens. Eur Urol. 2013;63(2):321–32.
5. Kamat AM, Gee JR, Dinney CP, et al. The case for early cystectomy in the treatment of non-muscle invasive micropapillary bladder carcinoma. J Urol. 2006;175(3 Pt 1):881–5.
6. Ghoneim IA, Miocinovic R, Stephenson AJ, et al. Neoadjuvant systemic therapy or early cystectomy? Single-center analysis of outcomes after therapy for patients with clinically localized micropapillary urothelial carcinoma of the bladder. Urology. 2011;77(4):867–70.
7. Comperat E, Roupret M, Yaxley J, et al. Micropapillary urothelial carcinoma of the urinary bladder: a clinicopathological analysis of 72 cases. Pathology. 2010;42(7):650–4.
8. Vourganti S, Harbin A, Singer EA, Shuch B, Metwalli AR, Agarwal PK. Low grade micropapillary urothelial carcinoma, does it exist? – analysis of management and outcomes from the Surveillance, Epidemiology and End Results (SEER) database. J Cancer. 2013;4(4):336–42.
9. Amin A, Epstein JI. Noninvasive micropapillary urothelial carcinoma: a clinicopathologic study of 18 cases. Hum Pathol. 2012;43(12):2124–8.
10. Wright JL, Black PC, Brown GA, et al. Differences in survival among patients with sarcomatoid carcinoma, carcinosarcoma and urothelial carcinoma of the bladder. J Urol. 2007;178(6):2302–6; discussion 2307.
11. Shapur NK, Katz R, Pode D, et al. Is radical cystectomy mandatory in every patient with variant histology of bladder cancer. Rare Tumors. 2011;3(2):e22.
12. Jozwicki W, Domaniewski J, Skok Z, Wolski Z, Domanowska E, Jozwicka G. Usefulness of histologic homogeneity estimation of muscle-invasive urinary bladder cancer in an individual prognosis: a mapping study. Urology. 2005;66(5):1122–6.
13. Monn MF, Kaimakliotis HZ, Pedrosa JA, et al. Contemporary bladder cancer: variant histology may be a significant driver of disease. Urol Oncol. 2015;33(1):18 e15–20.
14. Turker P, Bostrom PJ, Wroclawski ML, et al. Upstaging of urothelial cancer at the time of radical cystectomy: factors associated with upstaging and its effect on outcome. BJU Int. 2012;110(6):804–11.
15. Kassouf W, Agarwal PK, Grossman HB, et al. Outcome of patients with bladder cancer with pN+ disease after preoperative chemotherapy and radical cystectomy. Urology. 2009;73(1):147–52.
16. Domanowska E, Jozwicki W, Domaniewski J, et al. Muscle-invasive urothelial cell carcinoma of the human bladder: multidirectional differentiation and ability to metastasize. Hum Pathol. 2007;38(5):741–6.
17. Rogers CG, Palapattu GS, Shariat SF, et al. Clinical outcomes following radical cystectomy for primary nontransitional cell carcinoma of the bladder compared to transitional cell carcinoma of the bladder. J Urol. 2006;175(6):2048–53; discussion 2053.
18. Scosyrev E, Ely BW, Messing EM, et al. Do mixed histological features affect survival benefit from neoadjuvant platinum-based combination chemotherapy in patients with locally advanced bladder cancer? A secondary analysis of Southwest Oncology Group-Directed Intergroup Study (S8710). BJU Int. 2011;108(5):693–9.
19. Weizer AZ, Wasco MJ, Wang R, Daignault S, Lee CT, Shah RB. Multiple adverse histological features increase the odds of under staging T1 bladder cancer. J Urol. 2009;182(1):59–65; discussion 65.
20. El-Sebaie M, Zaghloul MS, Howard G, Mokhtar A. Squamous cell carcinoma of the bilharzial and non-bilharzial urinary bladder: a review of etiological features, natural history, and management. Int J Clin Oncol. 2005;10(1):20–5.
21. Kamat AM, Dinney CP, Gee JR, et al. Micropapillary bladder cancer: a review of the University of Texas M. D. Anderson Cancer Center experience with 100 consecutive patients. Cancer. 2007;110(1):62–7.
22. Zhai QJ, Black J, Ayala AG, Ro JY. Histologic variants of infiltrating urothelial carcinoma. Arch Pathol Lab Med. 2007;131(8):1244–56.
23. Sung MT, Wang M, MacLennan GT, et al. Histogenesis of sarcomatoid urothelial carcinoma of the urinary bladder: evidence for a common clonal origin with divergent differentiation. J Pathol. 2007;211(4):420–30.

24. Lopez-Beltran A, Pacelli A, Rothenberg HJ, et al. Carcinosarcoma and sarcomatoid carcinoma of the bladder: clinicopathological study of 41 cases. J Urol. 1998;159(5):1497–503.
25. Wang J, Wang FW, Lagrange CA, Hemstreet Iii GP, Kessinger A. Clinical features of sarcomatoid carcinoma (carcinosarcoma) of the urinary bladder: analysis of 221 cases. Sarcoma. 2010;2010:454792, 7.
26. Black PC, Brown GA, Dinney CP. The impact of variant histology on the outcome of bladder cancer treated with curative intent. Urol Oncol. 2009;27(1):3–7.
27. Froehner M, Gaertner HJ, Manseck A, Wirth MP. Durable complete remission of metastatic sarcomatoid carcinoma of the bladder with cisplatin and gemcitabine in an 80-year-old man. Urology. 2001;58(5):799.
28. Keck B, Wach S, Stoehr R, et al. Plasmacytoid variant of bladder cancer defines patients with poor prognosis if treated with cystectomy and adjuvant cisplatin-based chemotherapy. BMC Cancer. 2013;13:71.
29. Keck B, Stoehr R, Wach S, et al. The plasmacytoid carcinoma of the bladder – rare variant of aggressive urothelial carcinoma. Int J Cancer. 2011;129(2):346–54.
30. Shiota M, Song Y, Yokomizo A, et al. Foxo3a suppression of urothelial cancer invasiveness through Twist1, Y-box-binding protein 1, and E-cadherin regulation. Clin Cancer Res. 2010;16(23):5654–63.
31. Topalak O, Saygili U, Soyturk M, et al. Serum, pleural effusion, and ascites CA-125 levels in ovarian cancer and nonovarian benign and malignant diseases: a comparative study. Gynecol Oncol. 2002;85(1):108–13.
32. Dayyani F, Czerniak BA, Sircar K, et al. Plasmacytoid urothelial carcinoma, a chemosensitive cancer with poor prognosis, and peritoneal carcinomatosis. J Urol. 2013;189(5):1656–61.
33. Hayashi T, Tanigawa G, Fujita K, et al. Two cases of plasmacytoid variant of urothelial carcinoma of urinary bladder: systemic chemotherapy might be of benefit. Int J Clin Oncol. 2011;16(6):759–62.
34. Holmang S, Thomsen J, Johansson SL. Micropapillary carcinoma of the renal pelvis and ureter. J Urol. 2006;175(2):463–6; discussion 466–7.
35. Johansson SL, Borghede G, Holmang S. Micropapillary bladder carcinoma: a clinicopathological study of 20 cases. J Urol. 1999;161(6):1798–802.
36. Alvarado-Cabrero I, Sierra-Santiesteban FI, Mantilla-Morales A, Hernandez-Hernandez DM. Micropapillary carcinoma of the urothelial tract. A clinicopathologic study of 38 cases. Ann Diagn Pathol. 2005;9(1):1–5.
37. Baschinsky DY, Chen JH, Vadmal MS, Lucas JG, Bahnson RR, Niemann TH. Carcinosarcoma of the urinary bladder – an aggressive tumor with diverse histogenesis. A clinicopathologic study of 4 cases and review of the literature. Arch Pathol Lab Med. 2000;124(8):1172–8.
38. Sangoi AR, Beck AH, Amin MB, et al. Interobserver reproducibility in the diagnosis of invasive micropapillary carcinoma of the urinary tract among urologic pathologists. Am J Surg Pathol. 2010;34(9):1367–76.
39. Samaratunga H, Khoo K. Micropapillary variant of urothelial carcinoma of the urinary bladder; a clinicopathological and immunohistochemical study. Histopathology. 2004;45(1): 55–64.
40. Lopez-Beltran A, Cheng L. Histologic variants of urothelial carcinoma: differential diagnosis and clinical implications. Hum Pathol. 2006;37(11):1371–88.
41. Wang JK, Boorjian SA, Cheville JC, et al. Outcomes following radical cystectomy for micropapillary bladder cancer versus pure urothelial carcinoma: a matched cohort analysis. World J Urol. 2012;30(6):801–6.
42. Fairey AS, Daneshmand S, Wang L, et al. Impact of micropapillary urothelial carcinoma variant histology on survival after radical cystectomy. Urol Oncol. 2014;32(2):110–6.
43. Willis DL, Flaig TW, Hansel DE, et al. Micropapillary bladder cancer: current treatment patterns and review of the literature. Urol Oncol. 2014;32(6):826–32.
44. Meeks JJ, Taylor JM, Matsushita K, et al. Pathological response to neoadjuvant chemotherapy for muscle-invasive micropapillary bladder cancer. BJU Int. 2013;111(8):E325–30.
45. Willis DL, Fernandez MI, Dickstein RJ, et al. Clinical outcomes of cT1 micropapillary bladder cancer. J Urol. 2015;193(4):1129–34.

46. Spaliviero M, Dalbagni G, Bochner BH, et al. Clinical outcome of patients with T1 micropapillary urothelial carcinoma of the bladder. J Urol. 2014;192(3):702–7.
47. Porten SP, Willis D, Kamat AM. Variant histology: role in management and prognosis of non-muscle invasive bladder cancer. Curr Opin Urol. 2014;24(5):517–23.
48. Choi W, Porten S, Kim S, et al. Identification of distinct basal and luminal subtypes of muscle-invasive bladder cancer with different sensitivities to frontline chemotherapy. Cancer Cell. 2014;25(2):152–65.
49. Choi W, Czerniak B, Ochoa A, et al. Intrinsic basal and luminal subtypes of muscle-invasive bladder cancer. Nat Rev Urol. 2014;11(7):400–10.
50. Eble JN, Sauter G, Epstein JI, Sesterhenn IA. Pathology and genetics of tumours of the urinary system and male genital organs. World Health Organization Classification of Tumours, IARC Press, Lyon, France. 2004. p. 1–354.

Primary Sarcomas and Other Sarcomatoid Tumors of the Bladder

7

Jue Wang, Midhun Malla, and Jeffrey Wang

Introduction

Primary bladder sarcoma [1, 2] (PBS) and sarcomatoid carcinoma (formerly carcinosarcoma) [2] of the urinary bladder (SCUB) are both rare types of malignancy occurring in the urinary bladder. Although these tumors are widely considered to have a poor prognosis, the body of literature is limited to case reports and small, single institutional series. Because of the rarity of these tumors, there is no consensus on their optimal management.

In this article, we aim to summarize the current understanding of PBS and SCUB and to provide an overview of epidemiology, and clinical features, as well as management options of these variants of bladder cancer.

Primary Bladder Sarcoma

Genitourinary sarcomas account for approximately 5 % of all sarcomas, representing about 1–2 % of genitourinary malignancies [3–6]. Russo [6] identified 43 cases of genitourinary sarcomas from 1,583 adults (2.7 %) with soft tissue sarcoma admitted to the Memorial Sloan Kettering Cancer Center (MSKCC) from July 1982 to December 1989. The most common site of origin of the tumor was paratesticular (33 %), followed by the prostate/seminal vesicle (28 %), bladder (23 %), and kidney (16 %).

J. Wang, MD (✉)
Genitourinary Oncology Division, University of Arizona Cancer Center at St. Joseph's Hospital and Medical Center, 625 N. 6th Street, Phoenix, AZ 85004, USA
e-mail: Jue.Wang@DignityHealth.org

M. Malla, MD
Internal Medicine, St. Joseph's Hospital and Medical Center, 500 W. Thomas Road, Suite 720, Phoenix, AZ 85013, USA

J. Wang
Baylor University, College of Arts and Sciences, Waco, TX, USA

L. Pagliaro (ed.), *Rare Genitourinary Tumors*,
DOI 10.1007/978-3-319-30046-7_7

Histology, Epidemiology, and Risk Factors

Leiomyosarcoma is the most common malignant mesenchymal tumor of the urinary bladder in adults [5–11]. In a review of 19 patients with PBS at the University of Texas MD Anderson Cancer Center [8], the most common histological type of bladder sarcoma was leiomyosarcoma (74 %), followed by angiosarcoma (16 %), and unclassified sarcoma (11 %). We identified 470 cases of PBS treated in1973–2012 using the Surveillance, Epidemiology, and End Results (SEER) national cancer registries, with the most common histological type being leiomyosarcoma (38.9 %), followed by embryonal rhabdomyosarcoma (18.5 %), sarcoma NOS (15.7 %), rhabdomyosarcoma NOS (3.8 %), and other histological sarcoma categories (23 %). Figure 7.1 shows the histological distribution of PBS reported in the SEER database (1973–2012).

Approximately 100 cases of leiomyosarcoma have been reported in the medical literature so far [4–10]. Rosser et al. [7] reported one of the largest series, consisting of 36 adult patients with leiomyosarcoma of the urinary bladder treated at MD Anderson between 1986 and 1998. The mean age of the patients was 63 years. Twenty-six patients were white men in their seventh decade. The most common presenting symptoms were gross hematuria (81 %), urinary frequency (28 %), and dysuria (19 %).

Information on the pathogenesis and risk factors of leiomyosarcoma is limited. Leiomyosarcomas have reportedly developed in patients 5–20 years after

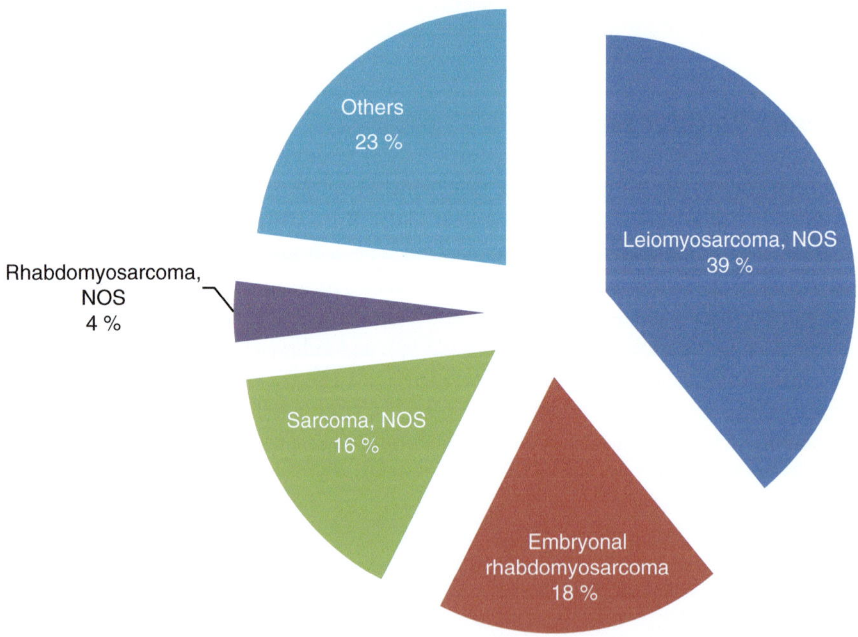

Fig. 7.1 Histologic distribution of primary bladder sarcoma reported in the SEER database (1973–2012)

cyclophosphamide treatment [12, 13]. It was hypothesized that accumulation of acrolein, a metabolite of cyclophosphamide, in the bladder increases the risk of bladder cancers, including epithelial and the rare nonepithelial cancers. Multiple cases also suggest an association between the hereditary retinoblastoma and urinary bladder leiomyosarcoma [14]. Several reports have demonstrated abnormalities in the p53 pathway [14] as well as in the Rb-cyclin D pathway [15] in leiomyosarcoma.

Rhabdomyosarcoma (RMS) is a tumor of childhood, and adult RMS in the urinary bladder is rare [16]. RMS is classified into embryonal (ERMS), alveolar (ARMS), and pleomorphic (PRMS) subtypes. ERMS, including botryoid variants, typically occurs in young children, ARMS typically occurs in older children and young adults, and PRMS occurs in older adults. Risk factors of RMS include a history of local irradiation, prior cyclophosphamide treatment, and schistosomiasis. Most cases of RMS appear to be sporadic, but the disease has been associated with familial syndromes (neurofibromatosis, the Li-Fraumeni, Beckwith-Wiedemann, and Costello syndromes) [17].

Angiosarcoma occurs very rarely in the genitourinary tract as either a primary or metastatic malignancy and can present great diagnostic difficulty [18–21]. A literature search using PubMed revealed less than 20 cases of angiosarcoma affecting the bladder. This tumor is more frequent in older men with a history of radiotherapy to the pelvis. Prior radiation is a well-documented risk factor [19, 20] and should raise suspicion of angiosarcoma in patients with hematuria without evidence of urothelial carcinoma. Patients usually present with muscle invasive disease, and the prognosis is dismal.

Diagnosis and Management of Primary Bladder Sarcoma

Cystoscopy is the gold standard for the diagnostic evaluation of a patient with suspected bladder cancer, regardless of subtype. Effort should be made to ensure that the tissue is processed properly. Review of the biopsy samples by a pathologist with special expertise in sarcoma should be strongly considered because of the profound implications of a precise diagnosis on treatment outcome.

Because of the rarity of PBS, there is no single accepted staging system. A staging system developed at the Sloan Kettering Cancer Center (MSKCC) constituting tumor grade, size (< or >5 cm), depth of invasion, presence of metastatic disease, and retinoblastoma gene product has proved useful in terms of prognosis and predicting survival rates [5].

The treatment of pediatric soft tissue sarcoma has evolved considerably over the past several decades, largely due to the use of multimodal therapy and effort of large international cooperative groups [22]. By comparison, the literature on treatment of adult PBS is sparse. Currently, management of PBS follows principles of sarcoma management in other sites [3].

In general, surgery is the mainstay of therapy [4–9]. In an MD Anderson series, the majority of patients (97 %) had a radical cystectomy, and 63 % of patients received either neoadjuvant or adjuvant chemotherapy [7]. In a SEER registry study of leiomyosarcoma [23], most patients (92.9 %) received cancer-directed surgery (CDS), with 34 % having radical or partial cystectomy, 38 % having a transurethral resection, and 20 % having unspecified CDS. 7.7 % of patients received radiation therapy in combination with surgery.

For patient with very large primary tumors, neoadjuvant chemotherapy is often recommended if the tumor has a histology for which a reasonable response is anticipated [7, 22]. Adjuvant chemotherapy and radiation therapy as a means to decrease the risk for disease recurrence in patients with localized soft tissue sarcoma at diagnosis has also been investigated [22, 24]. The available reports have been limited by patient heterogeneity, short follow-up, and low patient accrual. In cases of metastatic disease, combination chemotherapy (doxorubicin, ifosfamide, cisplatinum, and docetaxel) is frequently used [22–25].

Prognosis

Poor prognosis associated with undifferentiated grade and advanced stage has been reported in previous studies [5, 7, 11, 23, 25]. In the MD Anderson Cancer Center series [7], the disease-specific survival rates at 1, 3, and 5 years were 88.6 %, 62.0 %, and 62.0 %, respectively. Multivariate analyses demonstrated that only the MSKCC disease stage system was a significant predictor of survival for patients with bladder leiomyosarcoma. Russo reported their 25-year MSKCC experience in adult genitourinary sarcoma [5]. On a univariate analysis, unfavorable prognostic variables for disease-specific survival were metastasis at presentation, high tumor grade, a lack of leiomyosarcoma and liposarcoma histological subtypes, prostate sarcoma, large tumor size, incomplete surgical resection, and positive surgical margin. On multivariate analysis, tumor size and metastasis at diagnosis remained significant predictors of disease-specific survival. Rodríguez et al. identified several poor prognostic factors including advanced age, undifferentiated tumor grade, distant disease, and failure to undergo CDS in their multivariate analysis [22]. In our analysis of 470 PBS cases, we found histological subtypes of PBS, along with patient age, gender, tumor stage, and CDS, which are significant predictors of disease-specific survival (Table 7.1).

Sarcomatoid Carcinoma of the Urinary Bladder

Sarcomatoid carcinoma of the urinary bladder (SCUB) is an unusual malignancy composed of both carcinomatous and sarcomatous components. It is a rare but aggressive form of bladder cancer, comprising less than 1 % of all bladder cancers [7, 26]. In most reported cases of SCUB, the epithelial component is urothelial carcinoma (UC), although squamous cell and small cell carcinoma components are also reported [27–34]. The mesenchymal component varies from homogeneous sarcoma to more heterotopic elements such as malignant bone, cartilage, and other mesenchymal tissues [27, 32, 33, 35].

Table 7.1 Multivariate analyses of factors associated with cancer-specific mortality in patients with primary bladder sarcoma (PBS)

Characteristics		Hazard ratio	95 % confidence interval	*p*-value
Age	≥65	3.10	1.73–5.55	<0.001
Gender	Female	2.05	1.22–3.43	0.01
Histology	EMS	1.00		
	LMS	3.44	1.19–9.98	0.03
	RMS NOS	3.09	0.82–11.6	0.10
	SC NOS	5.46	1.76–17.0	0.003
SEER stage	Distant	3.23	1.80–5.78	<0.001
CDS	Yes	0.26	0.09–0.79	0.02

LMS leiomyosarcoma, *RMS* rhabdomyosarcoma, not otherwise specified, *EMS* embryonal rhabdomyosarcoma, *SC NOS* sarcoma, not otherwise specified, *CDS* cancer-directed surgery

Multiple terms have been used to describe SCUB, including *malignant mesodermal mixed tumor, spindle cell carcinoma, giant cell carcinoma, carcinosarcoma, pseudosarcomatous transitional cell carcinoma, and malignant teratoma* [29, 31–34]. The current World Health Organization classification recommends the usage of the term *sarcomatoid carcinoma (SC)* for all biphasic malignant neoplasms of the urinary tract exhibiting morphologic and/or immunohistochemical evidence of epithelial and mesenchymal differentiation [26].

Clinical observation suggests that tumors with larger proportion of sarcomatoid component appear to correlate with poorer outcomes. However, no published studies have looked at the effect of the percentage of sarcomatoid transformation on the prognosis of SCUB so far. In addition, there is no agreed-upon cutoff point for risk stratification at this time. This highlights the need for developing a standardized pathological reporting system for SC to compare results across studies.

Epidemiology

Although the reported incidence of SCUB in single institutional studies has ranged from 0.3 to 4.3 % of all the histological types of bladder carcinoma [27, 44], the incidence reported in an analysis of the SEER database is much lower [35, 36]. Evidence from a contemporary cohort revealed that the incident of variants of bladder cancer can increase over time [40]. Our analysis of SCUB in SEER databases showed that this is also true for SCUB (Fig. 7.2). This observation is likely due to heightened awareness of this aggressive subtype and improved immunohistochemistry techniques.

Similar to the conventional urothelial carcinomas (UC), SCUB is a disease of advancing age. Lopez-Beltran et al. [26] reported that SCUB usually presents between the age of 50 and 77 years with a mean age of presentation at 66 years. The male preponderance (male to female ratio, 1.8:1) and age distribution were similar to those of ordinary UC. Wang and associates [36] reported a large cohort of 221 patients with a median age at diagnosis of 75 years (range of 41–96 years).

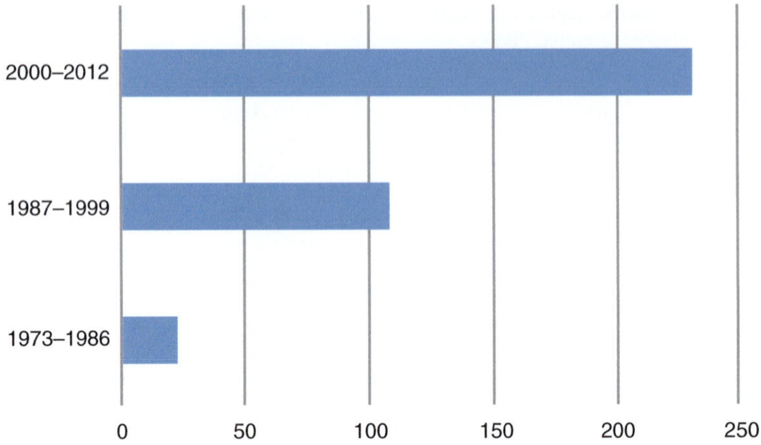

Fig. 7.2 Cases of sarcomatoid carcinoma of urinary bladder (SCUB) reported in the SEER database (1973–2012)

Etiology and Histogenesis

While no definite risk factors have been identified to date, SCUB is usually associated with cigarette smoking; between 50 and 79 % of patients with SCUB are current or former smokers [29, 31, 37, 38]. History of intravesical cyclophosphamide and radiation therapy for a prior conventional urothelial carcinoma has been reported to result in sarcomatoid transformation [27, 45].

Several theories exist as to histogenesis of SCUB. Some investigators suggest that these tumors may develop as a result of undifferentiated, totipotent neoplastic cells that undergo multiple pathways of terminal differentiation into either mesenchymal or epithelial elements [46, 52]. Others conclude that SC might arise as multiclonal collision tumors [47]. Recently, the results of molecular/genetic studies have provided strong support for a common monoclonal origin of both epithelial and mesenchymal components in SCUB [39, 41, 49–51].

Clinical Presentation

The clinical presentation of patients with SCUB is similar to those with typical urothelial carcinoma. Hematuria is the most common presenting symptom [27, 37, 38, 45]. Other frequently reported symptoms and signs of SCUB include dysuria, acute urinary retention, lower abdominal pain, and urinary tract infection [27, 38]. The diagnosis of SCUB should be considered in a clinical scenario of large bladder mass and rapid clinical progression. Cystoscopy usually shows one or more broad-based, often polypoid mass(es) with ulcerated and hemorrhagic surface(s). Macroscopically, SCUB is identical to transitional cell carcinoma, with tumor size typically ranging from 1.5 to 13.0 cm. The most common sites of SCUB are the lateral wall and fundus of the bladder, though in some cases, the trigone may be involved [27, 30, 31, 36, 37]. Histologically, these tumors show a mixture of carcinomatous and sarcomatoid components in varying ratios. Many studies have defined a tumor as SCUB if even a small amount of sarcomatoid differentiation is present, whereas other studies have excluded tumors with a sarcomatoid component less than 20 % of the tumor volume or less than one microscopic low-power (10 xs) field in size. However, some evidence indicates that even small amounts of sarcomatoid differentiation may be clinically relevant and should be included in the pathology report [35–37].

SCUB typically presents at advanced stage and with more frequent regional and distant metastases compared with UC. In a SEER study, 98 % of tumors were graded as poorly differentiated or undifferentiated. The stage distribution was observed to be localized cancer in 25 % of the cases, regional spread in 52 %, distant metastasis in 15 %, and stage unknown in 8 % of the cases. In a retrospective review from the University of Nebraska Medical Center [37], 85 % of the patients had muscle invasive disease and 50 % of the patients presented with stage IV disease.

Management of SCUB

Owing to the rareness of SCUB, and in the absence of randomized controlled trials, there is no standardized treatment protocol for this disease. Therefore, management for SCUB is usually extrapolated from the approach to patients with UC. Several retrospective studies have provided some insight into therapy for this disease [27, 31, 32, 36–38, 42, 43].

For non-muscle invasive SCUB, TURBT (transurethral resection for bladder tumor) or partial cystectomy carries very high risk of incomplete tumor removal [35]. Black et al. recommended forgoing transurethral bladder tumor resection and intravesical therapy, proceeding directly to cystectomy in patients well enough to undergo this procedure, an approach that was also supported by others [36, 42].

For muscle invasive disease, multimodal therapy including radical cystectomy whenever possible was advocated [35–37, 42]. In a review of 221 patients with SCUB, the 2-year survival rate in patients treated with partial cystectomy was 14 % when compared with 52 % in patients treated with radical cystectomy [36].

Given the high rate of local recurrence and metastasis of the tumor after radical cystectomy, various combinations of neoadjuvant or adjuvant chemotherapy and/or radiotherapy after radical surgery were advocated [35, 36]. Black et al. [42] reported that 45 % patients who were administered neoadjuvant chemotherapy for clinical stage T2 or T3 disease were downstaged to pT0. However, this finding could not be correlated to survival benefit because of insufficient sample size. Spiess et al. [32] reported 17 patients with SCUB, out of which seven patients were treated with neoadjuvant chemotherapy followed by surgery. There are a few case reports that demonstrated complete remission after multimodality treatment [37, 53–58].

The hypothesis of common monoclonal origin of both epithelial and mesenchymal components in SCUB [46, 50, 52] would support the use of platinum-based regimens, which are active in the treatment of UC. Several retrospective case reports and series showed that gemcitabine/cisplatin regimen is well tolerated and effective given its ability to induce complete remission in selected patients [11, 32, 36, 48, 54, 59] and long-term survival has been reported in selected patients who were treated with multimodality therapy [27, 30, 37, 48, 53, 54]. However, response to chemotherapy has been variable in the current literature. For example, Baseskioglu et al. reported that most of their patients died before completing the chemotherapy protocol due to the rapid progression of the disease [38]. Multi-institutional clinical trials are needed to establish a better therapeutic protocol for this rare but aggressive cancer.

Prognosis

Most investigators have reported poor outcomes for patients with SCUB, regardless of the type of treatment [27, 35, 36]. Black et al. [42] also demonstrated that patients with SCUB have worse disease-specific and overall survival, even after adjusting for stage of tumor, in comparison with patients with high-grade pure UC. In the largest SEER cohort of SCUB, pathologic stage was identified as the best predictor of survival. Patients with regional and distant spread of disease have a twofold and eightfold increased risk of mortality from SCUB, respectively [35, 36].

Multidisciplinary Approach

Significant variation in treatment pattern (cystectomy, radiation, and chemotherapy) and outcomes was observed, when comparing single-institution studies to the SEER cohorts [60]. This discrepancy is likely related to differences in practice patterns. In consideration of the rarity of this tumor, a multidisciplinary approach in referral centers is highly recommended. The close collaboration between medical oncologists, urologists, radiation oncologists, radiologists, and pathologists is essential for optimal management of this rare disease.

Future Directions

The diagnostic classification of PBS and SCUB is traditionally based on histological features as defined by the World Health Organization (WHO) classification [26]. Emerging technology including next-generation sequencing will continue to further our understanding of saromagenesis, enable more precise classification and diagnosis of sarcomas, and identify actionable target therapies in the future [61–63].

SCUB represents a complete phenotype with various pathways of epithelial-mesenchymal transition (EMT) [8]; conceivably, targeting EMT program could become a valid therapeutic strategy for these life-threatening tumors. Recently, the findings of high EMT scores in mesenchymal non-small cell lung cancer (NSCLC) associated with distinct immune phenotypes with increased expression of immune inhibitory molecules [64] provide a potential mechanism for EMT-associated immunosuppression. The higher PD-L1 expression levels in SC of lung cancer [65] support the potential use of anti-PD-1/PD-L1 targeted therapies.

Conclusion

PBS and SCUB are heterogeneous groups of tumors that pose significant diagnostic and therapeutic challenge. The continuous evolution of radiographic imaging and molecular biology has led to a better diagnostic definition for these complex tumors. Multidisciplinary approach in tertiary centers is highly recommended for optimal management. Future efforts should be directed at the early detection of these tumors and the development of more effective systemic therapies including target therapy and immunotherapy.

References

1. Carver J. Sarcoma of bladder. Proc R Soc Med. 1938;31(9):1079–80.
2. Sen SE, Malek RS, Farrow GM, Lieber MM. Sarcoma and carcinosarcoma of the bladder in adults. J Urol. 1985;133(1):29–30.
3. Yang JC, Rosenberg SA, Glastein EJ, et al. Sarcomas of soft tissue. In: DeVita VT, Hellman S, Rosenberg SA, editors. Cancer: principles and practice of oncology. 4th ed. Philadelphia: Lippincott; 1993. p. 1436–55.
4. Dotan ZA, Tal R, Golijanin D, Snyder ME, Antonescu C, Brennan MF, Russo P. Adult genitourinary sarcoma: the 25-year Memorial Sloan-Kettering experience. J Urol. 2006;176(5):2033–8.
5. Russo P, Brady MS, Conlon K, et al. Adult urological sarcoma. J Urol. 1992;147:1032–7.
6. Russo P. Urologic sarcoma in adults. Memorial Sloan-Kettering Cancer Center experience based on a prospective database between 1982 and 1989. Urol Clin N Am. 1991;18(3):581–8.
7. Rosser CJ, Slaton JW, Izawa JI, et al. Clinical presentation and outcome of high-grade urinary bladder leiomyosarcoma in adults. Urology. 2003;61:1151–5.
8. Spiess PE, Kassouf W, Steinberg JR, Tuziak T, Hernandez M, Tibbs RF, Czerniak B, Kamat AM, Dinney CP, Grossman HB. Review of the M.D. Anderson experience in the treatment of bladder sarcoma. Urol Oncol. 2007;25(1):38–45.
9. Izumi K, Mizokami A, Sugimoto K, Narimoto K, Miyagi T, Maeda Y, Kitagawa Y, Kadono Y, Konaka H, Namiki M. Role of surgical resection in adult urological soft tissue sarcoma: 25-year experience. Urol Int. 2010;84(3):309–14.
10. Mills SE, Bova GS, Wick MR, Young RH. Leiomyosarcoma of the urinary bladder. A clinicopathologic and immunohistochemical study of 15 cases. Am J Surg Pathol. 1989;13(6):480–9.
11. Martin SA, Sears DL, Sebo TJ, Lohse CM, Cheville JC. Smooth muscle neoplasms of the urinary bladder: a clinicopathologic comparison of leiomyoma and leiomyosarcoma. Am J Surg Pathol. 2002;26:292–300.
12. Parekh DJ, Jung C, O'Conner J, Dutta S, Smith Jr ER. Leiomyosarcoma in urinary bladder after cyclophosphamide therapy for retinoblastoma and review of bladder sarcomas. Urology. 2002;60(1):164.
13. Kawamura J, Sakurai M, Tsukamoto K, Tochigi H. Leiomyosarcoma of the bladder eighteen years after cyclophosphamide therapy for retinoblastoma. Urol Int. 1993;51(1):49–53.
14. Konomoto T, Fukuda T, Hayashi K, Kumazawa J, Tsuneyoshi M. Leiomyosarcoma in soft tissue: examination of p53 status and cell proliferating factors in different locations. Hum Pathol. 1998;29:74–81.

15. Cohen JA, Geradts J. Loss of RB and MTS1/CDKN2 (p16) expression in human sarcomas. Hum Pathol. 1997;28:893–8.
16. Dagher R, Helman L. Rhabdomyosarcoma: an overview. Oncologist. 1999;4:34.
17. Anderson J, Gordon A, Pritchard-Jones K, Shipley J. Genes, chromosomes, and rhabdomyosarcoma. Genes Chromosomes Cancer. 1999;26:275.
18. Aragona F, Ostardo E, Prayer-Galetti T, et al. Angiosarcoma of the bladder: a case report with regard to histologic and immunohistochemical findings. Eur Urol. 1991;20:161.
19. Engel JD, Kuzel TM, Moceanu MC, et al. Angiosarcoma of the bladder: a review. Urology. 1998;52:778–84.
20. Kulaga A, Yilmaz A, Wilkin RP, et al. Epithelioid angiosarcoma of the bladder after irradiation for endometrioid adenocarcinoma. Virchows Arch. 2007;450:245–6.
21. Matoso A, Epstein JI. Epithelioid angiosarcoma of the bladder: a series of 9 cases. Am J Surg Pathol. 2015;39:1377–82.
22. Mondaini N, Palli D, Saieva C, Nesi G, Franchi A, Ponchietti R, Tripodi S, Miracco C, Meliani E, Carini M, Livi L, Zanna I, Trovarelli S, Marino V, Vignolini G, Pomara G, Orlando V, Giubilei G, Selli C, Rizzo M. Clinical characteristics and overall survival in genitourinary sarcomas treated with curative intent: a multicenter study. Eur Urol. 2005;47(4):468–73.
23. Rodríguez D, Preston MA, Barrisford GW, Olumi AF, Feldman AS. Clinical features of leiomyosarcoma of the urinary bladder: analysis of 183 cases. Urol Oncol. 2014;32(7):958–65.
24. O'Sullivan B, Ward I, Catton C. Recent advances in radiotherapy for soft-tissue sarcoma. Curr Oncol Rep. 2003;5:274–81.
25. Lee TK, Miyamoto H, Osunkoya AO, Guo CC, Weiss SW, Epstein JI. Smooth muscle neoplasms of the urinary bladder: a clinicopathologic study of 51 cases. Am J Surg Pathol. 2010;34(4):502–9.
26. Wick MR, Swanson PE. Carcinosarcomas: current perspectives and an historical review of nosological concepts. Semin Diagn Pathol. 1993;10(2):118–27.
27. Lopez-Beltran A, Pacelli A, Rothenberg HJ, Wollan PC, Zincke H, Blute ML, Bostwick DG. Carcinosarcoma and sarcomatoid carcinoma of the bladder: clinicopathological study of 41 cases. J Urol. 1998;159(5):1497–503.
28. Jones EC, Young RH. Myxoid and sclerosing sarcomatoid transitional cell carcinoma of the urinary bladder: a clinicopathologic and immunohistochemical study of 25 cases. Mod Pathol. 1997;10(9):908–16.
29. Perret L, Chaubert P, Hessler D, Guillou L. Primary heterologous carcinosarcoma (metaplastic carcinoma) of the urinary bladder: a clinicopathologic, immunohistochemical, and ultrastructural analysis of eight cases and a review of the literature. Cancer. 1998;82(8):1535–49.
30. Ikegami H, Iwasaki H, Ohjimi Y, Takeuchi T, Ariyoshi A, Kikuchi M. Sarcomatoid carcinoma of the urinary bladder: a clinicopathologic and immunohistochemical analysis of 14 patients. Hum Pathol. 2000;31(3):332–40.
31. Young RH, Wick MR, Mills SE. Sarcomatoid carcinoma of the urinary bladder. A clinicopathologic analysis of 12 cases and review of the literature. Am J Clin Pathol. 1988;90(6):653–61.
32. Spiess PE, Tuziak T, Tibbs RF, Bassett R, Tamboli P, Brown GA, Grossman HB, Ayala AG, Czerniak B. Pseudosarcomatous and sarcomatous proliferations of the bladder. Hum Pathol. 2007;38(5):753–61.
33. Cheng L, Zhang S, Alexander R, Maclennan GT, Hodges KB, Harrison BT, Lopez-Beltran A, Montironi R. Sarcomatoid carcinoma of the urinary bladder: the final common pathway of urothelial carcinoma dedifferentiation. Am J Surg Pathol. 2011;35(5):e34–46.
34. Torenbeek R, Blomjous CE, de Bruin PC, Newling DW, Meijer CJ. Sarcomatoid carcinoma of the urinary bladder. Clinicopathologic analysis of 18 cases with immunohistochemical and electron microscopic findings. Am J Surg Pathol. 1994;18(3):241–9.
35. Wright JL, Black PC, Brown GA, Porter MP, Kamat AM, Dinney CP, Lin DW. Differences in survival among patients with sarcomatoid carcinoma, carcinosarcoma and urothelial carcinoma of the bladder. J Urol. 2007;178(6):2302–6.
36. Wang J, Wang FW, Lagrange CA, Hemstreet Iii GP, Kessinger A. Clinical features of sarcomatoid carcinoma (carcinosarcoma) of the urinary bladder: analysis of 221 cases. Sarcoma. 2010. pii: 454792. doi:10.1155/2010/454792.

37. Wang J, Gillaspie C, Kunadharaju R, Talmon G, Enke C. Sarcomatoid urothelial carcinoma: a single cancer center experience. World J Oncol. 2011;4:175–80.
38. Başeskioglu B, Duman BB, Kara IO, Can C, Yildirim M, Açikalin M. Early detection and gemcitabine/cisplatin combination positively effect survival in sarcomatoid carcinoma of the urinary bladder. Asian Pac J Cancer Prev. 2012;13(11):5729–33.
39. Armstrong AB, Wang M, Eble JN, MacLennan GT, Montironi R, Tan PH, Lopez-Beltran A, Zhang S, Baldridge LA, Spartz H, Cheng L. TP53 mutational analysis supports monoclonal origin of biphasic sarcomatoid urothelial carcinoma (carcinosarcoma) of the urinary bladder. Mod Pathol. 2009;22(1):113–8.
40. Monn MF, Kaimakliotis HZ, Pedrosa JA, Cary KC, Bihrle R, Cheng L, Koch MO. Contemporary bladder cancer: variant histology may be a significant driver of disease. Urol Oncol. 2015;33(1):18.e15–20.
41. Cheng L, Lopez-Beltran A, MacLennan GT, et al. Neoplasms of the urinary bladder. In: Bostwick DG, Cheng L, editors. Urologic surgical pathology. 2nd ed. Philadelphia: Elsevier/Mosby; 2008. p. 259–352.
42. Black PC, Brown GA, Dinney CP. The impact of variant histology on the outcome of bladder cancer treated with curative intent. Urol Oncol. 2009;27(1):3–7.
43. Wang J, Wang FW, Lagrange CA, Hemstreet GP. Clinical features and outcomes of 25 patients with primary adenosquamous cell carcinoma of the prostate. Rare Tumor. 2010;2(3):e47.
44. Chalasani V, Chin JL, Izawa JI. Histologic variants of urothelial bladder cancer and nonurothelial histology in bladder cancer. Can Urol Assoc J. 2009;3(6 Suppl 4):S193–8.
45. Sigal SH, Tomaszewski JE, Brooks JJ, Wein A, LiVolsi VA. Carcinosarcoma of bladder following long-term cyclophosphamide therapy. Arch Pathol Lab Med. 1991;115(10):1049–51.
46. Völker HU, Zettl A, Schön G, Heller V, Heinrich E, Rosenwald A, Handwerker M, Müller-Hermelink HK, Marx A, Ströbel P. Molecular genetic findings in two cases of sarcomatoid carcinoma of the ureter: evidence for evolution from a common pluripotent progenitor cell? Virchows Arch. 2008;452(4):457–63.
47. Gorstein F, Anderson TL. Malignant mixed mesodermal tumors: carcinoma, sarcoma, or both? Hum Pathol. 1991;22(3):207–9.
48. Froehner M, Gaertner HJ, Manseck A, Wirth MP. Durable complete remission of metastatic sarcomatoid carcinoma of the bladder with cisplatin and gemcitabine in an 80-year-old man. Urology. 2001;58(5):799.
49. Halachmi S, DeMarzo AM, Chow NH, Halachmi N, Smith AE, Linn JF, Nativ O, Epstein JI, Schoenberg MP, Sidransky D. Genetic alterations in urinary bladder carcinosarcoma evidence of a common clonal origin. Eur Urol. 2000;37(3):350–7.
50. Thompson L, Chang B, Barsky SH. Monoclonal origins of malignant mixed tumors (carcinosarcomas). Evidence for a divergent histogenesis. Am J Surg Pathol. 1996;20(3):277–85.
51. Sung MT, Wang M, MacLennan GT, Eble JN, Tan PH, Lopez-Beltran A, Montironi R, Harris JJ, Kuhar M, Cheng L. Histogenesis of sarcomatoid urothelial carcinoma of the urinary bladder: evidence for a common clonal origin with divergent differentiation. J Pathol. 2007;211(4):420–30.
52. McCluggage WG. Malignant biphasic uterine tumours: carcinosarcomas or metaplastic carcinomas? J Clin Pathol. 2002;55(5):321–5.
53. Antonelli A, Simeone C, Ferrari V, Tardanico R, Cunico SC. Durable and complete remission of a metastatic bladder sarcomatoid carcinoma with chemotherapic and surgical treatments. Arch Ital Urol Androl. 2006;78(2):67–70.
54. Damiano R, D'Armiento M, Cantiello F, Amorosi A, Tagliaferri P, Sacco R, Venuta S. Gemcitabine and cisplatin following surgical treatment of urinary bladder carcinosarcoma. Tumori. 2004;90(5):458–60.
55. Onal C, Pehlivan B, Bal N, Topkan E, Kilinc F, Topuk S. Sarcomatoid carcinoma of the urinary bladder treated with adjuvant radiotherapy: a case report. Clin Med Case Rep. 2009;2:39–42.
56. Tazi FM, Ahallal Y, Benlemlih A, Khallouk A, Elfassi MJ, Farih MH. Urinary bladder carcinosarcoma: a complete pathological response after neoadjuvant chemotherapy. Turkish J Urol. 2012;38(2):114–6.

57. Hoshi S, Sasaki M, Muto A, Suzuki K, Kobayashi T, Tukigi M, Ono K, Sugano O, Saso S. Case of carcinosarcoma of urinary bladder obtained a pathologically complete response by neoadjuvant chemoradiotherapy. Int J Urol. 2007;14(1):79–81.
58. Wallach JB, Wang B, Sanfilippo N. High-grade hyperinvasive sarcomatoid urothelial bladder carcinoma demonstrating complete response to bladder-preserving chemoradiation. Curr Oncol. 2009;16(3):55–7.
59. Guo AT, Huang H, Wei LX. Clinicopathological characteristics and prognosis of Chinese patients with sarcomatoid carcinoma of the bladder. Histol Histopathol. 2013;28(9):1167–74.
60. Malla M, Wang J. The natural history, treatment pattern, and survival of the patients with sarcomatoid bladder carcinoma: a pooled analysis. J Clin Oncol. 2015;33(suppl; abstr e15532).
61. Lauer S, Gardner JM. Soft tissue sarcomas – new approaches to diagnosis and classification. Curr Probl Cancer. 2013;37(2):45–61.
62. Paniz Mondolfi AE, Jour G, Johnson M, Reidy J, Cason RC, Barkoh BA, Benaim G, Singh R, Luthra R. Primary cutaneous carcinosarcoma: insights into its clonal origin and mutational pattern expression analysis through next-generation sequencing. Hum Pathol. 2013;44(12):2853–60.
63. Paniz-Mondolfi A, Singh R, Jour G, Mahmoodi M, Diwan AH, Barkoh BA, Cason R, Huttenbach Y, Benaim G, Galbincea J, Luthra R. Cutaneous carcinosarcoma: further insights into its mutational landscape through massive parallel genome sequencing. Virchows Arch. 2014;465(3):339–50.
64. Velcheti V, Rimm DL, Schalper KA. Sarcomatoid lung carcinomas show high levels of programmed death ligand-1 (PD-L1). J Thorac Oncol. 2013;8(6):803–5.
65. Lou Y, Diao L, Byers LV, Gibbons DL, Warren Denning W, Jing Wang J, Vassiliki Papadimitrakopoulou V, Wistuba I, Goswami S, Cortez MA, Welsh J, Kurie JM, Heymach J. Association of epithelial-mesenchymal transition status with PD1/PDL1 expression and a distinct immunophenotype in non-small cell lung cancer: implications for immunotherapy biomarkers. J Clin Oncol. 2014;32:5s (suppl; abstr 3018).

8 Neuroendocrine and Small Cell Carcinoma of the Urinary Tract

Richard Meijer and Axel Bex

Introduction

Neuroendocrine and small cell carcinoma of the bladder (SCCB) are rare conditions, accounting for approximately 0.5–0.7 % of urothelial malignancies [1, 2, 11, 26] Due to this low incidence, the published single-institution reports on this topic contain limited numbers of patients (ranging from 5 to 125) and are mainly retrospective. A consensus on the optimal treatment strategy has not been reached [5, 36, 57], though attempts at national guidelines have been made. Initially radical cystectomy was considered the standard of care for patients with clinically localized disease. However, the high rate of metastases has led to the introduction of multimodality approaches with systemic chemotherapy combined with either surgery or radiotherapy [2, 5, 8, 36, 57].

In the 1980s it was recognized that the biological and clinicopathological features of SCCB are similar to those of small cell lung carcinoma (SCLC) [24, 43]. Thus the treatment approach to this rare tumor has been greatly influenced by the treatment of the far more common SCLC. In the approach of SCLC, a distinction is made between patients with limited disease (tumor confined to the hemithorax, mediastinum, or supraclavicular lymph nodes) and patients with extensive disease (tumor outside these areas) [55]. Patients with limited disease (LD) SCLC are generally treated with a combination of systemic chemotherapy and local radiotherapy [22, 32, 59, 60]. This multimodality treatment is applied to address the risk of occult micrometastases at the time of diagnosis. Patients

R. Meijer
Department of Urology, University Medical Center Utrecht, Utrecht, The Netherlands
e-mail: rmeijer6@umcutrecht.nl

A. Bex, MD, PhD (✉)
Division of Surgical Oncology, Department of Urology, The Netherlands Cancer Institute, Plesmanlaan 121, Amsterdam 1066 CX, The Netherlands
e-mail: a.bex@nki.nl

L. Pagliaro (ed.), *Rare Genitourinary Tumors*,
DOI 10.1007/978-3-319-30046-7_8

with extensive disease (ED) SCLC are treated with palliative chemotherapy only [55]. Considering the similar tumor biology of SCCB and SCLC, some authors define limited (LD) and extensive disease (ED) SCCB in analogy to SCLC to guide treatment decisions [8, 35, 44]. It has been suggested by some institutions that the treatment approach for LD-SCCB should follow the multimodality treatment applied for LD-SCLC (i.e., systemic chemotherapy combined with external beam radiotherapy) rather than cystectomy subsequent to neoadjuvant therapy [8, 36].

Definition of Neuroendocrine and Small Cell Carcinoma of the Bladder

The first case of primary small cell bladder cancer (SCCB) was reported in 1981 [16]. Since then approximately 800–1,000 cases diagnosed according to World Health Organization (WHO) criteria [23, 24] have been published in small single-arm prospective studies, retrospective series, and case reports. Based on the WHO classification, SCCB is defined as appearance of typical oat cell-shaped tumor cells at light microscopy. SCCB may consist of additional other bladder cancer subtypes and neuroendocrine cells but the diagnostic leading feature is the presence of small cells. In the literature, neuroendocrine tumors and SCCB are occasionally grouped together to describe outcome of treatment approaches [10]. However, they are not a single disease entity. SCCB may often contain neuroendocrine cells, but not exclusively and not consistently [21] (see also chapter "Diagnosis" and Table 8.1). The concomitant occurrence of other bladder cancer subtypes and neuroendocrine cells has prompted several theories about the origin of SCCB of which the theory of a common pluripotent stem cell in the urothelium leading to heterogeneity of tumor subtypes and a variety of epithelial and endocrine markers is favored [11]. Large cell neuroendocrine carcinoma (LCNC) is defined in the urinary bladder, as in other sites, as a high-grade neoplasm exhibiting neuroendocrine features at light microscopy with hematoxylin-eosin staining (H&E), high mitotic activity, and evidence of neuroendocrine differentiation by immunohistochemistry [15, 53]. Paraganglioma (PG) of the urinary bladder is a rare neuroendocrine neoplasm, accounting for <0.1 % of all bladder tumors [42].

Table 8.1 Neuroendocrine markers in small cell bladder cancer

Marker	Number of studies and patients per study (range)	% of SCCB	Reference
Neuron specific enolase (NSE)	4 (18–51)	25–100	[3, 11, 21, 28]
Serotonin	1 (22)	78	[21]
Synaptophysin	3 (18–51)	67–76	[3, 11, 28]
Chromogranin A	4 (2–51)	22–89	[3, 11, 28, 45]

Epidemiology

Neuroendocrine bladder carcinoma and SCCB are rare diseases. Of all bladder cancers, their frequency is less than 1 %. Based on the WHO definition of small cell carcinoma, which includes neuroendocrine variants, SCCB is a form of extrapulmonary small cell carcinoma (ESPCC). Small cell carcinoma accounts for one fifth of lung cancer cases but is rarely observed in extrapulmonary tumors [27]. In a recent Surveillance, Epidemiology and End Results (SEER) Program analysis, 55,722 cases of small cell carcinoma were diagnosed among the analyzed population between 1992 and 2010 (incidence rate = 81.8/million patient years). The incidence of SCLC (n=51,959; incidence rate=76.3) was 22 times more than that of extrapulmonary SCC (n=2,438; incidence rate=3.5). While SCLC accounted for 93 % of cases of small cell carcinoma, the urinary bladder seems to be among the most common extrapulmonary site. Of the extrapulmonary sites, incidence rates were low for the renal pelvis and ureter (incidence rate of urinary bladder 1.48 for men and 0.30 for women versus 0.07 for men and not assessable for women in the upper urinary tract). Small cell carcinoma IR was 35 % higher among men than women, with the greatest gender disparities for urinary bladder (male-to-female incidence rate ratio = 4.91) [18].

Extrapulmonary neuroendocrine tumors are rare. Neuroendocrine bladder cancer has been reported in only eight cases over a period of 3 years (2010–2012) in collective data from ten oncological centers in Germany [39]. This report did not distinguish between LCNC and neuroendocrine SCCB. Pure LCNC seems to be a rare disease and possibly underreported in the literature. A recent case report reviewed the literature and found only 12 cases of pure LCNC. The authors hypothesized that prior to the introduction of immunohistochemistry, most of these tumors which have a very aggressive course of disease were probably being diagnosed as high-grade undifferentiated urothelial cell carcinoma [51]. Due to the rarity of LCNC and absence of treatment recommendations, this chapter will predominantly focus on SCCB.

Clinical Presentation

SCCB often presents with large bladder tumors (Fig. 8.1a) and, in elderly patients, gross hematuria in up to 94 % and early metastasis [21]. This is similar to the presentation of neuroendocrine bladder tumors, both SCCB or LCNC. A case series demonstrated that neuroendocrine bladder cancer is predominantly a disease of the elderly, who present with distant metastatic disease at the time of diagnosis in up to 50 % cases [10]. Patients with SCCB are typically elderly men and in some series more than half of the patients were over 70 years of age [13, 14]. A SEER study of SCCB (n=642) confirmed the predominance of elderly Caucasian men with a median age of 73 years. Thirty-six percent of the patients presented with distant metastatic disease at the time of diagnosis [35]. Advanced disease stage in an elderly population poses particular problems regarding treatment options. In a series of 32

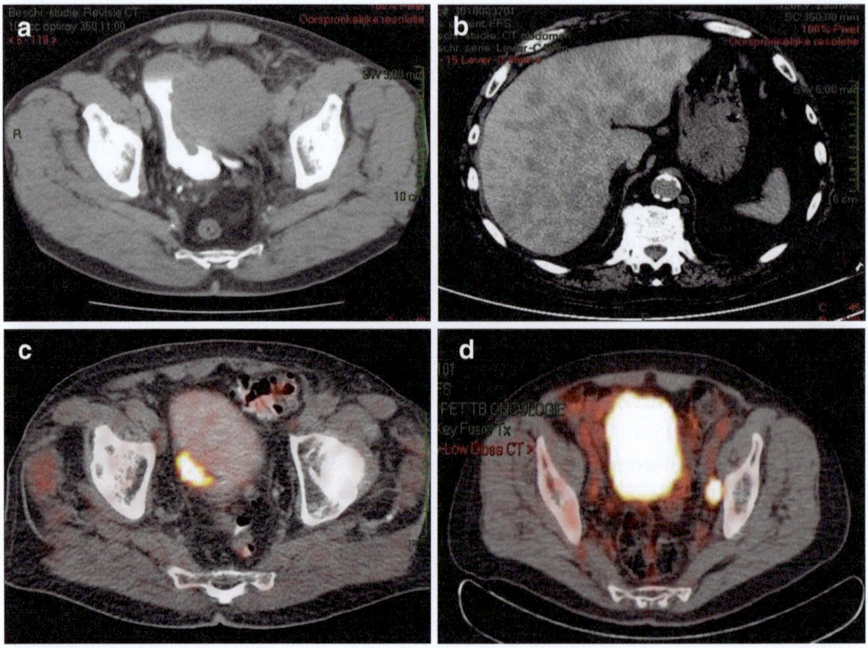

Fig. 8.1 Computed tomography (CT) of the abdomen demonstrating a large small cell carcinoma of the bladder (SCCB) with extravesical extension (**a**); CT of the abdomen with extensive liver metastasis at diagnosis in a patient with extensive disease stage (**b**); fluorodeoxyglucose (FDG)-positron emission tomography (PET) of a primary SCCB after image attenuation for physiological excretion in the urine (**c**); FDG-PET in a patient with limited disease stage demonstrating pelvic lymph node metastasis

patients with LD-SCCB, 4 patients (12.5 %) with a median age of 80 years (range 79–87 years) did not receive chemotherapy due to age-related comorbidity and were treated with radiotherapy only. One patient refused any treatment [7]. Preferred metastatic sites are the pelvic and retroperitoneal lymph nodes (Figs. 8.1d and 8.2b), liver, lung, bone, and brain [44]. With up to 12 % brain metastases, intracranial secondaries are more common than in conventional transitional cell carcinoma but less common than in SCLC [9]. In comparison to the already high percentage of clinically evident metastatic disease, occult micrometastases are a very common feature of SCCB and responsible for the poor outcome reported.

Another difference between SCLC and SCCB is observed in the percentage of patients with extensive disease. Sixty to 70 % have extensive SCLC at presentation, whereas some authors reported only 30 % in SCCB. This may be due to a difference in definition or clinical signs such as hematuria leading to an early diagnosis, but it is known that extent of disease and prognosis is partially depending on the primary disease site [38]. Whether this is due to distinct anatomical features of a particular site or underlying differences in genetic patterns remains to be determined.

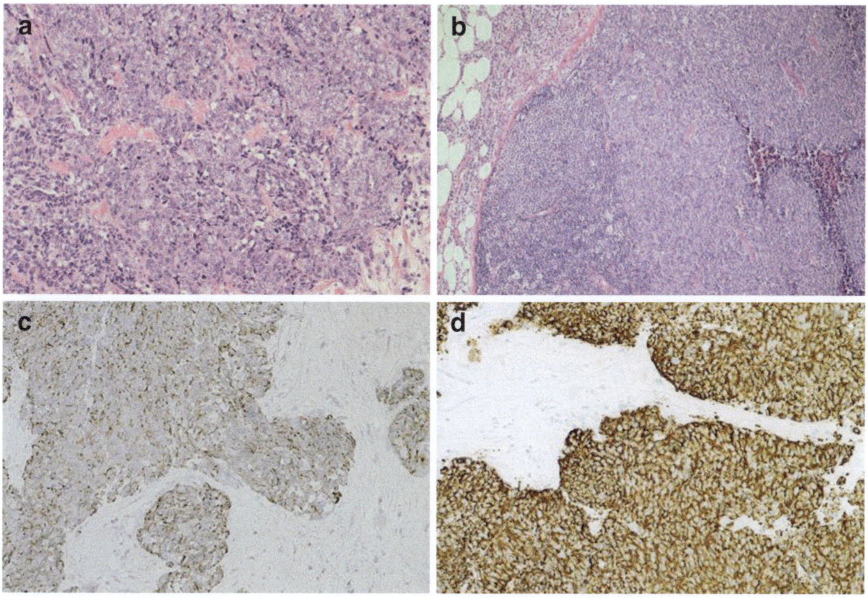

Fig. 8.2 Typical oat cell-shaped appearance of small cell bladder cancer in a transurethral resection (TUR) specimen (20×) (**a**); lymph node metastasis of SCCB with peripheral remnants of lymph node tissue (10×) (**b**); TUR specimen of SCCB staining positive for chromogranin A (20×) (**c**); TUR specimen of SCCB positive for synaptophysin (20×) (**d**)

Paraneoplastic symptoms have been described such as hypercalcemia, Lambert-Eaton myasthenic syndromes, or symptoms originating from ectopic ACTH secretion [14, 44, 54].

Diagnosis

Usually the diagnosis is made by histopathological examination of the transurethral resection (TUR) specimen revealing appearance of typical oat cell-shaped tumor cells at light microscopy (Fig. 8.2a). This can be challenging in case of smaller tumors and non-muscle invasive bladder cancer (NMIBC) because of limited tissue sample sizes and because the clinical appearance does not suggest the presence of a more aggressive variant [56]. In these cases immunohistochemistry may be of additional value as SCCB expresses a variety of neuroendocrine markers (Table 8.1, Fig. 8.2c–d). The presence of neuroendocrine and small cell components is of poor prognostic relevance with increased risk for recurrence and progression. However, the prognostic significance of neuroendocrine marker expression in addition to an existing small cell cancer type remains controversial. Nevertheless, patients with small cell NMIBC need to be clearly identified as they are not candidates for bladder instillation therapies but should receive treatment as outlined in the following sections. Unfortunately, this is often not the case in both non-muscle invasive and muscle-invasive bladder cancer. Paraganglioma or LCNC of the bladder may be misdiagnosed as undifferentiated high-grade urothelial cell carcinoma [42]. Often small cell components are not recognized in the specimen collected at TUR or are not part of the resected material. In a series of 32 patients with LD-SCCB, 7 patients (21.9 %) were treated with cystectomy without neoadjuvant chemotherapy because the small cell component was only revealed in the final specimen and not at TUR [7]. Combined SCCB is observed between 23 % and 75 % and the transitional cell carcinoma, adenocarcinoma, or squamous cell components have no apparent prognostic influence [11, 13, 21, 26]. The proportion of the non-SCCB component may exceed the resected volume. There are several reports in the literature suggesting that the presence of SCCB in combined bladder tumors is the leading prognosticator and that these combined tumors should be managed like pure SCCB [6, 38].

Staging and Prognosis

Bladder cancer, including neuroendocrine and SCCB, is staged according to the UICC TNM classification. Clinical staging depends on imaging with computed tomography (CT) of the chest and abdomen. Fluorodeoxyglucose (FDG)-positron emission tomography (PET) may further help to identify systemic disease (Fig. 8.1c–d). Several TNM versions have been used in the past and differences need to be taken into account when evaluating the reported outcome in the literature. However, in a large retrospective analysis of SCCB [38], tumor stage was not independently associated with survival suggesting that micrometastases are often present in clinically localized disease. Due to very early micrometastasis at diagnosis, some authors favor the division of patients with SCCB into groups with limited (LD-SCCB) and extensive disease (ED-SCCB) in analogy to the far more common SCLC [44].

In this staging approach patients with tumor confined to the pelvis are defined as limited disease. Furthermore, it provides a useful classification for both treatment and prognosis. Patients with LD-SCCB have a significantly better outcome compared to patients with ED-SCCB.

In general the prognosis of SCCB is poor, with 5-year OS ranging from 8 % to 44 % for limited disease [2, 7, 36]. In earlier reports only platinum-based combination chemotherapy has been associated with significant improvement of survival regardless of the regimen used [37, 38, 57].

Neuroendocrine variants and SCCB with components of other bladder tumor subtypes have been studied with regard to a different prognosis. Evidence from the literature supports that the presence of SCCB in combined bladder tumors is the leading prognosticator [21, 38] and that it should be managed like pure SCCB with cisplatin-based chemotherapy. If the component obtained at TUR was predominantly transitional cell carcinoma (>50 %), some authors applied MVAC as suggested in the literature [7, 8, 41]. The transitional cell carcinoma, adenocarcinoma, or squamous cell components have no apparent prognostic influence, although a retrospective series in which patients were treated with cystectomy only suggested that mixed subtypes tended to have a better outcome than pure SCCB ($p=0.064$) [52]. However, this series of 25 patients also included 5 LCNC. In a more recent series of 18 neuroendocrine tumors, 14 of which were SCCB including other various subtypes, an OS analysis revealed no difference between pure neuroendocrine tumors and those with mixed subtypes [10].

Due to the paucity of LCNC bladder cancer, there is considerable uncertainty regarding the prognosis of this disease in comparison to SCCB or neuroendocrine SCCB. A retrospective analysis of 572 bladder tumors revealed 14 cases of neuroendocrine SCCB and 4 LCNC bladder cancers [10]. The authors compared the course of disease and outcome of these patients. Interestingly, one patient had SCCB on the primary site and large LCNC on the metastatic site. Overall survival did not differ between SCCB and LCNC; however, the study was limited by different treatment modalities and very low numbers of patients with LCNC [10].

Treatment

The paucity of SCCB has not encouraged to design and conduct prospective randomized trials and the optimal therapeutic strategy is still unknown. Sufficient data demonstrate a similarity of the clinical course of SCCB and SCLC which in the past has been used as a rationale to introduce chemotherapy into the treatment algorithm of SCCB [6]. In SCLC survival increased only after the introduction of multi-agent chemotherapy regimens. Most of the benefit occurred in patients less than 65 years of age [22]. The definition of limited SCLC takes early metastasis into account with tumor confined to the hemithorax of origin, the mediastinum, or the supraclavicular lymph nodes [32]. All patients with tumor beyond these limits are considered to have extensive disease. The current treatment of limited SCLC consists of a combination of cisplatin and etoposide plus irradiation of the chest preferably during the first or second cycle of chemotherapy [25, 49]. Prophylactic brain radiation follows in patients with a complete response [32]. This strategy leads to median survival of 18–24 months and 50 % 2-year survival. Due to early micrometastasis, the overall survival of SCLC remains poor with 5–10 % after 5 years [55].

Currently, there is no consensus regarding the optimal treatment for limited disease SCCB. A 12-year National Cancer Database analysis on clinical characteristics and treatment patterns of 625 patients with SCCB revealed that most patients were treated with a multimodal bladder-preserving approach [48]. Upfront cystectomy with adjuvant chemotherapy has been propagated [21] as well as combinations of neoadjuvant chemotherapy with transurethral resection (TUR), cystectomy, and partial cystectomy and radiotherapy [26, 38, 43]. A contemporary report on 107 cases from an International Rare Cancer Network revealed a broad range of surgical or bladder-sparing approaches with or without adjuvant or neoadjuvant chemotherapy in the current era [47]. A Canadian consensus guideline from 2013 established the evidence base in a robust narrative review from the English language literature from 1946 until 2013 for the role of neoadjuvant chemotherapy in combination with either cystectomy or radiotherapy of the bladder [44]. Retrospective series suggest that platinum-based chemotherapy is essential. The benefit of cisplatin-based chemotherapy for SCCB has been observed in early studies [36, 38, 57]. Conversely, in SCLC, two or more drugs are needed for maximal effect but most regimens produced similar survival outcomes regardless of cisplatin [25]. In SCCB, combinations without cisplatin were not associated with prolonged survival [38], though this should be interpreted with caution. Good performance status required for cisplatin-based chemotherapy may explain the observed association of this drug with improved survival in retrospect. Chemotherapy is the only treatment option for patients with distant metastatic disease (extensive SCCB).

Limited Disease SCCB

Cystectomy as Single Treatment Modality

Historically, cystectomy was the preferred treatment for SCCB although the poor prognosis of the disease became rapidly apparent after its first description in 1981. Due to early micrometastases, cystectomy only is no longer recommended in reviews of the literature or national consensus documents [44]. This applies mainly to SCCB but is probably also true for LCNC of the bladder. There are patients, particularly in earlier stages (pT1–2 N0M0) in whom cure has been reported after cystectomy only [34]. In a retrospective analysis of the Mayo Clinic on 44 patients with SCCB, 12 patients had pT1–2 N0M0. Five-year survival for this group was reported at 63.3 % and six of eight who underwent cystectomy only were considered cured [14]. Finally, retrospective studies that compared patients with neoadjuvant chemotherapy and cystectomy to those with cystectomy only or adjuvant chemotherapy clearly suggest that cystectomy as single treatment modality or followed by adjuvant chemotherapy is far inferior in terms of survival and downstaging, including lower stages who are often clinically understaged [57] (Table 8.2).

Neoadjuvant Chemotherapy

Due to the inferior results with cystectomy, only some institutions have propagated neoadjuvant chemotherapy as an essential modality in the treatment of SCCB. Neoadjuvant chemotherapy has been chosen in analogy to regimens accepted in the treatment of SCLC (Table 8.3). Some institutions chose methotrexate 30 mg/m^2, vinblastine 3 mg/m^2, doxorubicin 30 mg/m^2, and cisplatin 70 mg/m^2 (M-VAC) for patients with <50 % SCCB in combination with urothelial carcinoma in the primary TUR-BT specimen. The number of courses differs, but often four courses were given with response evaluation after the first two courses. The optimal number of cycles of neoadjuvant chemotherapy is currently unknown. In a clinical trial of neoadjuvant chemotherapy for SCCB [58], 18 patients received four cycles of alternating chemotherapy. While patients with cT2N0 disease had a high likelihood of cure with this approach, those with stage cT3a-4 N0 did not fare as well, with SCCB remaining at cystectomy. This may reflect either poor biology or the need for additional chemotherapy in the setting of more bulky disease. Over the past years the cisplatin-based SCLC regimens changed. Four courses of ifosfamide 1.2 g/m^2

Table 8.2 Outcome after cystectomy with or without adjuvant or neoadjuvant chemotherapy

Reference	Study design	Number of patients[a]	TNM stage/extent of disease	Treatment modality	Median OS/CSS	5-year OS/ DSS[a]
Neoadjuvant chemotherapy plus cystectomy						
Lynch [37]	Retrospective	48	≤cT4aN0M0/ LD-SCCB	Neoadjuvant CTx + cystectomy	159.5	79 %
Siefker-Radtke [58]	Prospective	18	≤cT4aN0M0/ LD-SCCB [cT2N0M0] {cT3a-4}	Neoadjuvant CTx + cystectomy	58 [80] {38}	NR
Siefker-Radtke [57]	Retrospective	21	cT2-T4N0M0	Neoadjuvant CTx + cystectomy	Not reached[a]	78 %[a]
Cystectomy plus adjuvant chemotherapy						
Ismaili [29]	Retrospective	4	LD-SCCB	Cystectomy + adjuvant CTx	38.6	NR
Kaushik [34]	Retrospective	18	cT2b-T4bN0-1M0	Cystectomy + adjuvant CTx	NR	43 %
(Majority) cystectomy only						
Kaushik [34]	Retrospective	50	cT1-T4bN0-N1M0	Cystectomy	NR	20 %
Cheng [13]	Retrospective	37	cT1-T4N0-N1M0	Cystectomy	20	16 %[a]
Ismaili [29]	Retrospective	5	LD-SCCB	Cystectomy	22.5	NR
Siefker-Radtke [57]	Retrospective	25	cT2-4N0M0	Cystectomy (+ adjuvant CTx in 7)	23[a]	36 %[a]
Lynch [37]	Retrospective	47	≤ cT4aN0M0/ LD-SCCB	Cystectomy (+ adjuvant CTx in 21)	18.3	20 %

[a]Actual number of patients receiving the described treatment; the total number reported in the respective publications may differ
NR not reported

Table 8.3 Recommended chemotherapy regimen for SCCB

Regimen	Drug and dose	Schedule
EP	Etoposide 100–120 mg/m^2 on days 1–3, cisplatin 60–100 mg/m^2 on day 1	Days 1–3, repeated after 21 days
ECa in patients where cisplatin is contraindicated	Etoposide 100–120 mg/m^2 on days 1–3, carboplatin AUC 5–6 on day 1	Days 1–3, repeated after 21 days

(maximum 1.75 g), VP-16 (etoposide) 75 mg/m^2, and cisplatin 20 mg/m^2 (VIP) on days 1–4 repeated after 21 days were later replaced by 4 courses of cisplatin 75 mg/m^2 day 1 with etoposide 100 mg/m^2 intravenous (CE) on days 1–3, repeated after 21 days [32]. In one study patients with SCCB and contraindications for cisplatin but a performance score of WHO ≤2 received five courses of cyclophosphamide 1 g/m^2 (day 1), doxorubicin 45 mg/m^2 (day 1), and etoposide 100 mg/m^2 (days 1–3) (CDE) repeated after 21 days. Later that regimen was changed to carboplatin AUC 5 (day 1) with etoposide 100 mg/m^2 intravenous (CaE) on days 1–3, repeated after 21 days [7]. One prospective phase II trial investigated alternating chemotherapy with cisplatin/etoposide and doxorubicin/ifosfamide until cystectomy [58].

Response to neoadjuvant chemotherapy should be evaluated according to RECIST 1.1 and based on CT scan and cystoscopy. In doubtful cases TUR-BT or biopsy should be performed [19].

Two strategies are currently followed and recommended with level 3, grade C according to Oxford Centre of Evidence-Based Medicine (OCEBM) [44].

Neoadjuvant Chemotherapy and Cystectomy

Several studies including a prospective single-arm phase II trial revealed that for LD-SCCB, neoadjuvant chemotherapy followed by surgery can result in a 5-year survival of up to 80 % as reported in a subset of patients with resectable LD-SCCB [57, 58] (Table 8.2). In a series of 88 patients with neuroendocrine SCCB, 46 underwent cystectomy including 21 after neoadjuvant chemotherapy. Of the 25 patients with cystectomy, only 7 were treated with adjuvant chemotherapy. Independent of the fact that adjuvant therapy did not improve outcome, median cancer-specific survival (CSS) for initial cystectomy was 23 months, with only 36 % disease-free at 5 years. Contrary, for patients receiving neoadjuvant chemotherapy, median CSS had not been reached ($p = 0.026$) at the time the study reported, with a CSS at 5 years of 78 % and no cancer-related deaths observed beyond 2 years [57]. The most impressive outcome was reported in a large retrospective comparison performed by the authors of the prospective phase II trial. In a series of 95 patients with LD-SCCB who underwent cystectomy, 48 received neoadjuvant chemotherapy, and 47 underwent initial cystectomy. Neoadjuvant treatment was associated with improved OS and disease-specific survival compared with patients who underwent initial cystectomy. Median OS was 159.5 months versus 18.3 months, ($p < 0.001$) and the 5-year disease-specific survival (DSS) 79 % versus 20 % ($p < 0.001$). Moreover, neoadjuvant chemotherapy resulted in pathologic downstaging to ≤ pT1N0 in 62 % of tumors compared with only 9 % in patients treated with initial cystectomy and lymphadenectomy. Even in patients with clinically node-positive disease, neoadjuvant therapy and cystectomy led to clinical complete responses by chemotherapy and surgery in eight patients with a median OS of 23.3 months and 5-year OS of 38 % [37]. The majority of patients in these studies received cisplatin/etoposide or ifosfamide/doxorubicin alternating with cisplatin/etoposide [37, 57, 58]. Of note, these impressive survival outcomes are better than those reported after neoadjuvant chemotherapy for conventional urothelial bladder cancer and may be due to selection. In the randomized phase three trial of neoadjuvant chemotherapy for bladder cancer, the median OS for those receiving chemotherapy was 56 months at inclusion of cT1–4a cN0/x cM0 patients [20].

However, the results clearly suggest the beneficial roles of neoadjuvant chemotherapy in combination with cystectomy. Neoadjuvant chemotherapy results in significant pathological downstaging which may not only improve outcome but facilitate surgery [37]. Conversely, adjuvant chemotherapy following cystectomy was not shown to be superior to cystectomy alone although the numbers of patients receiving adjuvant therapy were small (7 of 25 and 21 of 47) [37, 57] (Table 8.2). In a retrospective SEER database analysis, chemotherapy improved outcome across all stages, but not in addition to cystectomy [35].

Bladder Preservation with Chemoradiotherapy

Despite cystectomy after neoadjuvant chemotherapy, SCCB remains to portend a dismal prognosis. Most institutions have reported a median OS for nonmetastatic SCCB of 13–23 months [44], although exceptional median OS of 58 months has been reported with this approach [58]. This has prompted investigation of bladder preservation with chemoradiotherapy (Table 8.4). Sequential chemoradiation for LD-SCCB results in a reasonable outcome with a high bladder preservation rate [4]. In general in SCLC patients, radiotherapy is applied concomitantly with the chemotherapy [29]. However, experience with an increased risk for local toxicity in the bladder after concurrent chemoradiation has led some institutions to schedule external beam radiotherapy (EBRT) after the neoadjuvant chemotherapy. EBRT has been applied using 8–18 MV photons with a three- or four-field technique. The median

Table 8.4 Outcome of bladder-sparing chemoradiotherapy series

Reference	Study design	Number of patients	TNM stage/ extent of disease	Treatment modality	Median OS/CSS[a]	5-year OS/DSS
Bex [7]	Retrospective	17	LD-SCCB	TURB + CTx + RT	32.5	36 %
Meijer [41]	Retrospective	27	LD-SCCB	TURB + CTx + RT	47[a]	39.6 %
Lohrisch [36]	Retrospective	10	LD-SCCB [ED 1]	TURB + CTx + RT	41	44 %
Ismaili [29]	Retrospective	1	LD-SCCB	TURB + CTX + RT	49.7	NR
Bastus [5]	Retrospective	5	cT2N0M0 cT3bN1M0	TURB + CTX + RT	45	NR
Asmis [4]	Retrospective	8	LD-SCCB	TURB + CTX + RT	19.8	NR

[a]Actual number of patients receiving the described treatment; the total number reported in the respective publications may differ

NR not reported

dose was 60 Gy. The target area consisted of the bladder and the tumor. When the total dose was 70 Gy, 50 Gy was given to the bladder and tumor with a 20 Gy boost to the tumor area only [7]. Early reports of small patient series with LD-SCCB reported long-term survival with three of five patients alive and free of disease 60, 48, and 27 months after diagnosis [5]. In another series of ten patients treated with sequential chemoradiation from British Columbia, five patients were alive and disease-free an average of 82 months following diagnosis [36].

Neoadjuvant Chemotherapy Followed by Cystectomy Versus Bladder Sparing with Sequential Chemoradiation

There are no prospective randomized studies comparing treatment modalities for SCCB. Recently Koay et al. reported on a large subset of patients from the Surveillance, Epidemiology, and End Results (SEER) Medicare database with SCCB treated with chemotherapy and radiotherapy versus cystectomy with chemotherapy, showing no significant differences in OS between the two treatment modalities [35]. Chemotherapy was shown to improve outcome in all stages of disease including those patients who were treated with TUR as their only surgical procedure. A bladder-sparing approach involving TUR combined with chemotherapy and radiation showed no significant difference in OS compared with patients undergoing at least a cystectomy (of whom over 90 % received radical cystectomy) with chemotherapy ($p>0.05$). However, this report has several limitations and did not distinguish between neoadjuvant or adjuvant chemotherapy in combination with cystectomy. Nevertheless, outcome data of several studies suggest that upfront chemotherapy may be the most important therapeutic modality with local therapeutic treatment options such as cystectomy, radiotherapy, or even complete TUR being secondary.

As with conventional transitional cell carcinoma of the bladder, the risk of bladder sparing has to be balanced against the local recurrence rate. The risk of local recurrence of transitional cell carcinoma after primary mixed tumors has been reported in several studies, especially in long-term survivors after chemoradiation [5, 36]. Though 5-year OS following bladder sparing with chemoradiation has been reported in a small case series [36], this approach has been criticized for the relatively high rate of local recurrences. Local recurrence rates of 20–69 % have been reported [5, 36] in small series of five and eight patients, respectively. In a larger retrospective analysis of 27 LD-SCCB treated with sequential chemoradiation, local recurrence in the bladder was seen in 29.6 % of patients [41]. Histopathology of the recurrences in the bladder revealed small cell carcinoma in two patients (7.4 %) and transitional cell carcinoma in six patients (22.2 %). The median time to local recurrence was 29 months. In some cases local recurrence in the bladder can be treated with conservative therapy (e.g., TUR-BT and adjuvant intravesical BCG instillations). In the group with LD-SCCB and sequential chemoradiation, the bladder preservation rate was 85.2 %.

Considering the nature of retrospective analyses with their inherent bias which influences the comparability of data, it appears that overall and progression-free survival is similar for local therapies such as cystectomy and radiotherapy as long as systemic chemotherapy had been applied. Cheng et al. retrospectively analyzed 64 cases and found no survival difference between those who had cystectomy and those who had not. Interestingly, none of the parameters age, gender, presenting symptoms, smoking history, the presence of a non-small cell carcinoma component, chemotherapy, or radiation therapy were associated with survival. Consequently, the authors raised doubt about the effectiveness of cystectomy as treatment modality. The 1- and 5-year survival times of those who had a cystectomy were 57 % and 16 % versus 55 % and 18 % for those who had no cystectomy [13]. However, the chemotherapy in those who underwent cystectomy was applied as adjuvant therapy which does not appear to be as effective as the neoadjuvant approach. As has been discussed in the previous paragraph, the majority of retrospective studies and one prospective study support neoadjuvant therapy when cystectomy is planned. Consequently, these data should be compared to the bladder-sparing chemoradiotherapy data. In a retrospective series of 17 patients with LD-SCCB treated with sequential chemoradiation, the 1- and 5-year survival estimate was 82 % (C.I. 0.56–0.92) and 36 % (C.I. 0.14–0.61), respectively [7].

Treatment Options for Elderly Comorbid Patients

Patients with SCCB are predominantly elderly men and in some series more than half of the patients were over 70 years of age [48]. Though there have been reports that chemotherapy for SCLC is feasible in elderly patients, a high rate of age-related comorbidity among patients older than 70 years has been observed [8]. In a series of 25 patients with SCCB, 48 % of patients were older than 70 years (12/25). In patients with limited disease unfit for chemotherapy, radiotherapy subsequent to a macroscopically complete TUR can be considered as a treatment option, especially if the disease is localized. Long-term survivors have been reported in a retrospective series with this strategy [26]. A more recent SEER database analysis of 533 patients with SCCB revealed that the majority of patients (54 %) received a TUR as their only surgical treatment [35]. A subset analysis of these patients indicated that chemotherapy played a role in all stages of disease ($p<0.05$) whereas radiation improved overall survival in regional-stage disease ($p<0.05$) [35]. These data however are retrospective and prone to selection bias. Exceptionally, cystectomy as single treatment modality can be considered if severe locoregional symptoms and/or contraindications for radiotherapy were present. In a series of 17 patients with LD-SCCB, ultimately 9 patients (52.9 %) could not be treated with chemotherapy and sequential radiotherapy, mostly because of PS WHO 3 ($n=7$) [8].

Distant Metastatic SCCB (Extensive Disease)

Patients with clinically evident extensive disease or distant metastasis have a poor outcome. The mainstay of therapy is systemic chemotherapy in analogy with the regimen given for SCLC described in the section on neoadjuvant chemotherapy. Reported median OS in the literature does not exceed 5–8 months and palliation is the main objective of therapy [30, 35].

Follow-Up and Prophylactic Cranial Irradiation

Due to frequent and late local recurrences in case of a bladder-sparing approach, regular follow-up with cystoscopy is mandatory for a prolonged period. In some instances, recurrences were diagnosed after almost 5 years of follow-up. No general imaging recommendations exist but cross-sectional imaging with computed tomography of chest and abdomen as for conventional bladder carcinoma is suggested. Patients with SCLC have a significant risk for the development of brain metastases (up to 60 % within 2–3 years after starting treatment). Therefore patients with complete response to chemotherapy are offered prophylactic cranial irradiation [32]. Similarly patients with SCCB show a risk for the development of brain metastases. Siefker-Radtke et al. reported up to 26.7 % brain metastases in patients with SCCB [58]. In a retrospective long-term analysis of patients with SCCB, 12.1 % developed symptomatic brain metastases [41]. An earlier analysis and review of the literature reported a pooled estimate of cumulative incidence of symptomatic brain metastases of 10.5 % [9]. This incidence is higher than brain metastases from transitional cell carcinoma of the bladder (approximately 3 %) but far lower than for SCLC. Differences in frequency of brain metastasis reported in the literature can be explained by routine brain scanning during follow-up versus cross-sectional imaging performed in symptomatic patients only. There are no studies indicating superiority of prophylactic cranial irradiation to cranial irradiation in SCCB patients with symptomatic brain metastases.

Conclusion: Future Therapeutic Strategies

There have been reports on the beneficial effects of concurrent administration of radiosensitizing agents (e.g., chemotherapy) potentiating the cytotoxic effect of radiotherapy for bladder cancer [31]. As the techniques of EBRT have evolved in recent years and the risks of local toxicity have been further reduced, the use of concurrent chemoradiation may be expected to gain terrain. Regarding chemotherapy for SCCB, new regimens are primarily investigated in the more common SCLC. Some authors suggest that PEI (platinum, etoposide, ifosfamide) is more effective than PE based on a randomized trial [12] but this is not supported by a systematic review [61]. Somatostatin may increase the efficacy of chemotherapy in SCLC [17].

There are very limited data on the second-line therapeutic options for patients who fail platinum-based chemotherapy. In a series including three patients with SCCB, single-agent weekly vinorelbine had shown promising safety and efficacy profile [33]. Targeted agents are being investigated but the paucity of the disease may require comparison with SCLC [50]. Expression of c-kit was investigated in 52 cases of SCCB [46]. Overall, 14 of 52 (27 %) SCCB were positive for c-kit expression when defining less than 10 % staining as negative. Outcome in the entire series was as reported previously. During a median follow-up of 11 months, 60 % of the patients died of disease. While no association was found between c-kit expression and survival or other clinicopathological parameters, 27 % of SCCB expressed c-kit, which may be a therapeutic target for imatinib. In addition, mTOR inhibitors have been investigated in preclinical models as has been the mechanism of resistance to everolimus [40].

Acknowledgments We thank Dr. J. de Jong, Department of Pathology of the Netherlands Cancer Institute, Amsterdam, for providing high-power field photomicrographs of SCCB.

References

1. The World Health Organization histological typing of lung tumours. 2nd ed. Am J Clin Pathol. 1982;77(2):123–36.
2. Abbas F, Civantos F, Benedetto P, Soloway MS. Small cell carcinoma of the bladder and prostate. Urology. 1995;46:617–30.
3. Abrahams NA, Moran C, Reyes AO, Siefker-Radtke A, Ayala AG. Small cell carcinoma of the bladder: a contemporary clinicopathological study of 51 cases. Histopathology. 2005;46:57–63.
4. Asmis TR, Reaume MN, Dahrouge S, Malone S. Genitourinary small cell carcinoma: a retrospective review of treatment and survival patterns at the Ottawa Hospital Regional Cancer Center. BJU Int. 2006;97:711–5.
5. Bastus R, Caballero JM, Gonzalez G, Borrat P, Casalots J, Gomez De Segura G, Marti LI, Ristol J, Cirera L. Small cell carcinoma of the urinary bladder treated with chemotherapy and radiotherapy: results in five cases. Eur Urol. 1999;35:323–6.
6. Bex A. Review: treatment of small cell carcinoma of the urinary bladder: can we learn from small cell lung cancer? Clin Adv Hematol Oncol. 2008;6:385–6.
7. Bex A, DE Vries R, Pos F, Kerst M, Horenblas S. Long-term survival after sequential chemoradiation for limited disease small cell carcinoma of the bladder. World J Urol. 2009;27:101–6.
8. Bex A, Nieuwenhuijzen JA, Kerst M, Pos F, Van Boven H, Meinhardt W, Horenblas S. Small cell carcinoma of bladder: a single-center prospective study of 25 cases treated in analogy to small cell lung cancer. Urology. 2005;65:295–9.
9. Bex A, Sonke GS, Pos FJ, Brandsma D, Kerst JM, Horenblas S. Symptomatic brain metastases from small-cell carcinoma of the urinary bladder: the Netherlands Cancer Institute experience and literature review. Ann Oncol. 2010;21:2240–5.
10. Bhatt VR, Loberiza Jr FR, Tandra P, Krishnamurthy J, Shrestha R, Wang J. Risk factors, therapy and survival outcomes of small cell and large cell neuroendocrine carcinoma of urinary bladder. Rare Tumor. 2014;6:5043.
11. Blomjous CE, Vos W, de Voogt HJ, van der Valk P, Meijer CJ. Small cell carcinoma of the urinary bladder. A clinicopathologic, morphometric, immunohistochemical, and ultrastructural study of 18 cases. Cancer. 1989;64:1347–57.
12. Boni C, Pagano M, Baldi L, Gnoni R, Braglia L, Savoldi L, Zanelli F. Pei regimen: a therapeutic option in small cell lung cancer? A retrospective monoinstitutional analysis of 46 consecutive cases. J Transl Med. 2015;13:130.
13. Cheng L, Pan CX, Yang XJ, Lopez-Beltran A, Maclennan GT, Lin H, Kuzel TM, Papavero V, Tretiakova M, Nigro K, Koch MO, Eble JN. Small cell carcinoma of the urinary bladder: a clinicopathologic analysis of 64 patients. Cancer. 2004;101:957–62.
14. Choong NW, Quevedo JF, Kaur JS. Small cell carcinoma of the urinary bladder. The Mayo Clinic experience. Cancer. 2005;103:1172–8.
15. Coelho HM, Pereira BA, Caetano PA. Large cell neuroendocrine carcinoma of the urinary bladder: case report and review. Curr Urol. 2013;7:155–9.
16. Cramer SF, Aikawa M, Cebelin M. Neurosecretory granules in small cell invasive carcinoma of the urinary bladder. Cancer. 1981;47:724–30.

17. Domvri K, Bougiouklis D, Zarogoulidis P, Porpodis K, Xristoforidis M, Liaka A, Eleutheriadou E, Lampaki S, Lazaridis G, Organtzis J, Kyriazis G, Hohenforst-Schmidt W, Tsirgogianni K, Karavasilis V, Baka S, Darwiche K, Freitag L, Trakada G, Zarogoulidis K. Could somatostatin enhance the outcomes of chemotherapeutic treatment in SCLC? J Cancer. 2015;6:360–6.
18. Dores GM, Qubaiah O, Mody A, Ghabach B, Devesa SS. A population-based study of incidence and patient survival of small cell carcinoma in the United States, 1992–2010. BMC Cancer. 2015;15:185.
19. Eisenhauer EA, Therasse P, Bogaerts J, Schwartz LH, Sargent D, Ford R, Dancey J, Arbuck S, Gwyther S, Mooney M, Rubinstein L, Shankar L, Dodd L, Kaplan R, Lacombe D, Verweij J. New response evaluation criteria in solid tumours: revised RECIST guideline (version 1.1). Eur J Cancer. 2009;45:228–47.
20. Griffiths G, Hall R, Sylvester R, Raghavan D, Parmar MK. International phase III trial assessing neoadjuvant cisplatin, methotrexate, and vinblastine chemotherapy for muscle-invasive bladder cancer: long-term results of the BA06 30894 trial. J Clin Oncol. 2011;29:2171–7.
21. Grignon DJ, Ro JY, Ayala AG, Shum DT, Ordonez NG, Logothetis CJ, Johnson DE, MacKay B. Small cell carcinoma of the urinary bladder. A clinicopathologic analysis of 22 cases. Cancer. 1992;69:527–36.
22. Hand S, Baker J, Smith AP, Macbeth FR. Outpatient intensive chemotherapy for small cell lung cancer: five years experience of modified 'ICE' ifosfamide carboplatin and etoposide. Clin Oncol (R Coll Radiol). 2002;14:367–71.
23. Hirsch FR, Matthews MJ, Aisner S, Campobasso O, Elema JD, Gazdar AF, MacKay B, Nasiell M, Shimosato Y, Steele RH, et al. Histopathologic classification of small cell lung cancer. Changing concepts and terminology. Cancer. 1988;62:973–7.
24. Hirsch FR, Matthews MJ, Yesner R. Histopathologic classification of small cell carcinoma of the lung: comments based on an interobserver examination. Cancer. 1982;50:1360–6.
25. Holbrechts S, Roelandts M. Treatment of small cell lung cancer: limited disease. Guidelines of clinical practice made by the European Lung Cancer Working Party. Rev Med Brux. 2014;35:160–3.
26. Holmang S, Borghede G, Johansson SL. Primary small cell carcinoma of the bladder: a report of 25 cases. J Urol. 1995;153:1820–2.
27. Ibrahim NB, Briggs JC, Corbishley CM. Extrapulmonary oat cell carcinoma. Cancer. 1984;54:1645–61.
28. Iczkowski KA, Shanks JH, Allsbrook WC, Lopez-Beltran A, Pantazis CG, Collins TR, Wetherington RW, Bostwick DG. Small cell carcinoma of urinary bladder is differentiated from urothelial carcinoma by chromogranin expression, absence of CD44 variant 6 expression, a unique pattern of cytokeratin expression, and more intense gamma-enolase expression. Histopathology. 1999;35:150–6.
29. Ismaili N, Elkarak F, Heudel PE, Flechon A, Droz JP. Small cell cancer of the bladder: the Leon-Berard cancer centre experience. Indian J Urol. 2008;24:494–7.
30. Ismaili N, Heudel PE, Elkarak F, Kaikani W, Bajard A, Ismaili M, Errihani H, Droz JP, Flechon A. Outcome of recurrent and metastatic small cell carcinoma of the bladder. BMC Urol. 2009;9:4.
31. James ND, Hussain SA, Hall E, Jenkins P, Tremlett J, Rawlings C, Crundwell M, Sizer B, Sreenivasan T, Hendron C, Lewis R, Waters R, Huddart RA. Radiotherapy with or without chemotherapy in muscle-invasive bladder cancer. N Engl J Med. 2012;366:1477–88.
32. Jett JR, Schild SE, Kesler KA, Kalemkerian GP. Treatment of small cell lung cancer: diagnosis and management of lung cancer, 3rd ed: American College of Chest Physicians evidence-based clinical practice guidelines. Chest. 2013;143:e400S–19.
33. June RR, Dougherty DW, Reese CT, Harpster LE, Hoffman SL, Drabick JJ. Significant activity of single agent vinorelbine against small-cell cancer of the bladder as second line chemotherapy: a case series and review of the literature. Urol Oncol. 2012;30:192–5.
34. Kaushik D, Frank I, Boorjian SA, Cheville JC, Eisenberg MS, Thapa P, Tarrell RF, Thompson RH. Long-term results of radical cystectomy and role of adjuvant chemotherapy for small cell carcinoma of the bladder. Int J Urol. 2015;22:549–54.

35. Koay EJ, Teh BS, Paulino AC, Butler EB. A surveillance, epidemiology, and end results analysis of small cell carcinoma of the bladder: epidemiology, prognostic variables, and treatment trends. Cancer. 2011;117:5325–33.
36. Lohrisch C, Murray N, Pickles T, Sullivan L. Small cell carcinoma of the bladder: long term outcome with integrated chemoradiation. Cancer. 1999;86:2346–52.
37. Lynch SP, Shen Y, Kamat A, Grossman HB, Shah JB, Millikan RE, Dinney CP, Siefker-Radtke A. Neoadjuvant chemotherapy in small cell urothelial cancer improves pathologic downstaging and long-term outcomes: results from a retrospective study at the MD Anderson Cancer Center. Eur Urol. 2013;64:307–13.
38. Mackey JR, Au HJ, Hugh J, Venner P. Genitourinary small cell carcinoma: determination of clinical and therapeutic factors associated with survival. J Urol. 1998;159:1624–9.
39. Maschmeyer G, Mugge LO, Kampfe D, Kreibich U, Wilhelm S, Assmann M, Schwarz M, Kahl C, Kohler S, Grobe N, Niederwieser D. A retrospective review of diagnosis and treatment modalities of neuroendocrine tumors (excluding primary lung cancer) in 10 oncological institutions of the East German Study Group of Hematology and Oncology (OSHO), 2010–2012. J Cancer Res Clin Oncol. 2015.
40. Matsumoto M, Seike M, Noro R, Soeno C, Sugano T, Takeuchi S, Miyanaga A, Kitamura K, Kubota K, Gemma A. Control of the MYC-eIF4E axis plus mTOR inhibitor treatment in small cell lung cancer. BMC Cancer. 2015;15:241.
41. Meijer RP, Meinhardt W, van der Poel HG, van Rhijn BW, Kerst JM, Pos FJ, Horenblas S, Bex A. Local control rate and prognosis after sequential chemoradiation for small cell carcinoma of the bladder. Int J Urol. 2013;20:778–84.
42. Menon S, Goyal P, Suryawanshi P, Tongaonkar H, Joshi A, Bakshi G, Desai S. Paraganglioma of the urinary bladder: a clinicopathologic spectrum of a series of 14 cases emphasizing diagnostic dilemmas. Indian J Pathol Microbiol. 2014;57:19–23.
43. Mills SE, Wolfe 3rd JT, Weiss MA, Swanson PE, Wick MR, Fowler Jr JE, Young RH. Small cell undifferentiated carcinoma of the urinary bladder. A light-microscopic, immunocytochemical, and ultrastructural study of 12 cases. Am J Surg Pathol. 1987;11:606–17.
44. Moretto P, Wood L, Emmenegger U, Blais N, Mukherjee SD, Winquist E, Belanger EC, Macrae R, Balogh A, Cagiannos I, Kassouf W, Black P, Czaykowski P, Gingerich J, North S, Ernst S, Richter S, Sridhar S, Reaume MN, Soulieres D, Eisen A, Canil CM. Management of small cell carcinoma of the bladder: consensus guidelines from the Canadian Association of Genitourinary Medical Oncologists (CAGMO). Can Urol Assoc J. 2013;7:E44–56.
45. Oesterling JE, Brendler CB, Burgers JK, Marshall FF, Epstein JI. Advanced small cell carcinoma of the bladder. Successful treatment with combined radical cystoprostatectomy and adjuvant methotrexate, vinblastine, doxorubicin, and cisplatin chemotherapy. Cancer. 1990;65:1928–36.
46. Pan CX, Yang XJ, Lopez-Beltran A, Maclennan GT, Eble JN, Koch MO, Jones TD, Lin H, Nigro K, Papavero V, Tretiakova M, Cheng L. c-kit expression in small cell carcinoma of the urinary bladder: prognostic and therapeutic implications. Mod Pathol. 2005;18:320–3.
47. Pasquier D, Barney B, Sundar S, Poortmans P, Villa S, Nasrallah H, Boujelbene N, Ghadjar P, Lassen-Ramshad Y, Senkus E, Oar A, Roelandts M, Amichetti M, Vees H, Zilli T, Ozsahin M. Small cell carcinoma of the urinary bladder: a retrospective, multicenter rare cancer network study of 107 patients. Int J Radiat Oncol Biol Phys. 2015;92:904–10.
48. Patel SG, Stimson CJ, Zaid HB, Resnick MJ, Cookson MS, Barocas DA, Chang SS. Locoregional small cell carcinoma of the bladder: clinical characteristics and treatment patterns. J Urol. 2014;191:329–34.
49. Pietanza MC, Byers LA, Minna JD, Rudin CM. Small cell lung cancer: will recent progress lead to improved outcomes? Clin Cancer Res. 2015;21:2244–55.
50. Puglisi M, Dolly S, Faria A, Myerson JS, Popat S, O'Brien ME. Treatment options for small cell lung cancer – do we have more choice? Br J Cancer. 2010;102:629–38.
51. Pusiol T, Morichetti D, Zorzi MG. "Pure" primary large cell neuroendocrine carcinoma of the urinary bladder: case report, literature review and diagnostic criteria. Pathologica. 2014;106:82–5.

52. Quek ML, Nichols PW, Yamzon J, Daneshmand S, Miranda G, Cai J, Groshen S, Stein JP, Skinner DG. Radical cystectomy for primary neuroendocrine tumors of the bladder: the university of southern California experience. J Urol. 2005;174:93–6.
53. Radović N, Turner R, Bacalja J. Primary "Pure" large cell neuroendocrine carcinoma of the urinary bladder: a case report and review of the literature. Clin Genitourin Cancer. 2015;13(5):e375–7. doi: 10.1016/j.clgc.2015.03.005. Epub 2015 Mar 30.
54. Reyes CV, Soneru I. Small cell carcinoma of the urinary bladder with hypercalcemia. Cancer. 1985;56:2530–3.
55. Rudin CM, Ismaila N, Hann CL, Malhotra N, Movsas B, Norris K, Pietanza MC, Ramalingam SS, Turrisi 3rd AT, Giaccone G. Treatment of small-cell lung cancer: American Society of Clinical Oncology Endorsement of the American College of Chest Physicians Guideline. J Clin Oncol. 2015;33:4106–11.
56. Seisen T, Comperat E, Leon P, Roupret M. Impact of histological variants on the outcomes of nonmuscle invasive bladder cancer after transurethral resection. Curr Opin Urol. 2014;24:524–31.
57. Siefker-Radtke AO, Dinney CP, Abrahams NA, Moran C, Shen Y, Pisters LL, Grossman HB, Swanson DA, Millikan RE. Evidence supporting preoperative chemotherapy for small cell carcinoma of the bladder: a retrospective review of the M. D. Anderson cancer experience. J Urol. 2004;172:481–4.
58. Siefker-Radtke AO, Kamat AM, Grossman HB, Williams DL, Qiao W, Thall PF, Dinney CP, Millikan RE. Phase II clinical trial of neoadjuvant alternating doublet chemotherapy with ifosfamide/doxorubicin and etoposide/cisplatin in small-cell urothelial cancer. J Clin Oncol. 2009;27:2592–7.
59. Turrisi 3rd AT. Limited stage small cell lung cancer: treatment and therapy. Curr Treat Options Oncol. 2003;4:61–4.
60. Wolff AC, Ettinger DS, Neuberg D, Comis RL, Ruckdeschel JC, Bonomi PD, Johnson DH. Phase II study of ifosfamide, carboplatin, and oral etoposide chemotherapy for extensive-disease small-cell lung cancer: an Eastern Cooperative Oncology Group pilot study. J Clin Oncol. 1995;13:1615–22.
61. Yang H, Ma Y, Liu Z, Wang Z, Han B, Ma L. Benefit from ifosfamide treatment in small-cell lung cancer: a meta-analysis. Mol Clin Oncol. 2015;3:420–4.

Urachal and Non-urachal Adenocarcinomas of the Bladder

9

Arlene O. Siefker-Radtke

Primary Bladder Adenocarcinoma (Non-urachal)

Background

Pure adenocarcinomas of the bladder are a very rare entity. It is important to understand the distinctions between the different types of adenocarcinomas that may be found in the bladder, as it may have an impact on their treatment. Urachal carcinomas, traditionally found in the mid-line or dome of the bladder, require a surgical procedure that is different from the typical cystectomy. Metastatic adenocarcinomas can occur from direct extension of local organs including colon and rectum, from drop implants/peritoneal seeding from other adenocarcinomas of the abdominal cavity, and even from hematogenous metastases from primary sites both within and outside the abdominal cavity. Often, a careful medical history of previous cancer, clinical symptoms which are not typically associated with a bladder primary, and radiological findings suggestive of other potential primaries, can aid in diagnosing a metastasis to the bladder. Adenocarcinomas of the urethra, which are addressed in a separate chapter, can also invade the bladder base and trigone secondarily. Only when none of these above findings are present, should one consider the patient a true primary adenocarcinoma of the bladder.

Introduction

Primary adenocarcinomas of the bladder account for 0.5–2.0 % of bladder tumors [1] and have a similar age of onset as conventional urothelial cancer with an

A.O. Siefker-Radtke, MD
Department of Genitourinary Medical Oncology, The University of Texas MD Anderson Cancer Center, 1155 Pressler, Unit 1374, Houston, TX 77030, USA
e-mail: asiefker@mdanderson.org

L. Pagliaro (ed.), *Rare Genitourinary Tumors*,
DOI 10.1007/978-3-319-30046-7_9

estimated male-to-female ratio of at least 2:1 [2]. It is the most common cancer in patients with bladder exstrophy [3], a rare developmental anomaly affecting less than 1 out of 50,000 births. They may be associated with the presence of intestinal metaplasia or cystitis cystica [1], which is felt to arise from metaplasia of Von Brunn nests resulting in columnar mucin-producing cells. Chronic irritation and infection in the bladder is also felt to play a role in the development of these lesions and is also felt to account for the higher incidence of bladder adenocarcinomas among patients with bilharziasis [4, 5].

The clear cell variant observed in bladder adenocarcinomas has a more distinct phenotype, most commonly arising in females with a 2:1 female predominance. A large number of these cases appear to arise from the urethra or periurethral glands, with some evidence suggesting a Mullerian etiology [6]. These tumors may be more responsive to taxane-based chemotherapy, similar to other gynecologic malignancies. Since these clear cell adenocarcinomas most commonly arise in the urethra and invade the bladder secondarily, they will be discussed more fully in the urethral chapter.

Pathology

Adenocarcinomas of the bladder are often classified based upon their histologic appearance [1]. Enteric adenocarcinomas have architectural characteristics including glandular features seen in adenocarcinomas of the colon. Mucinous adenocarcinomas often have single cells or nests of cells floating in lakes of extracellular mucin. Signet ring cell histology has been reported as well, with one large series suggesting adverse outcomes when present [7]. Plasmacytoid tumors, which also have a poor prognosis [8], may also be mistaken for the signet ring cell variant. However, the eccentric nucleus in plasmacytoid tumors contains an eosinophilic cytoplasm [9] as compared to the clear cytoplasmic vacuole seen in signet ring cell adenocarcinomas [1]. Hepatoid adenocarcinoma of the bladder, an extremely rare and aggressive variant primarily affecting elderly men, derives its name from the resemblance to hepatocellular carcinoma and positive staining for alpha-fetoprotein [10]. Hyaline globules and bile production have been observed on microscopy. Adenocarcinoma, not otherwise specified, is used when the pattern does not fit into the characteristics of the abovementioned types. An additional important feature is the absence of transitional cell/urothelial histology. When transitional cell histology is present, it is unlikely that one is dealing with an adenocarcinoma of the bladder.

Immunohistochemical Markers

Adenocarcinomas of the bladder often share immunohistochemical markers similar to adenocarcinomas of the gastrointestinal tract. CK7 and CK20 are not useful in distinguishing primary adenocarcinomas of the bladder from colonic adenocarcinoma. These two markers have been reported positive in over 50 % of primary adenocarcinomas of the bladder [11, 12]. The typical CK7-negative and CK20-positive panel seen in colonic adenocarcinomas unfortunately may be positive in up to 29 % of adenocarcinomas of the urothelium [11]. CDX-2, a homeobox gene implicated in the regulation of cell growth and differentiation of intestinal cells which was initially thought to be specific for colonic adenocarcinomas, was found to be positive in nearly 100 % of adenocarcinomas of the bladder [13]. Nuclear versus membranous staining for beta-catenin has been reported as a good marker for distinguishing between colon and bladder adenocarcinomas, with the nuclear staining pattern restricted to adenocarcinomas of the colon and membranous staining in both [11, 14]. Given the significant overlap in marker staining, often "clinical correlation" is advised. The presence of cystitis cystica in the bladder may also be helpful in determining bladder origin.

Clinical Presentation/Diagnosis

Many patients experience urinary symptoms including dysuria and frequency. The progression to gross hematuria often motivates the patient to seek medical care. The presence of gastrointestinal symptoms predating the urinary symptoms may be more suggestive of a gastrointestinal primary. A history of other malignancies will also aid in determining the possibility of metastases to the bladder. Radiographic imaging is an important aid in the diagnosis. The presence of a tumor in the midline or the dome of the bladder should suggest the possibility of this being a urachal carcinoma. Likewise, occurrence among the urethra, especially in women, would be consistent with a clear cell adenocarcinoma of the urethra. Diffuse thickening of the bladder on imaging may be consistent with "linitis plastica" which has been observed in this disease. However, radiographic imaging alone cannot confirm the diagnosis. A cystoscopy and urethroscopy may be extremely helpful in determining site of origin. The absence of tumor inside the bladder on cystoscopy would be much more consistent with a metastasis to the bladder. However, the presence of tumor inside the bladder is less helpful, since metastases, drop implants, or locally invading tumors can invade the bladder.

Staging and Prognostic Classification

Non-urachal adenocarcinomas of the bladder are believed to arise from the urothelial lining; therefore, the current TNM staging system appears appropriate when staging non-urachal adenocarcinomas. One large study using the Surveillance, Epidemiology, and End Results (SEER) database did not observe any significant difference in stage- or grade-adjusted cancer-specific mortality when comparing primary adenocarcinomas of the bladder with urothelial cancer patients [2]. The authors did note that patients with adenocarcinomas of the bladder were more likely to have advanced disease at radical cystectomy. In addition, they reported a higher frequency of bladder adenocarcinomas among female patients and non-Caucasian patients. Tumor grade and stage have been adverse prognostic factors [1, 2, 7, 15].

Treatment

Surgery

There are currently no published clinical trials regarding the optimal treatment for non-urachal adenocarcinomas of the bladder. Radical cystectomy remains the mainstay of treatment for these tumors. However, the survival rates remain poor with a treatment failure occurring in at least 50 % of patients undergoing cystectomy [1, 2, 7, 15]. Even in the setting of non-organ-confined, node-positive disease, the long-term survival rate may be as high as 15–30% [1, 2, 7, 15] in patients with clinically negative lymph nodes. These results should not be used to encourage surgical debulking procedures in patients with clinical evidence of lymph node disease where cure is not likely. Patients with organ-confined disease have a much better prognosis with a cure fraction that may be as high as 70 % at 5 years [1, 2, 7, 15].

Radiotherapy

Zaghloul et al. [16] reported that the use of postoperative radiation impacted the local control of adenocarcinomas of the bladder with a 5-year disease-free survival (DFS) rate of 56 % compared to 38 % in the cystectomy alone group ($p=0.066$). Since the two-thirds of patients in this study had grade 2 or less disease, it is not clear whether the use of radiation therapy would impact the treatment of high-grade disease as the 5-year DFS in patients with grade 3 disease undergoing cystectomy was 40 % as compared to 10.8 % in patients receiving radiation therapy ($p=0.34$) [16]. Distant metastases remained the leading cause of death in those receiving radiation. A larger series by Zaghloul et al. [7] published 3 years later showed a similar survival fraction that achieved a significant p-value with postoperative radiation, although 78 % of patients in this series had grade 2 or less disease.

Systemic Chemotherapy

The literature on non-urachal adenocarcinomas of the bladder has focused mainly on the role of surgery and a potential role for radiation. Most retrospective series have included any non-urothelial cancer histology for treatment and are not relevant to the pure adenocarcinomas of the bladder. In practice, patients with metastatic adenocarcinoma of the bladder commonly receive a cisplatin-based chemotherapy regimen, as they would for the more typical urothelial carcinoma. Given the limited information available, this author's preference would be to consider a 5-fluorouracil/cisplatin combination based upon the experience observed with urachal adenocarcinomas where a response rate has been observed in approximately 30 % of patients [17]. Combinations including 5-fluoruracil, leucovorin, gemcitabine, and cisplatin (GEM-FLP), or other adenocarcinoma regimens including FOLFOX (5-fluoruracil with oxaliplatin) and FOLFIRI (5-flurouracil with irinotecan), with the addition of bevacizumab, or cetuximab, used in the treatment of adenocarcinomas of the colon may be relevant. There are also limited data with respect to taxane-cisplatin combinations, such as paclitaxel, methotrexate, and cisplatin (TMP) [17] and ifosfamide, paclitaxel, and cisplatin (ITP) [18] in urachal adenocarcinomas of the bladder, where the response rate is estimated to be approximately 15 % of patients. These data may be potentially relevant to the non-urachal adenocarcinomas of the bladder as well.

Urachal Adenocarcinomas of the Bladder

Introduction

Urachal adenocarcinomas of the bladder are also a very rare form of carcinoma arising from the ligament which connects from the midline dome of the bladder to the umbilicus. The pathogenesis of this malignancy is distinct from a typical urothelial carcinoma of the bladder which has an implication on staging and surgical procedures. Urachal tumors arise from the ligament outside the bladder and invade the bladder secondarily; therefore, the traditional bladder cancer TNM staging which was derived from tumors arising from the urothelial lining is not applicable in this disease. A definitive resection should include en bloc resection of the urachal ligament with the umbilicus and bladder dome and a node dissection. Partial cystectomies are appropriate when there is adequate functional bladder remaining. There is also evidence suggesting that a 5-fluoruracil/cisplatin-based chemotherapy regimen is more likely to be active as compared to the typical urothelial cancer regimens. Therefore, it is important to recognize these tumors prior to surgery and chemotherapy in order to achieve the best clinical outcomes.

Epidemiology

Urachal cancers arise in a much younger patient population with several series suggesting a median age of diagnosis in the fifth decade [17, 19–21], with a fairly even distribution between the male and female gender. There have been rare reports of urachal tumors in a pediatric population [22]. Since most estimates suggest urachal tumors occur in less than 1 % of all bladder tumors, the available literature is comprised mostly of small case series. There are currently no definitive risk factors associated with the development of this cancer. However, one small case series suggested microsatellite instability in six out of seven cases of urachal carcinoma [23].

Anatomy

Urachal tumors arise from the urachal ligament which connects to the dome of the bladder inferiorly and superiorly connects via the ligamentum commune to the umbilicus [19]. This ligament is a vestigial structure which is formed during embryogenesis when the cloaca divides both anteriorly and posteriorly, with the anterior portion developing into the sexual organs and bladder and the posterior portion developing into the rectum. When the bladder descends into the pelvis, the lumen of the allantois is obliterated, forming the urachal ligament. However, in up to one-third of adults, there remains luminal continuity between urachal ligament and bladder [24]. This luminal continuity may even extend superiorly to the umbilicus. However, the low overall incidence of urachal tumors despite this finding suggests that there is no definitive association between a urachal cyst and the ultimate development of urachal carcinoma.

Pathology

Urachal tumors are nearly always adenocarcinomas and appear histologically identical to adenocarcinomas of the gastrointestinal tract [1, 19]. Enteric, mucinous, glandular, and even signet ring cell features can be found in urachal tumors. Other features of colorectal cancer, including microsatellite instability and KRAS mutations, have been reported in urachal cancers as well [23]. Rarely, transformation of these adenocarcinomas to sarcomatoid and small cell tumors has been reported [19, 21]. The presence of transitional cell histology or carcinoma in situ should raise the clinical suspicion that this is not a urachal tumor but rather a urothelial carcinoma that is involving the urachal ligament secondarily. The presence of cystitis cystica or cystitis glandularis transitioning between the tumor and the urothelium would raise the clinical suspicion that this is a non-urachal adenocarcinoma of the bladder. There is often a sharp demarcation between the tumor and normal urothelium which will aid in the diagnosis. Remnants of normal or even ulcerated urothelium may overlie a urachal tumor as well.

Two theories have been proposed regarding the development of urachal adenocarcinomas. With their similarities to adenocarcinomas of the GI tract, one theory is that these tumors may arise from enteric rests which did not migrate to the hindgut during embryogenesis. An alternate hypothesis is that these tumors may arise from a metaplastic pathway, since adenocarcinomas have been seen to arise from cystitis glandularis and bladder exstrophy.

Diagnostic Criteria

Sheldon et al. initially proposed strict criteria regarding the diagnosis of the urachal tumor [19] (Table 9.1), acknowledging that "strict application of these criteria would exclude early or far advanced urachal carcinomas." Cystitis cystica occasionally may be encountered in bladders with urachal tumors [25]. Urachal tumors may also arise anywhere along the midline of the bladder and not necessarily at the bladder dome [24]. Furthermore, a residual urachal remnant may not be easily found even with surgical resection [21]. Additional criterion requiring the exclusion of a primary adenocarcinoma located outside the bladder [25] with endoscopic procedures of the gastrointestinal tract and mammograms also seems rather extreme, especially when there is no clinical evidence or history of an alternate primary tumor. A more practical approach has been adopted at the MD Anderson Cancer Center (Table 9.1) [26].

Table 9.1 Sheldon and MD Anderson Cancer Center criteria for the diagnosis of urachal carcinoma

Sheldon criteria	MD Anderson criteria
1. Tumor located in the dome of the bladder	1. Location in the bladder dome or elsewhere in the midline of the bladder
2. Absence of cystitis glandularis and cystitis cystica	2. Sharp demarcation between the tumor and normal surface epithelium
3. Predominant invasion of the muscularis or deeper tissues with a sharp demarcation between tumor and the surface epithelium which is free of glandular of polypoid proliferation	Supportive criteria
4. Presence of a urachal remnant in association with the neoplasm	Adenocarcinoma histology
5. Tumor invading the bladder wall with extension to the space of Retzius, anterior abdominal wall, or umbilicus	Absence of urothelial dysplasia or transitional cell histology
	Absence of cystitis cystica or cystitis glandularis transitioning to the tumor
	Absence of primary adenocarcinoma of another organ

Clinical Presentation and Diagnostic Workup

Urachal tumors may arise anywhere along the urachal ligament. While the majority of patients present with hematuria and urinary symptoms once the tumor erodes into the bladder lining, there are patients who present instead with umbilical pain or umbilical discharge. Unfortunately, this also means that a large number of patients present with more advanced disease, since urachal tumors may remain relatively asymptomatic or with vague abdominal symptoms until invasion into a local structure occurs.

Diagnostic imaging studies including CT or magnetic resonance imaging of the abdomen and pelvis provide strong support in the clinical diagnosis of a urachal adenocarcinoma. The presence of a midline, cystic mass with calcifications is considered a pathognomonic finding (Fig. 9.1) [26]. Unfortunately peritoneal carcinomatosis [17] may occur frequently in this disease in addition to pseudomyxoma peritonei [27]. Serum tumor markers including CEA, CA-125, and CA19-9 may be elevated in 40–60 % of patients [17] and may be helpful in evaluating response and progression to treatment especially in the treatment of peritoneal carcinomatosis. A cystoscopy can be helpful in obtaining tumor tissue to confirm the presence of adenocarcinoma when invasion into the bladder has occurred. However, given the risk of rupture of these often cystic masses, this author would recommend against a percutaneous biopsy of the cystic mass when a potentially curative resection is being planned.

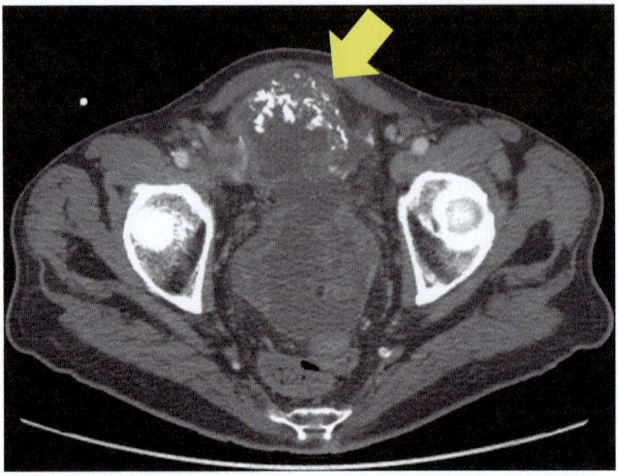

Fig. 9.1 A midline, cystic bladder mass with calcifications (*arrow*) is considered a pathognomonic finding in the diagnosis of urachal carcinoma

Table 9.2 Sheldon staging system for urachal carcinoma

Sheldon staging:
Stage I: No invasion beyond the urachal mucosa
Stage II: Invasion confined to the urachus
Stage III: Local extension into the:
Bladder (IIIA)
Abdominal wall (IIIB)
Peritoneum (IIIC)
Viscera other than bladder (IIID)
Stage IV: Metastases to the:
Regional lymph nodes (IVA)
Distant sites (IVB)

Staging

Since urachal tumors arise outside the bladder and invade the bladder secondarily, the typical TNM bladder cancer staging criteria are not applicable in this malignancy. Sheldon et al. initially proposed an extensive staging system for urachal carcinoma (Table 9.2) [19]. Unfortunately, most patients with urachal tumors present with stage III–IV diseases, since their symptoms may be vague or minimal until invasion into a local structure occurs. Given the lack of a confirmed staging system to date, it appears reasonable to use the Sheldon staging criteria until additional evidence is available suggesting a benefit from a more appropriate staging paradigm.

Surgical Management

Early recognition of a urachal carcinoma is extremely important as it requires planning for control of the primary site with an en bloc resection of the urachal ligament together with the bladder or bladder dome and umbilicus. Urachal tumors may occur anywhere along the urachal ligament and/or ligamentum commune, with one series suggesting involvement of the umbilicus in 8 % of cases [19]. Cystic communications along the extent of the urachal ligament/ligamentum commune can occur as well, which is another important reason to do a resection which is en bloc with the bladder dome and umbilicus. This author has seen operative reports where transection of the ligament at the umbilicus resulted in rupture of cystic contents contaminating the peritoneal cavity which was a likely contributor to the development of peritoneal carcinomatosis. Lack of complete resection of the umbilicus has been associated with an increased risk of relapse [17, 28].

A partial cystectomy with en bloc resection of the urachal ligament and umbilicus is most commonly used to treat surgically resectable urachal carcinomas. Long-term survival outcomes have been reported, including a median survival around 48 months and 5-year survival rates of 45–49 % [17, 28–30]. A complete cystectomy is indicated if it is impossible to have enough bladder remaining to maintain a functional reservoir. As with many cancers, margin status has been an important contributor to long-term cure. It is also important to achieve negative margins with the resection as the presence of positive margins has been associated with relapse. Contemporary series with the approach suggests median survival of around 48 months with fewer survival rates from 45 % to 49 %.

A lymph node dissection is also recommended due to the risk for occult metastasis in clinically negative lymph nodes. As one might anticipate, the presence of lymph node involvement has been associated with poor prognosis [17, 28, 29]. While the series at MD Anderson suggested no long-term survivors in the setting of node-positive disease [17], Herr et al. reported a 25 % 5-year survival at Memorial Sloan Kettering Cancer Center [30]. Currently, surgical debulking procedures of clinically involved lymph nodes cannot be routinely recommended as a curative procedure. However, this author has observed a few patients with clinically enlarged nodes treated with chemotherapy with an excellent response in their lymph nodes. There are now several cases treated with surgical consolidation with partial cystectomy and en bloc resection of the umbilicus and extended lymph node dissection who remain alive and cancer-free for more than 5 years [26].

Risk Factors for Relapse Following Surgery

An early retrospective study from the MD Anderson Cancer Center identified several factors increasing the risk for relapse of urachal cancer following surgery [17], with similar findings reported by other institutions as well [28–30]. While the likelihood of long-term survival is close to 50 % in all patients going to surgery, when any of these adverse risk factors are present, the likelihood of relapse appears to increase to 75 % or greater. As is common with many other cancers, the ability to achieve negative margins has had a strong impact in overall survival [17, 28, 30]. Lack of en bloc resection of the umbilicus with the ligament has also been shown to impact outcomes [17, 28], likely due to the risk of having tumor at the umbilicus [19] and/or cystic communications along the ligament. The presence of tumor involving the peritoneal lining [17, 28, 29, 31] and lymph node involvement have also been associated with a poor prognosis [17, 28–31]. Although there is no proven benefit for adjuvant chemotherapy, the presence of these factors appears to select for patients at high enough risk of relapse to justify the development of adjuvant therapy.

Systemic Chemotherapy for Urachal Carcinoma

Metastatic Setting

The lack of standard chemotherapy for urachal carcinoma in the historical literature is readily apparent, described by some as "invariably unsatisfactory" [32] or even has a "history of defeat." [33]. Standard urothelial cancer regimens such as gemcitabine with cisplatin and MVAC (methotrexate, vinblastine, doxorubicin, and cisplatin) have been rather unsatisfying with few responses reported [17]. In a series from the Mayo Clinic where the majority of patients with metastatic urachal carcinoma were treated with a urothelial cancer-type regimens, the median survival was less than 1 year [31]. There was early evidence of clinical activity with 5-FU-based combinations including 5-FU with doxorubicin and mitomycin-C [34] and 5-FU, cisplatin with alpha-interferon [17], an early regimen attempting to modulate the immune system which was too toxic for further development [35]. Another 5-FU-based regimen of 5-FU with leucovorin, gemcitabine, and cisplatin (Gem-FLP) suggested a response rate in around 33 % of patients [17]. This author has also seen activity with a combination of capecitabine and gemcitabine, a regimen initially developed in renal cell cancer [36]. Taxane-cisplatin combinations have a response rate around 15 %, for example, with ifosfamide, paclitaxel, and cisplatin (ITP) [18], or a combination of paclitaxel, methotrexate, and cisplatin (TMP) [17, 37]. Additional responses have been reported with FOLFOX6 [38], S-1/cisplatin [39], and irinotecan [40]. This author has also observed activity with other colorectal-like regimens including irinotecan with cetuximab and FOLFIRI. Although the survival with urothelial cancer-based regimens has been reportedly poor with a median survival less than 1 year by the Mayo Clinic [31], the historical experience at MD Anderson with 5-FU-/cisplatin-based options was around 24 months [17]. With the similarities in histology, response, and survival between urachal cancer and colorectal cancer, it seems that the use of 5-FU-based therapy is most appropriate given the limited data available.

Neoadjuvant and Adjuvant Setting

There currently is no proven role for the use of neoadjuvant or adjuvant chemotherapy for urachal carcinomas. Therefore, in a patient with node-negative, surgically resectable cancer (i.e., no invasion of the pelvic sidewall), the standard treatment would be a cystectomy or partial cystectomy with en bloc resection of the urachal ligament and umbilicus with a node dissection. Although there is no proven role for adjuvant chemotherapy, investigators at MD Anderson have been offering adjuvant Gem-FLP chemotherapy to patients in whom the risk of recurrence is high. When these high-risk features are present, the risk of relapse without any further intervention is high, likely around 75 % [17]. Adjuvant chemotherapy has had an impact in adenocarcinomas of the GI tract, which, as noted above, urachal cancer appears very similar. This author is currently advocating for five to six cycles of adjuvant Gem-FLP for patients with positive margins, lymph node involvement, peritoneal involvement, or when the umbilicus has not been resected en bloc.

Surgical Consolidation of Metastatic Disease

While the majority of patients with stage 4 metastatic tumors do ultimately succumb to their disease, there have been patients who benefited from surgical consolidation with resection of metastatic disease. These cases remain largely anecdotal; however, there is evidence supporting resection of solitary or low-volume metastatic sites in gastrointestinal cancer. Given the similarities between these two diseases, this may be relevant in some patients with urachal carcinomas as well. This has been most frequently offered to patients with slowly progressive disease with resection or metastasectomy in a solitary site such as lung metastases. These patients are typically given a trial of chemotherapy first to assess their sensitivity to chemotherapy and determine whether the biology of their urachal tumor suggests the potential for benefit. Surgical consolidation would be avoided for patients with bulky or rapidly progressive disease. This author has also observed anecdotal cases with patients presenting with bulky lymph nodes who responded well to chemotherapy and had surgical consolidation with partial (or complete) cystectomy with en bloc resection of the urachal ligament with umbilicus and an extended node dissection. We now have several patients who remain alive and disease-free for more than 5 years.

Conclusion

Urachal carcinomas and non-urachal adenocarcinomas of the bladder remain extremely rare malignancies. It is unlikely that there will be any randomized trials completed in this author's lifetime to confirm the benefit of different treatments. In the setting of surgically resectable disease, surgery may result in long-term disease-specific survival. It is important to note the differences in surgical planning when treating a urachal carcinoma. In the setting of metastatic disease, it appears that colorectal-like regimens, and in particular a combination of Gem-FLP, may have the most activity, with taxane-cisplatin combinations as a second-line option. A definitive role for neoadjuvant or adjuvant chemotherapy is as yet largely unknown. In the setting of urachal tumors, the presence of high risk factors associated with a high risk of relapse may help select the group of patient most likely to need adjuvant treatment. With the similarities between urachal carcinomas, non-urachal bladder adenocarcinomas, and adenocarcinomas of the colon, it seems reasonable to use regimens approved for the treatment of colorectal cancer as relevant options in this disease.

References

1. Grignon DJ, Ro JY, Ayala AG, et al. Primary adenocarcinoma of the urinary bladder. A clinicopathologic analysis of 72 cases. Cancer. 1991;67:2165–72.
2. Lughezzani G, Sun M, Jeldres C, et al. Adenocarcinoma versus urothelial carcinoma of the urinary bladder: comparison between pathologic stage at radical cystectomy and cancer-specific mortality. Urology. 2010;75:376–81.
3. Smeulders N, Woodhouse CR. Neoplasia in adult exstrophy patients. BJU Int. 2001;87:623–8.
4. Allen TD, Henderson BW. Adenocarcinoma of the bladder. J Urol. 1965;93:50–6.
5. Mostofi FK. Potentialities of bladder epithelium. J Urol. 1954;71:705–14.
6. Mai KT, Yazdi HM, Perkins DG, et al. Multicentric clear cell adenocarcinoma in the urinary bladder and the urethral diverticulum: evidence of origin of clear cell adenocarcinoma of the female lower urinary tract from Mullerian duct remnants. Histopathology. 2000;36:380–2.
7. Zaghloul MS, Nouh A, Nazmy M, et al. Long-term results of primary adenocarcinoma of the urinary bladder: a report on 192 patients. Urol Oncol. 2006;24:13–20.
8. Dayyani F, Czerniak BA, Sircar K, et al. Plasmacytoid urothelial carcinoma, a chemosensitive cancer with poor prognosis, and peritoneal carcinomatosis. J Urol. 2013;189:1656–61.
9. Ro JY, Shen SS, Lee HI, et al. Plasmacytoid transitional cell carcinoma of urinary bladder: a clinicopathologic study of 9 cases. Am J Surg Pathol. 2008;32:752–7.
10. Lopez-Beltran A, Luque RJ, Quintero A, et al. Hepatoid adenocarcinoma of the urinary bladder. Virchows Arch. 2003;442:381–7.
11. Wang HL, Lu DW, Yerian LM, et al. Immunohistochemical distinction between primary adenocarcinoma of the bladder and secondary colorectal adenocarcinoma. Am J Surg Pathol. 2001;25:1380–7.
12. Torenbeek R, Lagendijk JH, Van Diest PJ, et al. Value of a panel of antibodies to identify the primary origin of adenocarcinomas presenting as bladder carcinoma. Histopathology. 1998;32:20–7.
13. Werling RW, Yaziji H, Bacchi CE, et al. CDX2, a highly sensitive and specific marker of adenocarcinomas of intestinal origin: an immunohistochemical survey of 476 primary and metastatic carcinomas. Am J Surg Pathol. 2003;27:303–10.
14. Thomas AA, Stephenson AJ, Campbell SC, et al. Clinicopathologic features and utility of immunohistochemical markers in signet-ring cell adenocarcinoma of the bladder. Hum Pathol. 2009;40:108–16.
15. El-Mekresh MM, El-Baz MA, Abol-Enein H, et al. Primary adenocarcinoma of the urinary bladder: a report of 185 cases. Br J Urol. 1998;82:206–12.
16. Zaghloul MS, Abdel Aziz S. Primary adenocarcinoma of the urinary bladder: risk factors and value of postoperative radiotherapy. J Egypt Natl Canc Inst. 2003;15:193–200.
17. Siefker-Radtke AO, Gee J, Shen Y, et al. Multimodality management of urachal carcinoma: the M. D. Anderson Cancer Center experience. J Urol. 2003;169:1295–8.
18. Galsky MD, Iasonos A, Mironov S, et al. Prospective trial of ifosfamide, paclitaxel, and cisplatin in patients with advanced non-transitional cell carcinoma of the urothelial tract. Urology. 2007;69:255–9.
19. Sheldon CA, Clayman RV, Gonzalez R, et al. Malignant urachal lesions. J Urol. 1984;131:1–8.
20. Wright JL, Porter MP, Li CI, et al. Differences in survival among patients with urachal and nonurachal adenocarcinomas of the bladder. Cancer. 2006;107:721–8.
21. Henly DR, Farrow GM, Zincke H. Urachal cancer: role of conservative surgery. Urology. 1993;42:635–9.
22. Gupta S, Bhaijee F, Harmon EP. Mucinous neoplasm arising in a urachal cyst: a first in the pediatric population. Urology. 2014;83:455–6.
23. Sirintrapun SJ, Ward M, Woo J, et al. High-stage urachal adenocarcinoma can be associated with microsatellite instability and KRAS mutations. Hum Pathol. 2014;45:327–30.
24. Schubert GE, Pavkovic MB, Bethke-Bedurftig BA. Tubular urachal remnants in adult bladders. J Urol. 1982;127:40–2.

25. Johnson DE, Hodge GB, Abdul-Karim FW, et al. Urachal carcinoma. Urology. 1985;26:218–21.
26. Siefker-Radtke A. Urachal adenocarcinoma: a clinician's guide for treatment. Semin Oncol. 2012;39:619–24.
27. Takeuchi M, Matsuzaki K, Yoshida S, et al. Imaging findings of Urachal mucinous cystadenocarcinoma associated with pseudomyxoma peritonei. Acta Radiol. 2004;45:348–50.
28. Ashley RA, Inman BA, Sebo TJ, et al. Urachal carcinoma: clinicopathologic features and long-term outcomes of an aggressive malignancy. Cancer. 2006;107:712–20.
29. Bruins HM, Visser O, Ploeg M, et al. The clinical epidemiology of urachal carcinoma: results of a large, population based study. J Urol. 2012;188:1102–7.
30. Herr HW, Bochner BH, Sharp D, et al. Urachal carcinoma: contemporary surgical outcomes. J Urol. 2007;178:74–8. discussion 78.
31. Molina JR, Quevedo JF, Furth AF, et al. Predictors of survival from urachal cancer: a Mayo Clinic study of 49 cases. Cancer. 2007;110:2434–40.
32. Lane V. Prognosis in carcinoma of the urachus. Eur Urol. 1976;2:282–3.
33. Kakizoe T. Adenocarcinoma of urachus. Report of 7 cases and review of literature. Urology. 1983;21:360–6.
34. Logothetis CJ, Samuels ML, Ogden S. Chemotherapy for adenocarcinomas of bladder and urachal origin: 5-fluorouracil, doxorubicin, and mitomycin-C. Urology. 1985;26:252–5.
35. Siefker-Radtke AO, Millikan RE, Tu S-M, et al. Phase III trial of fluorouracil, interferon alpha-2b, and cisplatin versus methotrexate, vinblastine, doxorubicin, and cisplatin in metastatic or unresectable urothelial cancer. J Clin Oncol: Off J Am Soc Clin Oncol. 2002;20:1361–7.
36. Tannir NM, Thall PF, Ng CS, et al. A phase II trial of gemcitabine plus capecitabine for metastatic renal cell cancer previously treated with immunotherapy and targeted agents. J Urol. 2008;180:867–72. discussion 872.
37. Tu SM, Hossan E, Amato R, et al. Paclitaxel, cisplatin and methotrexate combination chemotherapy is active in the treatment of refractory urothelial malignancies. J Urol. 1995;154:1719–22.
38. Yanagihara Y, Tanji N, Miura N, et al. Modified FOLFOX6 chemotherapy in patients with metastatic urachal cancer. Chemotherapy. 2013;59:402–6.
39. Kojima Y, Yamada Y, Kamisawa H, et al. Complete response of a recurrent advanced urachal carcinoma treated by S-1/cisplatin combination chemotherapy. Int J Urol. 2006;13:1123–5.
40. Kume H, Tomita K, Takahashi S, et al. Irinotecan as a new agent for urachal cancer. Urol Int. 2006;76:281–2.

Primary Urethral Carcinomas

10

Kamran Zargar-Shoshtari, Pranav Sharma,
and Philippe E. Spiess

Background and Epidemiology

Primary urethral carcinomas (PUCs) account for <1 % of all genitourinary malignancies [1]. According to the Surveillance, Epidemiology, and End Results (SEER) database, over the past three decades, the annual incidence has ranged from 1.5 per million in women and a nearly threefold larger incidence in men (4.3 per million). The prevalence of all histological subtypes increases with age, with the peak annual incidence of 32 per million in men and 9.5 per million in women, seen in the 75–84-year age group, with disease being extremely uncommon in population younger than 55 years old (0.2 per million). The incidence of the disease has been reported to be twice as high in the African-American compared to the White population [2]. In Europe, the age standardized ratio is estimated as 1.6 per million in men and 0.6 per million in women, with a similar male-to-female ratio [3].

In men, chronic irritation associated with urethral stricture is identified as the cause of PUC in over 70 % of the cases. Other etiological factors include chronic inflammation associated with sexually transmitted disease, high-risk human papillomavirus (HPV) infections, intermittent catheterization, urethroplasty, and external beam and permanent seed radiation therapy. Chronic irritation is also attributed to the development of PUC in majority of female cases with urethra diverticula, leukoplakia, HPV infection, recurrent lower urinary tract infections, and child birth identified as other potential etiological factors [4–8].

K. Zargar-Shoshtari, MD
Department of Urology, Moffitt Cancer Center, Tampa, FL, USA

P. Sharma, MD • P.E. Spiess, MD (✉)
Department of Urology, Moffitt Cancer Center, 12902 Magnolia Dr., Tampa, FL 33612, USA
e-mail: Philippe.spiess@moffitt.org

L. Pagliaro (ed.), *Rare Genitourinary Tumors*,
DOI 10.1007/978-3-319-30046-7_10

Histological Variation

Table 10.1 summarizes the distribution of histological subtypes from various institutional reports. Traditionally, mainly single institution data have reported that in men, up to 80 % of urethral cancers are squamous cell in origin, with 15 % urothelial cell origin and the remaining 5 % being adenocarcinoma as well as other rare subtypes such as lymphoma, sarcoma, or melanoma.

In females, similarly it is often reported that squamous cell carcinoma is the most common histology (40–70 %), followed by adenocarcinoma (15–35 %) and urothelial carcinoma (15 %). In female, primary urethral carcinoma can affect the entire urethra in over 40 % of the cases; however, the majority of lesions involve the distal urethra (35–50 %) [9–11].

In men overall, 60 % of malignant lesions are seen in the bulbomembranous urethra, followed by a frequency of 30 % in the distal (penile) urethra and 10 % in the prostatic urethra. Squamous carcinoma is more common in the distal urethra, with 90 % of all distal urethral cancers being squamous in origin, followed by 80 % of all bulbar urethral and 10 % of all prostatic urethral malignancies. Urothelial carcinoma in seen in 10 %, 20 %, and 90 % of distal, bulbar, and prostatic urethral malignancies, respectively [10, 12].

More recent population-based reports from USA and Europe have suggested that urothelial carcinoma of the urethra is the predominant histologic type of primary UC (54–65 %), followed by squamous cell carcinoma (16–22 %) and adenocarcinoma (10–16 %). An analysis of SEER data from 1988 to 2006 reported that in men, urothelial carcinoma was the most common primary urethral carcinoma subtypes (78 %) followed by squamous cell carcinoma (12 %) and adenocarcinoma (5 %) [13]. SEER data report from 1983 to 2008 identified rates of 30 %, 29 %, and 28 % for urothelial, squamous cell, and adenocarcinoma in female patients, respectively [14]. A 1989–2008 report from the Netherlands National Cancer Registry reported that in female, urothelial carcinoma was the common histological subtypes (45 %), followed by adenocarcinoma (29 %), squamous cell carcinoma in (19 %), and other rare subtypes (6 %) [15].

Clinical Presentation and Diagnostic Workup

PUC often presents at a relatively advanced stage, with almost all lesions being symptomatic at presentation (Table 10.2) [10, 15, 16]. Unfortunately the majority of patients also present months after initiation of symptoms [17], with a median time to presentation of 4.5 months in female and 7.5 months in male patients [10, 17].

Patient evaluation should include physical examination of the genital region, pelvis, and the inguinal lymph nodes. In men, the size, location, and the mobility of the lesions have to be assessed, in order to evaluate the potential for organ preservation. Anterior urethra in men and the distal two-thirds of the female urethra drain into the inguinal lymph nodes. Therefore, assessment of regional lymph nodes is essential in patients presenting with primary UC, as unlike penile carcinoma, adenopathy in this

Table 10.1 Breakdown of histology in institutional reports of PUC

	Derksen [15]	Dalbagni [10]	DiMarco [16]	Garden [35]	Milosevic [32]	Dalbagni [17]	Cohen [33]	Smith [28]	Dayyani [19]	Gheiler [34]
Gender (no.)	F 91	F 72	F 63	F 97	F 34	M 46	M 18	M 18	F 28	F 10
									M 16	M 11
Study duration	1989–2008	1958–1994	1948–1999	1955–1989	1961–1990	1958–1996	1991–2006	5 years in 2000s	2005–2009	1980–1996
SCC	19	25	36	41	44	52	95	95	39	53
AC	29	35	26	36	18	2	5	0	30	31
UC	45	15	28	23	38	33	0	0	19	5
Others	7	25	10	0	0	13	0	5	12	11

SCC squamous cell carcinoma, *AC* adenocarcinoma, *UC* urothelial cell carcinoma, *No.* number, *F* female, *M* male

Table 10.2 Symptoms associated with PUC at presentation

Symptoms	Male (%)	Female (%)
Obstructive voiding	43	28
Irritative lower urinary tract symptoms	20	41
Spotting	20	35
Hematuria	17	16
Urethral mass	20	20
Discharge/abscess	31	7
Incidental	4	2

PUC primary urethral carcinoma

Table 10.3 Lymphatic drainage of the urethra [37]

Male	
Anterior urethra	The superficial and deep inguinal lymph nodes
Posterior urethra	Pelvic lymph nodes (external, obturator, and internal iliac)
Female	
Proximal third	Pelvic lymph nodes (external, obturator, and internal iliac)
Distal two-thirds	Superficial and deep inguinal nodes

group often indicates metastatic disease [17–19]. Table 10.3 summarizes the urethral lymphatic drainage.

Further assessment should include examination under anesthesia, urethrocystoscopy, biopsy, as well as cross-sectional radiological assessment of the chest, abdomen, and pelvis. Magnetic resonance imaging may provide excellent details for assessment of the local disease. In female patients, MRI with endovaginal coil has been used for the assessment of urethral disease extent with great effect. In men with PUC, experience in penile cancer has shown that MRI can provide excellent details with regard to local stage and invasion beyond corpus spongiosum which can assist in surgical planning [20–23]. Similarly, 18F-fluorodeoxyglucose PET/CT scan has been used for the evaluation of inguinal nodal metastases in patients with penile carcinoma with reported sensitivity of 88 % and a specificity of 98 % [24]. Based on these reports, 18F-FDG-PET/CT may also have utility in assessing patients with primary urethral carcinoma.

Staging

American Joint Committee for Cancer (AJCC) TNM staging system [25] described staging for primary urethral carcinoma, and this distinguished between prostatic or distal urethral lesions. In penile urethra and female urethra, invasion of subepithelial connective tissue is distinguished between Ta and T1 lesions. Invasion of deeper layers (corpus spongiosum in male and periurethral muscle in female) denotes stage T2 disease. Similar to penile carcinoma, invasion of corpus cavernosum is classified as T3 disease in male. In female, T3 disease involves anterior vaginal wall or the bladder neck. T4 tumors invade adjacent organs. Invasion of a single lymph node, less than two centimeters, is considered N1 disease, and any other nodal involvement is N2, and distant metastasis is classified as M1. There is no N3 defined for PUC.

In prostatic urethra, carcinoma in situ of the urethra (Tis pu) and carcinoma in situ of the prostatic ducts (Tis pd) are individually identified. Ta stage does not exist for prostatic PUC. Invasion of the subepithelial connective tissue (T1), prostatic stroma (T2), and beyond prostatic stroma (T3) denotes other stages, with similar definition of T4 disease as the penile urethra.

Treatment Options in Men with PUC

In men, distal urethral PUC, compared to more proximal disease, is associated with better clinical outcomes. It has been shown that compared to local tumor stage, nodal stage is a more important factor in predicting survival. Therefore, surgical strategies which aim to preserve penile length and function are oncologically acceptable as long as adequate assessment and treatment of nodal disease is performed [26].

In distal penile lesions, an organ-preserving approach, such as transurethral resection, local excision, or distal urethrectomy and perineal urethrostomy, may provide adequate treatment in selected patients with low-grade, noninvasive disease [27]. More locally advanced disease (T2 or higher), located at distal urethra and penis, may be treated with partial penectomy as long as negative margins can be achieved. However, carcinoma extending to the more proximal urethra, where resection-free margins are not possible, will require total penectomy. In men with anterior urethral pT1-3 N0-2 disease, following partial penectomy, local recurrence was not observed as long as surgical resection margins were negative, even if the tumor-free margin was less than 5 mm [28]. In older series, recurrence rates of 13 % have been reported following total penectomy [29].

Disease involving the bulbar urethra requires more careful assessment and planning. For limited, noninvasive disease, transurethral resection or partial excision of the urethra with primary anastomosis has been described. Although owing to relative late presentation and more advanced disease in men with bulbar urethral PUC, suitable candidates for these local therapies are not commonly encountered. Adequate surgical therapy in most men presenting with lesions at the bulbar urethra requires radical cystoprostatectomy and total penectomy, followed by adequate nodal staging [30].

Treatment Options in Females with PUC

The distal third of the female urethra may be excised without significant impact on the continence mechanism. Small distal lesions, near the meatus, may be amenable to circumferential excision of the urethra and the anterior vaginal wall. In these circumstances, adequate steps, such as frozen section sampling, must be taken to ensure complete excision and tumor-free margins. Incontinence rate of 42 % has been reported in a series of patients treated with partial urethrectomy [16].

In more advanced disease (T2–3), preservation of urethra may result in inadequate oncological control, with local recurrence rates of up to 21 % reported, even in T2 disease [16]. However, bladder-preserving strategies are still possible. In these circumstances, primary radical urethrectomy should be performed. This includes removal of all the periurethral tissue from the bulbocavernosus muscle bilaterally and distally, extending to the pubic symphysis and the bladder neck. Subsequently, the bladder neck is closed and proximal diversion can be accomplished with a catheterizable stoma (appendicovesicostomy or ileovesicostomy) [16, 26, 31]. More extensive disease will require cystectomy, with wide excision of the urethra and urinary diversion [16].

Management of Regional Lymph Nodes

There is no data supporting prophylactic inguinal or pelvic lymphadenectomy in PUC. As reported earlier, lymphadenopathy in PUC is often indicative of metastatic disease. Clinical examinations and cross-sectional anatomical and functional imaging as well as needle-guided biopsy can be used to confirm nodal metastases. In these patients, regional lymphadenectomy should be considered as part of the initial management. This approach may be curative in patients who have no evidence of distant metastases [26, 31].

Radiation therapy, combined with concurrent systemic chemotherapy, has also been used for the treatment of regional lymph nodes in both male and female patients. In this setting, the radiation fields were extended to include inguinal and pelvic nodes [32, 33]. Current National Comprehensive Cancer Network (NCCN) guidelines recommend concurrent chemoradiation or neoadjuvant chemotherapy followed by consolidative surgery for cN1-2 patients with PUC.

Radiation Therapy

Radiation therapy has been used both as the primary treatment and in combination with surgery and systemic therapies.

There are reports of primary radiation therapy in female for primary urothelial, squamous, as well as adenocarcinoma of the urethra. The administrated dose has ranged from 40 to 106 Gy and has included external beam radiation alone, brachytherapy alone, or combination of radiation modalities as well as radiation to the regional lymph nodes in selected patients [10, 32, 34, 35].

Reported local recurrence rates are 35 % with this approach, and relapse rates of around 30 % are also reported in patients with inguinal disease who had treatment to the nodes. One reported 38 % of patients were disease-free at median follow-up of 7.6 years, and another group reported a 5-year overall survival of 41 %, with local control rate of 64 % at 5 years [30, 32].

In patients who achieved local control, high rates of complications have been reported with severe complications rate of approximately 15 % including urethral stenosis, fistulae, necrosis, and radiation cystitis [32, 35].

Current recommendations for radiotherapy in primary PUC include 66–70 Gy of external beam radiation for cT2N0 disease. In cT3–4 or cN1–2 patients, it is recommended to deliver 45–50 Gy to the primary lesion and to the regional nodes with boost to the gross primary disease to 66–70 Gy and gross nodal disease to 54–66 Gy [36].

Systemic Chemotherapy

Contemporary cisplatin-based chemotherapy regimens have been associated with significant clinical response in PUC patients. A report of 44 PUC cases from 2005 to 2009 (39 % SCC, 30 % adenocarcinoma, 19 % UC, 18 % mixed/others; 98 % T3–T4, 43 % N+, and 16 % M+) demonstrated a 72 % response rate to neoadjuvant chemotherapy, with only a single patient advancing while on therapy. Table 10.4 summarizes the therapeutic regimens used in this study. In this cohort, patients with no metastatic disease who were treated with curative intent had a survival rate of 50 % at 42 months. Long-term survival was also observed in patients who presented with nodal disease, with over 40 % being alive at 3 years. Patients who underwent surgery after chemotherapy had significantly improved overall survival compared with those who were managed with chemotherapy alone [19].

Cohen and colleagues reported on their experience with combination of systemic chemo- and radiation therapy in 18 men. Fifty-five percent were cT3–T4 and 34 % were cN+. Majority of cases were SCC (95 %). Patients were concurrently treated with 5-fluorouracil and mitomycin-C as well as radiation therapy. The latter included 45–55 Gy in 25 fractions during 5 weeks to the genitalia, perineum, and inguinal and external iliac lymph nodes. Complete response rate was 83 % with 5-year overall and disease-specific survival rates of 60 and 83 %. Thirty percent of responder developed recurrence. Patients undergoing salvage surgery after chemoradiotherapy experienced a higher 5-year disease-free survival than those without salvage surgery (72 % vs. 54 %). All patients who did respond to chemoradiation developed urethral strictures requiring further management [33]. Others have also reported on the use of 5-fluorouracil and cisplatin for the management of adenocarcinoma and squamous cell carcinoma and MVAC in the treatment of urothelial carcinoma as part of multimodal therapies for the management of PUC in both male and female patients [34].

According to the current guidelines, in locally advanced disease (T3–T4, cN0), neoadjuvant therapy followed by consolidative therapy (surgery or radiation) is the recommended treatment. In cN1–2 patients, neoadjuvant chemotherapy followed by consolidative surgery or concurrent chemoradiation is recommended [36].

Table 10.4 Systemic chemotherapy for PUC

Urethral carcinoma histology	Systemic therapy regimen
SCC	Cisplatin, gemcitabine, and ifosfamide
Adenocarcinoma	5-fluorouracil, gemcitabine, and cisplatin
Urothelial	Methotrexate, vinblastine, doxorubicin, and cisplatin

Long-Term Results and Prognosis

Population-based data from Europe and USA estimated 5-year overall survival of 46–54 %, with a 5-year cancer-specific survival rate of 68 % in the USA [2, 3].

Reported overall survival rates in men range from 83 % in noninvasive disease to 36 % in invasive disease [17]. In female, low-stage disease has reported 5-year survival of 78 % and higher stage tumor reported survival of 22 % [10].

A number of factors have been identified as prognostic indicators, including tumor pathology (stage, histology, grade, nodal involvement, and metastatic disease), tumor size and location, as well as age, race, and treatment modality [3, 13–15].

Conclusion

Secondary to its low incidence, there is no prospective data on the management of PUC. All reports in the literature are based on single institutional experience spanning many decades. Subsequently there is a significant variation in reported patient selection, assessment, and management strategies. The reports suggest that all modalities may have similar overall treatment outcomes, with different long-term side effects. Potentially the best outcomes can be achieved with multimodal therapies that are individualized to a given patient.

References

1. Gatta G, van der Zwan JM, Casali PG, et al. Rare cancers are not so rare: the rare cancer burden in Europe. Eur J Cancer. 2011;47:2493.
2. Swartz MA, Porter MP, Lin DW, et al. Incidence of primary urethral carcinoma in the United States. Urology. 2006;68:1164.
3. Visser O, Adolfsson J, Rossi S, et al. Incidence and survival of rare urogenital cancers in Europe. Eur J Cancer. 2012;48:456.
4. Van de Voorde W, Meertens B, Baert L, et al. Urethral squamous cell carcinoma associated with urethral stricture and urethroplasty. Eur J Surg Oncol. 1994;20:478.
5. Mohan H, Bal A, Punia RP, et al. Squamous cell carcinoma of the prostate. Int J Urol. 2003;10:114.
6. Cupp MR, Malek RS, Goellner JR, et al. Detection of human papillomavirus DNA in primary squamous cell carcinoma of the male urethra. Urology. 1996;48:551.
7. Wiener JS, Liu ET, Walther PJ. Oncogenic human papillomavirus type 16 is associated with squamous cell cancer of the male urethra. Cancer Res. 1992;52:5018.
8. Chung DE, Purohit RS, Girshman J, et al. Urethral diverticula in women: discrepancies between magnetic resonance imaging and surgical findings. J Urol. 2010;183:2265.
9. Weghaupt K, Gerstner GJ, Kucera H. Radiation therapy for primary carcinoma of the female urethra: a survey over 25 years. Gynecol Oncol. 1984;17:58.
10. Dalbagni G, Zhang ZF, Lacombe L, et al. Female urethral carcinoma: an analysis of treatment outcome and a plea for a standardized management strategy. Br J Urol. 1998;82:835.
11. Anderson KA, McAninch JW. Primary squamous cell carcinoma of anterior male urethra. Urology. 1984;23:134.
12. Srinivas V, Khan SA. Male urethral cancer. A review. Int Urol Nephrol. 1988;20:61.
13. Rabbani F. Prognostic factors in male urethral cancer. Cancer. 2011;117:2426.
14. Champ CE, Hegarty SE, Shen X, et al. Prognostic factors and outcomes after definitive treatment of female urethral cancer: a population-based analysis. Urology. 2012;80:374.

15. Derksen JW, Visser O, de la Riviere GB, et al. Primary urethral carcinoma in females: an epidemiologic study on demographical factors, histological types, tumour stage and survival. World J Urol. 2013;31:147.
16. Dimarco DS, Dimarco CS, Zincke H, et al. Surgical treatment for local control of female urethral carcinoma. Urol Oncol. 2004;22:404.
17. Dalbagni G, Zhang ZF, Lacombe L, et al. Male urethral carcinoma: analysis of treatment outcome. Urology. 1999;53:1126.
18. Heyns CF, Fleshner N, Sangar V, et al. Management of the lymph nodes in penile cancer. Urology. 2010;76:S43.
19. Dayyani F, Pettaway CA, Kamat AM, et al. Retrospective analysis of survival outcomes and the role of cisplatin-based chemotherapy in patients with urethral carcinomas referred to medical oncologists. Urol Oncol. 2013;31:1171.
20. Kim B, Kawashima A, LeRoy AJ. Imaging of the male urethra. Semin Ultrasound CT MR. 2007;28:258.
21. Neitlich JD, Foster Jr HE, Glickman MG, et al. Detection of urethral diverticula in women: comparison of a high resolution fast spin echo technique with double balloon urethrography. J Urol. 1998;159:408.
22. Ryu J, Kim B. MR imaging of the male and female urethra. Radiographics. 2001;21:1169.
23. Hanchanale V, Yeo L, Subedi N, et al. The accuracy of magnetic resonance imaging (MRI) in predicting the invasion of the tunica albuginea and the urethra during the primary staging of Penile Cancer. BJU Int. 2016;117:439–43.
24. Schlenker B, Scher B, Tiling R, et al. Detection of inguinal lymph node involvement in penile squamous cell carcinoma by 18F-fluorodeoxyglucose PET/CT: a prospective single-center study. Urol Oncol. 2012;30:55.
25. Edge SB, American Joint Committee on Cancer, American Cancer Society. AJCC cancer staging handbook: from the AJCC cancer staging manual. 7th ed. New York: Springer; 2010. p. xix–718.
26. Gakis G, Witjes JA, Comperat E, et al. EAU guidelines on primary urethral carcinoma. Eur Urol. 2013;64:823.
27. Hakenberg OW, Franke HJ, Froehner M, et al. The treatment of primary urethral carcinoma – the dilemmas of a rare condition: experience with partial urethrectomy and adjuvant chemotherapy. Onkologie. 2001;24:48.
28. Smith Y, Hadway P, Ahmed S, et al. Penile-preserving surgery for male distal urethral carcinoma. BJU Int. 2007;100:82.
29. Kaplan GW, Bulkey GJ, Grayhack JT. Carcinoma of the male urethra. J Urol. 1967;98:365.
30. Dinney CP, Johnson DE, Swanson DA, et al. Therapy and prognosis for male anterior urethral carcinoma: an update. Urology. 1994;43:506.
31. Karnes RJ, Breau RH, Lightner DJ. Surgery for urethral cancer. Urol Clin North Am. 2010;37:445.
32. Milosevic MF, Warde PR, Banerjee D, et al. Urethral carcinoma in women: results of treatment with primary radiotherapy. Radiother Oncol. 2000;56:29.
33. Cohen MS, Triaca V, Billmeyer B, et al. Coordinated chemoradiation therapy with genital preservation for the treatment of primary invasive carcinoma of the male urethra. J Urol. 2008;179:536.
34. Gheiler EL, Tefilli MV, Tiguert R, et al. Management of primary urethral cancer. Urology. 1998;52:487.
35. Garden AS, Zagars GK, Delclos L. Primary carcinoma of the female urethra. Results of radiation therapy. Cancer. 1993;71:3102.
36. Clark PE, Agarwal N, Biagioli MC, et al. Bladder cancer. J Natl Compr Canc Netw. 2013;11:446.
37. Carroll PR, Dixon CM. Surgical anatomy of the male and female urethra. Urol Clin North Am. 1992;19:339.

Adenocarcinoma of the Urethra

11

Patricia J. Eifel

Epidemiology

Primary urethral carcinomas of any histologic type are very rare, constituting fewer than 1 % of genitourinary malignancies; from a SEER review for the years 1973–2002, the estimated annual age-adjusted incidence rates were 4.3 per million and 1.5 per million men and women, respectively [1]. Adenocarcinomas are even more rare, accounting for only 15 % of all primary urethral cancers.

The racial and gender distributions differ between adenocarcinomas and other subtypes. The most common histologic subtype of urethral cancer, transitional cell carcinoma, is much more common in men than women and has a similar incidence in African-Americans and Whites. However, in the United States, adenocarcinoma of the urethra is predominantly a disease of African-American women who have an annual incidence rate of 2.2 per million, approximately ten times the rate observed in White women and four times the rate observed in African-American men [1]. Differing racial demographics may explain the apparently lower incidence of female urethral cancer in Europe than in the United States [2, 3]; in an epidemiologic study of female urethral carcinomas in the Netherlands, the annual incidence of adenocarcinomas was only 0.2 per million [2]. For US women, the incidence of urethral adenocarcinoma peaks at about age 50 with a fairly constant incidence up to about age 75.

P.J. Eifel, MD
Department of Radiation Oncology, The University of Texas MD Anderson Cancer Center, 1515 Holcombe Blvd., Houston, TX 77030, USA
e-mail: peifel@mdanderson.org

L. Pagliaro (ed.), *Rare Genitourinary Tumors*,
DOI 10.1007/978-3-319-30046-7_11

Pathology and Differential Diagnosis

Clear Cell Carcinomas The most frequently reported subtype of urethral adenocarcinoma in women is clear cell carcinoma. Histologically, these cancers are characterized by abundant glycogen-rich clear cytoplasm and hobnail cells that are typically arranged in papillary structures although some cancers may have a tubular or diffuse architectural pattern [4]; in some cases, several growth patterns may be present in the same tumor [5]. The morphologic appearance of urethral and bladder clear cell carcinoma is virtually identical to that of clear cell carcinomas arising in the ovary or endometrium [4, 6–8].

Data regarding immunophenotyping of urethral clear cell carcinomas are sparse. However, clear cell carcinomas of the urethra appear to be similar to ovarian and endometrial clear cell carcinomas in that they usually express CA-125, an antigen that is expressed by many Müllerian carcinomas (although CA-125 is also expressed in a minority of urothelial transitional carcinomas) [9]. Vang et al. [8] compared tumor marker immunohistochemical expression of two urinary tract clear cell carcinomas (one urethral and one bladder) with that of 17 gynecologic clear cell carcinomas and found very similar patterns of expression in all of these tumors; nearly all (including the two urinary tract cancers) showed expression of CK7, CAM 5.2, 34βE12, CEA, Leu-M1, bcl-2, p53, and Ca-125, and most were negative for CK 20, estrogen receptor, and progesterone receptor. In a study that included ten clear cell carcinomas of the bladder, Oliva et al. [9] also reported a staining pattern similar to that of gynecologic clear cell carcinomas. Sun et al. [10] noted that urinary tract clear cell carcinomas tend to be positive for P504S and negative for p63, suggesting a non-urothelial origin. Finally, Brimo et al. [11] reported positive staining for hepatocyte nuclear factor-1β (a marker known to distinguish ovarian clear cell carcinomas from other Müllerian subtypes) in 18/18 clear cell carcinomas of the bladder and urethra; in contrast, only 1/35 transitional cell carcinomas and 1/21 non-clear cell adenocarcinomas expressed this marker.

Although more study is needed, the evidence suggests that the histogenesis of clear cell carcinomas of the urethra, bladder, ovary, endometrium, and cervix is similar. That said, the precise nature and origin of these cancers remains obscure. Although Fadare et al. [12] have reported finding potential benign precursor lesions with cleared cytoplasm in many endometrial clear cell carcinomas, the origin of these putative precursors is uncertain. To cloud the picture further, Sung et al. [5] described two cases of concurrent clear cell carcinoma and urothelial neoplasia (one invasive and one in situ); they reported finding identical patterns of nonrandom X chromosome inactivation in the clear cell and urothelial components, suggesting a common clonal origin.

In the late 1970s, a sharp increase was noted in the rate of clear cell carcinoma of the cervix and vagina in girls and young women; when investigated, nearly all of these patients were found to have had in utero exposure to diethylstilbestrol (DES), a drug commonly used in the 1950s and 1960s to prevent miscarriage.

There is currently no evidence that any clear cell carcinomas of the urethra have been associated with in utero DES exposure. Nearly all of the known cases of DES-associated clear cell carcinomas were in women less than 40 years of age, while non-DES-related genitourinary clear cell carcinomas almost always occur in women over the age of 40.

Although, in the past, the term "mesonephric" was sometimes used to describe urethral and bladder clear cell carcinomas, these cancers lack the typical features of mesonephric (wolffian) tumors, which generally form small glands and solid masses of cells with little or no glycogen [4]. Although renal cell clear cell carcinomas do in rare cases metastasize to the bladder or urethra, the histologic features are sufficiently different from primary clear cell carcinomas of the bladder or urethra that they should not be confused [8, 9]. The main differential diagnostic consideration is nephrogenic adenoma, a benign metaplastic condition that is usually associated with a history of trauma to the urethra [13]. Nephrogenic adenoma lesions generally lack the degree of nuclear pleomorphism characteristic of clear cell carcinoma; they also tend to be smaller, often incidental findings and often occur in younger individuals than typical for clear cell adenocarcinoma [4, 13]. Nephrogenic carcinomas also generally are negative for hepatocyte nuclear factor-1β expression [11].

Clear cell carcinomas are extremely rare in males, with fewer than ten cases reported in the literature [14].

Non-clear Cell Adenocarcinomas Extremely rare primary urethral adenocarcinomas having morphologic and immunohistochemical characteristics of colon carcinoma have been reported in males and females [15, 16]. It is thought that some of these may arise in areas of intestinal-type metaplasia of urinary tract epithelium [16]. More commonly seen (though still extremely rare) are colonic-type adenocarcinomas originating in the periurethral vagina or soft tissue, which may obstruct or secondarily involve the urethra [17–19]. Other very rare adenocarcinomas that have been reported to arise in the urethra include high-grade serous carcinoma [20], endometrioid adenocarcinoma [21], signet ring cell adenocarcinoma [22], and glassy cell carcinoma [23].

Secondary Involvement of the Urethra by Adenocarcinoma Adenocarcinomas of the vagina [24] or prostate can obstruct or secondarily involve the urethra. Adenocarcinomas can also, rarely, metastasize to the urethra from other sites [25].

Presenting Signs and Symptoms of Urethral Carcinoma

The most common presenting symptom is gross hematuria. However, patients with urethral adenocarcinomas may also present with dysuria, urgency, frequency, incontinence, or urethral obstruction [4, 6, 26, 27]. These symptoms may be associated with or confused with urinary tract infection. Tumors that arise in diverticula may achieve considerable size before producing symptoms of obstruction.

Anatomy and Natural History

Urethral adenocarcinomas are frequently found to be arising in urethral diverticula [4, 28, 29]. Although the exact proportion of cancers presenting with this feature is uncertain, there are many descriptions of the association in the literature. The precise nature of this relationship is unclear. Although most urethral diverticula are benign, a study of diverticula from 90 female patients revealed invasive adenocarcinoma in 5 (6 %), high-grade dysplasia in 3, villous adenoma in 1, intestinal metaplasia in 5, and nephrogenic adenoma in 10 [30].

Urethral cancers may extend proximally to involve the base of the bladder. In females, they can invade locally to involve paraurethral tissues including the vagina or vulva and may become fixed to pubic bone.

Adenocarcinomas frequently metastasize to lymph nodes. In general, tumors of the distal urethra in both females and males drain preferentially to the inguinal lymph nodes, while cancers involving the proximal urethra metastasize to the internal iliac, external iliac, or even presacral nodes.

Distant metastases can occur, most frequently to the lung but also to the bone, liver, supradiaphragmatic nodes, or other sites.

Diagnostic Evaluation and Staging

Because clear cell carcinomas may arise in the vagina, cervix, uterus, or ovaries, evaluation of women should include pelvic examination, including careful inspection of the external genitalia and urethral meatus; speculum examination of the vagina should be performed in a way that permits visualization of the entire vaginal mucosa and (if present) cervix; digital examination of the vagina and rectovaginal examination should also be performed. In men, the external genitalia should be palpated for evidence of nodularity or induration. In some cases, examination under anesthesia may be warranted to achieve a high-quality examination. The inguinal regions should also be palpated for evidence of lymphadenopathy.

Any patient suspected of having a urethral carcinoma should have a urethrocystoscopy with detailed description of the site and extent of tumor involvement and biopsy of any suspicious lesions. Voided urine cytology is an unreliable method of diagnosing invasive lesions [31].

For the evaluation of the extent of local tumor in the urethra and periurethral tissues, magnetic resonance imaging (MRI) is generally superior to computed tomography [32, 33]. A high-quality MRI study can provide important information about the size and location of tumor and about the extent of paraurethral tissue infiltration. However, the quality of the study is dependent on optimal preparation of the patient and the method of image acquisition. MRI also may not detect areas of superficial mucosal extension, particularly in the vagina. CT or MRI can provide valuable information about possible regional lymph node involvement; however, because the diagnostic criteria for nodal involvement by tumor are based primarily on tumor size, the accuracy of these studies is only modest, particularly in the groin where

Table 11.1 American Joint Committee on Cancer (AJCC) staging of urethral cancer

Stage 0	Limited to the mucosa
Stage I	Tumor invades subepithelial connective tissue (T1); nodes negative (N0)
Stage II	Tumor invades corpus spongiosum, prostate, or periurethral muscle (T2); nodes negative (N0)
Stage III	Tumor invades corpus cavernosum, beyond the prostatic capsule, anterior vagina or bladder neck (T3); or metastasis to a single lymph node ≤2 cm in diameter (N1)
Stage IV	Tumor invades other adjacent organs (T4); or metastasis in one node ≥2 cm or multiple nodes (N2); or distant metastases (M1)

inflammatory responses frequently cause benign enlargement. For groin nodes, ultrasound, sometimes accompanied by fine-needle aspiration biopsy, is a very accurate method for the detection of lymph node involvement. Few data are available about the value of FDG-PET in the management of urethral adenocarcinoma.

Cancers are usually staged using a TNM staging system designated by the American Joint Committee on Cancer (Table 11.1).

Treatment

Because most reports either include fewer than five cases, depend on pooled data lacking treatment-related details [6], or span many years [34–36], it is extremely difficult to draw meaningful conclusions about the relative benefits of different treatments. In four of the largest experiences, the Mayo Clinic had only 14 cases of urethral adenocarcinoma treated with primary surgery over 51 years (1948–1999) [34]; Garden et al. reported 34 cases treated at MD Anderson in 34 years (1955–1989) [35], Grigsby et al. reported 13 cases treated in 36 years at Washington University [27], and Princess Margaret Hospital had 6 cases treated over a 30-year period [36]. Because these experiences span many years of evolving radiation therapy technique, surgical practice, and chemotherapy recommendations, there tend to be almost as many treatment approaches used as there are patients treated.

However, several conclusions may be drawn from available data. Outcome seems to depend greatly on the ability to achieve local disease control. In the surgical series reported by DeMarco et al. [34], 7 of 14 patients treated with initial surgery recurred in the pelvis; the 5-year cause-specific survival rate for the series was 47 %, suggesting that local recurrence played a role in most disease-related deaths. Similarly, in a series of 97 urethral carcinomas treated with radiation [35], approximately two-thirds of treatment failures had a component of local recurrence; although recurrence patterns were not detailed for different histologic types, the results were said to be similar for the squamous and adenocarcinomas that made up most of the cases in this series.

Both radiation and primary surgery have been recommended to treat primary urethral carcinomas. However, the effectiveness of these treatments is difficult to compare, in part because surgery (usually radical cystourethrectomy) has tended to be used to treat smaller cancers, while radiation therapy is often recommended for large, unresectable cancers.

Retrospective studies of urethral cancer suggest that surgical treatment is most successful for early lesions. Overall, for patients treated with anterior exenteration for locally advanced disease, local recurrence rates are about 67 % and survival rates <20 % [37]. DiMarco et al. reported an overall 5-year relapse-free survival rate of 73 % for patients with T1–T2 cancers but only 36 % for T3–4 cancers and 15 % for N1–2 cancers treated with primary surgery. The results of surgery were about the same for patients treated throughout the study period from 1948 to 1999. Only 14 of the 54 patients included in the study by Dimarco et al. had adenocarcinomas; however, the overall relapse-free and disease-specific survival rates were similar for adenocarcinomas, squamous, and transitional cell carcinomas.

When early stage tumors are treated with radiation therapy, local control rates appear to be 80–90 % and most patients retain bladder function [27, 35, 38]; however, the number of reported cases (particularly adenocarcinomas) is very low. Even advanced cancers can often be cured with radiation alone. Although most of the 97 women reported by Garden et al. [35] appear to have had stage III or IV disease, the 5-year and 10-year disease-specific survival rates after primary treatment with radiation were 49 % and 45 %, respectively. Histologic type was not found to be a predictor of outcome. Milosevic et al. [36] reported no correlation between histologic type and outcome, although their series included only six adenocarcinomas. Although most authors have reported similar outcomes for adenocarcinomas as for other histologies, Grigsby et al. [27] found adenocarcinoma to be a poor prognostic factor for women with urethral cancer. All of these studies are severely limited by the outdated techniques used to treat with radiation. Few if any of the reported cases were treated with the modern, image-based conformal radiation therapy techniques that, when expertly applied, can improve the accuracy, conformality, and homogeneity of external beam treatments. Clinicians are increasingly exploring the use of concurrent chemotherapy for gynecologic cancers (including clear cell carcinomas) treated with definitive radiation therapy, and a few investigators have reported using this approach for urethral cancers [39, 40], but very few data are available to guide the use of such treatment for urethral adenocarcinoma.

Some clinicians have also explored the use of neoadjuvant chemotherapy before surgical resection of urethral carcinomas with encouraging results [37, 41]. However, the number of adenocarcinomas treated in this way is small. Clear cell carcinomas of the ovary are known to respond more poorly to chemotherapy than Müllerian carcinomas of other types [42], but the relevance of this finding to clear cell carcinomas of the urethra is uncertain. However, some urethral adenocarcinomas do respond to cisplatin-based chemotherapy (Fig. 11.1). Hong et al. reported a median time to progression of 8 months for advanced and recurrent urethral adenocarcinomas treated with chemotherapy; they reported one complete response in a patient treated with cisplatin and 5-fluouracil and 4 partial responses in 14 patients treated with various chemotherapy regimens. At least one complete clinical response

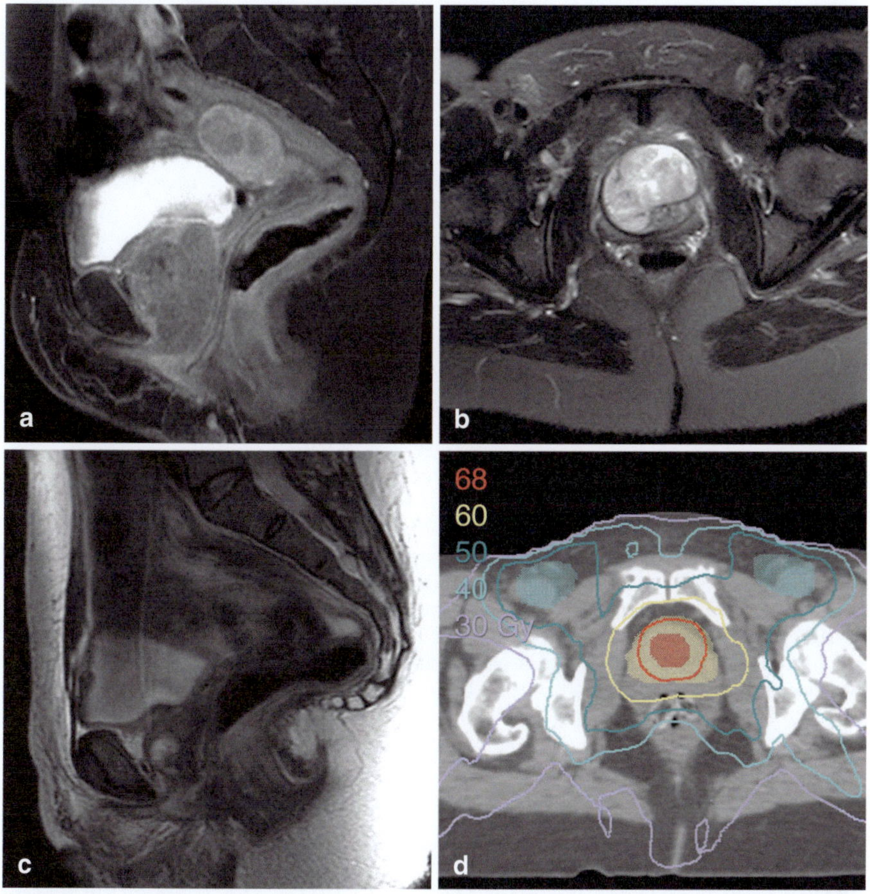

Fig. 11.1 A large T3N0M0 clear cell carcinoma of the urethra in a 60-year-old African-American woman with a past history of a resected urethral diverticulum. The patient presented with acute urinary retention after a several-month history of a weak urine stream. MRI (**a**) showed a 4.5 × 6 cm urethral mass that abutted but did not infiltrate the vaginal wall. She initially received neoadjuvant chemotherapy with cisplatin, paclitaxel, and methotrexate; this was changed to methotrexate, vinblastine, doxorubicin, and cisplatin because of paclitaxel-related neuropathy. After 14 weeks of chemotherapy, her MRI demonstrated an excellent partial response (**c**) and she was referred for radiation therapy. The primary site and inguinal and iliac lymph nodes were treated using intensity-modulated radiation therapy (IMRT) (**d**); she also received concurrent weekly cisplatin. At 4.5 years she has no evidence of disease and normal urinary function

to ifosfamide, carboplatin, and paclitaxel has been reported in a patient with colonic-type carcinoma [16], but data are extremely sparse for this subtype.

The prognosis of recurrent urethral adenocarcinoma is poor, but local recurrences are occasionally salvaged with pelvic exenteration [34] or radiation therapy (Fig. 11.2).

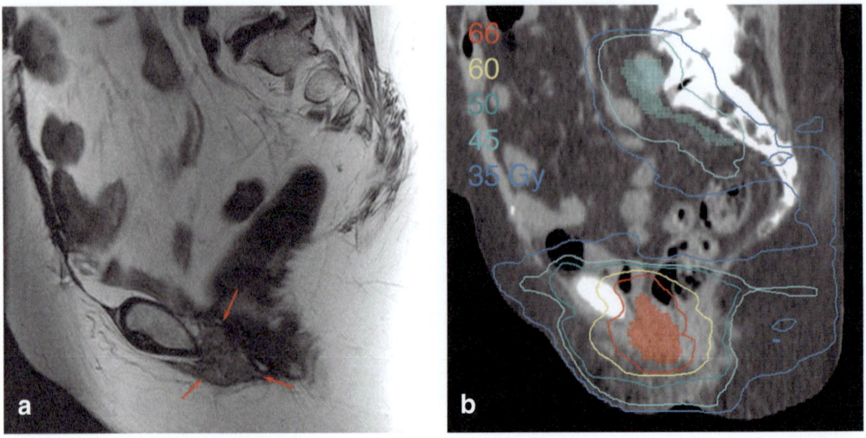

Fig. 11.2 Locally recurrent clear cell carcinoma of the urethra after surgical resection. A 73-year-old woman initially had a 3 cm urethral mass that was treated with cystourethrectomy, ileal conduit formation, and pelvic lymphadenectomy. Clear cell carcinoma involved the periurethral soft tissue, and there was lymphatic space invasion, but the surgical margins and all nodes were negative. Five years later, she noted a mass in the anterior vestibule of the vagina, which was biopsied showing recurrent clear cell carcinoma. On MRI, there was multifocal recurrence with a 3×4 cm mass in the right retropubic soft tissues (**a**) and 1.5×3 cm nodule in the left ischiorectal fossa. The patient was treated with concurrent weekly cisplatin and radiation therapy (**b**). At 2 years, she has no evidence of disease

References

1. Swartz MA, Porter MP, Lin DW, Weiss NS. Incidence of primary urethral carcinoma in the United States. Urology. 2006;68:1164–8.
2. Derksen JW, Visser O, de la Riviere GB, Meuleman EJ, Heldeweg EA, Lagerveld BW. Primary urethral carcinoma in females: an epidemiologic study on demographical factors, histological types, tumour stage and survival. World J Urol. 2013;31:147–53.
3. Gakis G, Witjes JA, Comperat E, et al. EAU guidelines on primary urethral carcinoma. Eur Urol. 2013;64:823–30.
4. Young RH, Scully RE. Clear cell adenocarcinoma of the bladder and urethra. A report of three cases and review of the literature. Am J Surg Pathol. 1985;9:816–26.
5. Sung MT, Zhang S, MacLennan GT, et al. Histogenesis of clear cell adenocarcinoma in the urinary tract: evidence of urothelial origin. Clin Cancer Res. 2008;14:1947–55.
6. Drew PA, Murphy WM, Civantos F, Speights VO. The histogenesis of clear cell adenocarcinoma of the lower urinary tract. Case series and review of the literature. Hum Pathol. 1996;27:248–52.
7. Fadare O, Parkash V, Dupont WD, et al. The diagnosis of endometrial carcinomas with clear cells by gynecologic pathologists: an assessment of interobserver variability and associated morphologic features. Am J Surg Pathol. 2012;36:1107–18.
8. Vang R, Whitaker BP, Farhood AI, Silva EG, Ro JY, Deavers MT. Immunohistochemical analysis of clear cell carcinoma of the gynecologic tract. Int J Gynecol Pathol. 2001;20:252–9.
9. Oliva E, Amin MB, Jimenez R, Young RH. Clear cell carcinoma of the urinary bladder: a report and comparison of four tumors of mullerian origin and nine of probable urothelial origin with discussion of histogenesis and diagnostic problems. Am J Surg Pathol. 2002;26:190–7.

10. Sun K, Huan Y, Unger PD. Clear cell adenocarcinoma of urinary bladder and urethra: another urinary tract lesion immunoreactive for P504S. Arch Pathol Lab Med. 2008;132:1417–22.
11. Brimo F, Herawi M, Sharma R, Netto GJ, Epstein JI, Illei PB. Hepatocyte nuclear factor-1beta expression in clear cell adenocarcinomas of the bladder and urethra: diagnostic utility and implications for histogenesis. Hum Pathol. 2011;42:1613–9.
12. Fadare O, Liang SX, Ulukus EC, Chambers SK, Zheng W. Precursors of endometrial clear cell carcinoma. Am J Surg Pathol. 2006;30:1519–30.
13. Herawi M, Drew PA, Pan CC, Epstein JI. Clear cell adenocarcinoma of the bladder and urethra: cases diffusely mimicking nephrogenic adenoma. Hum Pathol. 2010;41:594–601.
14. Gandhi JS, Khurana A, Tewari A, Mehta A. Clear cell adenocarcinoma of the male urethral tract. Indian J Pathol Microbiol. 2012;55:245–7.
15. Baldi A, Rossiello R, Di Marino M, et al. Colonic type adenocarcinoma of male urethra. In Vivo. 2000;14:487–92.
16. Hale CS, Huang H, Melamed J, et al. Urethral adenocarcinoma associated with intestinal-type metaplasia, case report and literature review. Int J Clin Exp Pathol. 2013;6:1665–70.
17. Heller DS, Merrell M, Sama J, Anderson J, Cracchiolo B. Periurethral vaginal adenocarcinoma of the intestinal type: report of two cases and review of the literature. Gynecol Oncol. 2000;77:478–81.
18. Kato H, Kobayashi S, Islam AM, Nishizawa O. Female para-urethral adenocarcinoma: histological and immunohistochemical study. Int J Urol. 2005;12:117–9.
19. Sebesta EM, Mirheydar HS, Parsons JK, Wang-Rodriguez J, Kader AK. Primary mucin-producing urothelial-type adenocarcinoma of the prostatic urethra diagnosed on TURP: a case report and review of literature. BMC Urol. 2014;14:39.
20. Flynn C, Oxley J, McCullagh P, McCluggage WG. Primary high-grade serous carcinoma arising in the urethra or urethral diverticulum: a report of 2 cases of an extremely rare phenomenon. Int J Gynecol Pathol. 2013;32:141–5.
21. Aydin F. Endometrioid adenocarcinoma of prostatic urethra presenting with anterior urethral implantation. Urology. 1993;41:91–5.
22. Suzuki T, Furuse H, Kurita Y, et al. Long-term survival of metastatic clear cell adenocarcinoma of the female urethra by multidisciplinary treatment: a case report. Nihon Hinyokika Gakkai Zasshi. 2013;104:549–53.
23. Weissbart SJ, Bianco Jr FJ, Sotelo T, Atalla MA, Sesterhenn IA, Jarrett TW. Glassy cell carcinoma of the urethra. Urology. 2009;73:60.
24. Frank SJ, Deavers MT, Jhingran A, Bodurka DC, Eifel PJ. Primary adenocarcinoma of the vagina not associated with diethylstilbestrol (DES) exposure. Gynecol Oncol. 2007;105: 470–4.
25. Chang YH, Chuang CK, Ng KF, Liao SK. Urethral metastasis from a colon carcinoma. Urology. 2007;69:575 e571–3.
26. Bagby CM, MacLennan GT. Clear cell adenocarcinoma of the bladder and urethra. J Urol. 2008;180:2656.
27. Grigsby PW. Carcinoma of the urethra in women. Int J Radiat Oncol Biol Phys. 1998;41:535–41.
28. Hruby G, Choo R, Lehman M, Herschorn S, Kapusta L. Female clear cell adenocarcinoma arising within a urethral diverticulum. Can J Urol. 2000;7:1160–3.
29. Patanaphan V, Prempree T, Sewchand W, Hafiz MA, Jaiwatana J. Adenocarcinoma arising in female urethral diverticulum. Urology. 1983;22:259–64.
30. Thomas AA, Rackley RR, Lee U, Goldman HB, Vasavada SP, Hansel DE. Urethral diverticula in 90 female patients: a study with emphasis on neoplastic alterations. J Urol. 2008;180:2463–7.
31. Touijer AK, Dalbagni G. Role of voided urine cytology in diagnosing primary urethral carcinoma. Urology. 2004;63:33–5.
32. Surabhi VR, Menias CO, George V, Siegel CL, Prasad SR. Magnetic resonance imaging of female urethral and periurethral disorders. Radiol Clin North Am. 2013;51:941–53.
33. Takeuchi M, Matsuzaki K, Nishitani H. Clear cell adenocarcinoma of the female urethra: magnetic resonance imaging. J Comput Assist Tomogr. 2009;33:142–4.

34. Dimarco DS, Dimarco CS, Zincke H, et al. Surgical treatment for local control of female urethral carcinoma. Urol Oncol. 2004;22:404–9.
35. Garden AS, Zagars GK, Delclos L. Primary carcinoma of the female urethra. Results of radiation therapy. Cancer. 1993;71:3102–8.
36. Milosevic MF, Warde PR, Banerjee D, et al. Urethral carcinoma in women: results of treatment with primary radiotherapy. Radiother Oncol. 2000;56:29–35.
37. Dalbagni G, Donat SM, Eschwege P, Herr HW, Zelefsky MJ. Results of high dose rate brachytherapy, anterior pelvic exenteration and external beam radiotherapy for carcinoma of the female urethra. J Urol. 2001;166:1759–61.
38. Koontz BF, Lee WR. Carcinoma of the urethra: radiation oncology. Urol Clin North Am. 2010;37:459–66.
39. Cohen SM. Comparative pathology of proliferative lesions of the urinary bladder. Toxicol Pathol. 2002;30:663–71.
40. Kent M, Zinman L, Girshovich L, Sands J, Vanni A. Combined chemoradiation as primary treatment for invasive male urethral cancer. J Urol. 2015;193:532–7.
41. Dayyani F, Pettaway CA, Kamat AM, Munsell MF, Sircar K, Pagliaro LC. Retrospective analysis of survival outcomes and the role of cisplatin-based chemotherapy in patients with urethral carcinomas referred to medical oncologists. Urol Oncol. 2013;31:1171–7.
42. Heintz AP, Odicino F, Maisonneuve P, et al. Carcinoma of the ovary. FIGO 26th Annual Report on the Results of Treatment in Gynecological Cancer. Int J Gynaecol Obstet. 2006;95 Suppl 1:S161–92.

Primary Urethral Melanoma

12

Austen Slade, Michael Tetzlaff, Van Anh Trinh, Wen-Jen Hwu, and Curtis A. Pettaway

Background

Urethral melanomas are an exceedingly rare malignancy. A recent review of collected patient information over the past 40 years yielded approximately 150 cases [1]. Most of what is known is derived from case reports, with the largest single series to date consisting of only 15 patients [2]. Urethral melanoma arises on a mucosal surface and shares many characteristics with mucosal melanomas at other sites. The overall prognosis tends to be worse when compared to cutaneous melanoma [3]. The difference in prognosis is believed to be multifactorial including delay in presentation or diagnosis, inadequate margins from surgical removal due to anatomic constraints or procedure choice, and the rich lymphatic and vascular supply to the urethra which may aid in early metastatic dissemination [4, 5]. It is important to note that these differences are likely not attributable to the intrinsic biology of urethral melanoma but rather its presentation at a higher stage. We expect that urethral and mucosal melanomas behave similarly when compared at similar stages of presentation.

A. Slade, BS • C.A. Pettaway, MD (✉)
Departments of Urology, The University of Texas MD Anderson Cancer Center, 1515 Holcombe Blvd., Unit 1373, Houston, TX 77030, USA
e-mail: Austen.Slade@uth.tmc.edu; CPettawa@mdanderson.org

M. Tetzlaff, MD, PhD
Department of Pathology, The University of Texas MD Anderson Cancer Center, 1515 Holcombe Blvd., Houston, TX 77030, USA
e-mail: MTetzlaff@mdanderson.org

V.A. Trinh, PharmD • W.-J. Hwu, MD, PhD
Department of Melanoma Medical Oncology, The University of Texas MD Anderson Cancer Center, 1515 Holcombe Blvd., Houston, TX 77030, USA
e-mail: VTrinh@mdanderson.org; WenJHwu@mdanderson.org

L. Pagliaro (ed.), *Rare Genitourinary Tumors*,
DOI 10.1007/978-3-319-30046-7_12

In females, melanomas comprise 5 % of all urethral malignancies with an incidence of roughly 1.5 per million [3]. Melanoma of the urethra is three times more common in women than in men; the overall incidence in both men and women is less than 1.5 per million [1, 2]. When considering all melanomas, mucosal melanoma represents less than 1 % [1–3]. Approximately 50 % of mucosal melanomas arise from the head and neck region, 25 % begin in the anorectal region and 20 % in the female genital tract [6]. The rarity of melanoma in the urethra is likely to be at least partially attributed to the embryologic origins of the urethra, which arises from endoderm, compared to the ectodermal origins of the skin that give rise to cutaneous melanomas [1]. Among females, the higher concentration of melanocytes in the area of the vulvar mucosa may in part explain why melanoma is more common in females than males [1].

Etiology

Little is known about the etiology of urethral melanomas. The relative rarity of urethral melanoma makes identifying the risk factors for the disease all the more challenging [7]. In contrast to its cutaneous counterpart, sun exposure is not a risk factor for urethral melanoma [3]. Aside from there being a higher occurrence in women, urethral melanomas also predominately occur in the white race [7]. Interestingly, BRAF, a serine/threonine kinase which has been shown to be mutated in 66 % of cutaneous malignant melanomas, is rarely mutated in mucosal and urethral melanomas [7, 8]. Conversely, c-KIT, a tyrosine kinase mutated in only 5 % of cutaneous melanomas, has a mutation rate of 15–20 % in mucosal melanomas and has emerged as a rational target for systemic therapies [9].

Presentation, Natural History, and Survival

The most common symptom leading to presentation is a urethral mass [1, 3]. Other symptoms include dysuria, local bleeding, hematuria, incontinence, and pain (Table 12.1) [1, 3, 4, 9]. As previously stated, patients often present with advanced disease [1, 3]. Indeed, one study found the mean delay from onset of symptoms to presentation to be 2 years [2]. This delay likely contributes to the fact that 50 % of patients have metastases at diagnosis [1] and have a mean thickness of melanoma at presentation of 7.1 mm which correlates with advanced stage (i.e., stage T4), metastases, and decreased survival [3, 10]. Common sites of metastasis in decreasing frequency include inguinal lymph nodes, lungs, central nervous system, and bones [1, 2]. Tumor sizes generally range from 0.8 to 6.0 cm with a mean size of 2.6 cm in the largest dimension [2]. The most common location of urethral melanomas in both males and females is at the meatus followed by the distal urethra [1–4, 11].

Late presentation has an adverse effect on survival; most patients do not survive beyond 3 years [2]. One study of 11 female patients found the overall and disease-specific survival at 3 years to be 27 % and 38 %, respectively [4]. A large review that

Table 12.1 Common presenting symptoms in males versus females

Males	Females
Palpable tumor, hematuria, bleeding, dysuria, obstruction, urethral pain, and incontinence	Hematuria, obstruction, spraying urinary stream, dysuria, and pain

included case reports of 112 female patients found the 5-year survival to be 10 % [3]. The reported median survival varies between around 1.5–2 years. El-Safadi et al. reported a median survival of 25.6 months, with only 12 patients alive beyond 4 years [1].

Average recurrence-free interval among all urethral melanoma patients has been estimated to be around 12.5 months [1]. Little is known about prognostic factors that predict survival; however, similar to its cutaneous counterpart, tumor thickness has been shown to influence prognosis [1]. Tumor thickness less than 2 mm is associated with better survival [2]. Unfortunately due to the prominent vertical growth phase found in most urethral melanoma, thickness >2 mm is more the rule than the exception [2]. Up to 71 % of patients with urethral melanoma will recur after initial surgery, and when they do, El-Safadi et al. found 55 % recur locally and 28 % recur as metastases in the inguinal lymph nodes, 38 % in the lungs, and 6 % in the bones [1, 11]. The same study also showed that surgical treatment of recurrence positively influenced survival and should be performed in eligible patients [1].

Tumor Characteristics and Pathologic Features

One of the challenges of diagnosing urethral melanomas is up to 25% are amelanotic and, thus, do not always share the hyper-pigment features typical of cutaneous melanoma [3]. Even when pigmentation is evident, there are also benign pigmented skin and mucosal lesions that may appear in the urethra that should be considered in evaluating a pigmented urethral lesion. These include genital lentiginosis, atypical lentiginous melanocytic hyperplasia, and melanocytic nevi of the genital type [2]. Of note, a diagnosis of atypical melanocytic hyperplasia/proliferation should be pursued in the context of the clinical presentation. In particular, if the biopsy represents a small portion of a larger pigmented lesion, additional biopsies or a complete excision should be considered to exclude melanoma. Furthermore, urethral melanomas only rarely arise in association with a preexisting nevus [2]. Urethral melanomas are frequently polypoid in appearance, leading to confusion with urethral polyps, caruncles, mucosal prolapse, or other tumors, including urothelial carcinoma [2].

Urethral melanomas often exhibit an intraepithelial pattern of growth reminiscent of that seen in acral lentiginous melanomas [12]. Namely, the epithelium often exhibits variable hyperplasia (Fig 12.1a). Within this hyperplastic epithelium, there is a contiguous proliferation of mostly single and occasionally nested melanocytes along the basilar epithelium. At its apex, these melanocytes can entirely replace the basilar epithelium. Upward pagetoid migration is frequently seen

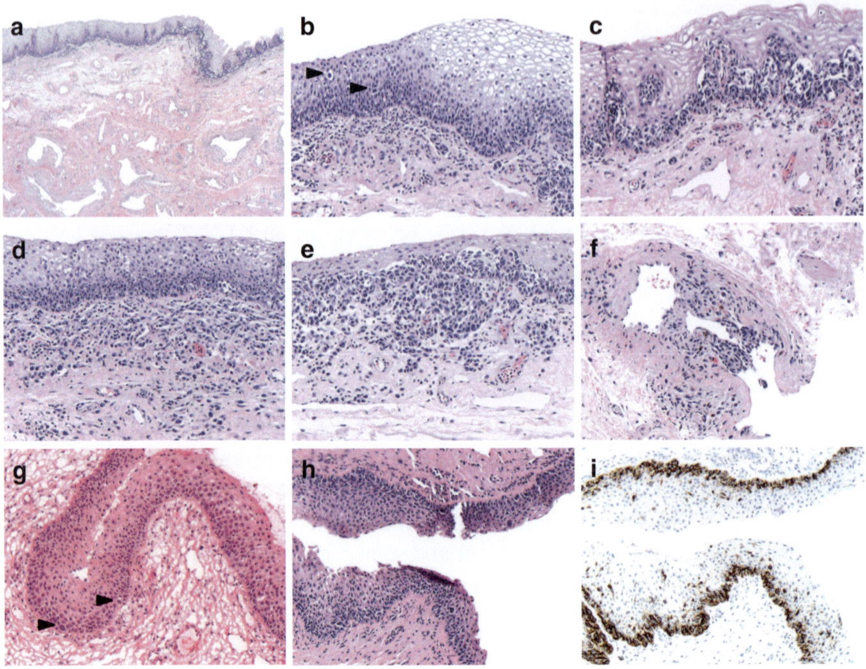

Fig. 12.1 Histopathologic features of urethral melanoma. (**a**) Low-power examination reveals urethral mucosa and subjacent rich vascular tissue (H&E, 4×). (**b**, **c**) There is a disorganized, continuous proliferation of single and nested melanocytes replacing the basilar epithelium (**c**) with focal areas of upward pagetoid migration (*arrows*; H&E, 100×). (**d**, **e**) Invasive melanoma consisting of atypical epithelioid melanocytes infiltrating the submucosa (H **c**: 100×, **d**: 200×). (**b**) Lymphovascular invasion by tumor cells. (**g**) Frozen section evaluation of urethral margin en face reveals only rare atypical epithelioid cells difficult to distinguish from surrounding epithelial cells (*arrows*; H&E, 100×). (**h**) Permanent section of same urethral melanoma margin reveals conspicuous melanoma in situ (H&E, 100×). (**i**) An immunohistochemical study on the same specimen using an anti-melanocytic cocktail (HMB45 and anti-tyrosinase) highlights the confluent intraepithelial proliferation of single and nested melanocytes along the basilar epithelium and confirms the diagnosis of melanoma in situ at the en face urethral margin (100×)

(Fig. 12.1b–f). The melanocytes typically exhibit prominent cytologic atypia including increased amphophilic cytoplasm and enlarged, irregular nuclei with prominent nucleoli. Two features of in situ urethral melanomas merit particular emphasis. First, frozen section evaluation can be challenging because the diagnostic features which are readily identified following formalin fixation and paraffin embedding are typically not apparent on frozen section slides (Fig. 12.1.g–i). Second, peripheral aspects of in situ mucosal melanomas may exhibit more subtle features than that seen toward the center of the lesion [13, 14]. These features emphasize the importance of avoiding frozen section analysis for marginal assessment as well as the need to perform multiple mucosal biopsies for accurate diagnosis and effective transparent communication with the pathologist regarding clinical features (e.g., size, color, borders).

Most invasive urethral melanomas display a vertical growth phase and may also have a prominent nodular architecture [2]. The invasive component may exhibit a wide histologic spectrum including diffuse, nested, fascicular, or storiform proliferations of usually markedly pleomorphic variably epithelioid and/or spindled tumor cells [2, 15]. In our experience, examination of mucosal melanoma resection specimens often reveals an associated lichenoid lymphohistiocytic inflammatory infiltrate, and the tendency for lymphohistiocytic exocytosis into the overlying squamous mucosa is an important mimic and pitfall, necessitating immunohistochemical characterization to exclude a melanocytic proliferation—especially when evaluating en face margins.

The histopathologic differential diagnosis most often confronted in mucosal sites is urothelial carcinoma. This is particularly true when lesions are either poorly differentiated with a solid growth pattern if there is papillary architecture (or a pseudopapillary pattern) and the cells are devoid of melanin [2]. Urethral melanoma may also resemble a small cell carcinoma although this would most likely have originated in the bladder or prostate with secondary involvement into the urethra [16]. A variety of immunohistochemical stains are available to confirm melanocytic differentiation including antibodies for S-100, Sox-10, HMB-45, and melan A. Together with cytokeratins and GATA-3, these stains may be necessary for distinguishing among cancer types [17].

Evaluation

Primary Urethral Tumor in Males and Females

It is critical to establish whether the urethral site represents the primary tumor or a metastasis from another site such as the bladder or regional spread from the vulva or vagina. As such, a thorough examination is essential for establishing the origin of the neoplasm and guiding subsequent treatment [2]. Many of the presenting symptoms such as hematuria and dysuria can be nonspecific, making a thorough initial evaluation all the more important.

Borrowing from the experience of patients with urethral carcinoma, the recommended process of evaluation in both males and females begins with a genital examination, seeking to identify protruding lesions or masses. A careful examination of the inguinal lymph nodes should follow, as clinical involvement carries important prognostic and therapeutic implications. Next, patients must undergo cystourethroscopy with biopsy of random sites along the urethra and bladder to map the extent of disease. Additionally, any other pigmented lesions in the area should also be biopsied to determine their histology and potential relationship to the index melanoma lesion. An exam under anesthesia in order to define the local extent of disease is an important part of the examination to determine the size of the lesion as well as involvement of surrounding structures [18]. Cross-sectional imaging of the pelvis and urethra with MRI is particularly useful in defining soft tissue anatomy and locoregional extent of disease at diagnosis [18].

Evaluation of Inguinal Region, Pelvis, and Distant Sites

Inguinal Palpation

Understanding the patterns of urethral lymphatic drainage plays an integral role in evaluating lymph node status. In males, preprostatic, prostatic, and membranous urethras correspond to lymphatic drainage of the prostate, which drains into pelvic lymph nodes associated with the iliac vessels and obturator fossa. Distally, the penile urethra and glans drain into the inguinal and subinguinal lymph nodes [9, 19]. In females, the proximal two thirds of the urethra drains to internal iliac (hypogastric) lymph nodes, whereas the distal one third drains to inguinal and subinguinal lymph nodes [20]. Given the extent of urethral lymphatic drainage depending on tumor location, inguinal palpation may detect some but not all involved nodes requiring additional techniques for complete evaluation.

Dynamic Sentinel Lymph Node Biopsy

The role of dynamic sentinel lymph node biopsy (DSNB) in the evaluation of urethral melanoma remains a controversial and largely unexplored topic. Unlike cutaneous melanoma where DSNB is recommended in all lesions >1 mm and selected pT1 lesions (lesions <1 mm with high-risk histopathologic features, including those with thickness >0.75, ulceration, mitotic figures, extensive regression, and thin lesions that are transected at the biopsy base), definite guidelines for the recommended use of DSNB sampling in urethral melanoma are lacking [21, 22]. Several studies and case reports have identified patients who underwent DSNB, but it was unclear if the information generated by DSNB improved the prognosis or enhanced survival [3, 4, 11, 23]. Currently, several authors believe that DSNB is technically feasible for urethral melanoma, may improve staging of the disease, and is preferred to inguinal lymph node dissection to limit morbidity [3, 11]. DSNB is known to improve survival in penile carcinoma over surveillance among patients with clinically negative nodes. Therefore, it is reasonable but as yet unproven to expect similar results in urethral melanoma [4, 24].

Ultrasound

The use of ultrasound for detecting lymph node involvement in cutaneous melanoma patients has been shown to have a sensitivity and specificity of 20–34 % and 87–90 %, respectively, and 4.7 % and 100 %, respectively, when combined with fine-needle aspiration [25, 26]. Although ultrasound can be used to identify involved lymph nodes, thus avoiding costlier and more invasive DSNB, its poor sensitivity limits its routine use. Therefore, ultrasound and biopsy of suspicious inguinal nodes are of benefit when metastases are discovered but negative results do not preclude DSNB. While the use of ultrasound in patients with urethral melanoma has yet to be studied, it likely shares a limited role as seen in cutaneous melanoma.

CT or CT/PET

Imaging with CT and PET and brain MRI are recommended prior to surgical management and allow for more accurate staging [3, 18]. Given the often-delayed presentation of urethral melanomas, these imaging modalities allow for the evaluation of potential occult metastatic lesions in regional or distant nodal sites, lung, bone, and brain.

Staging

Whereas the prognosis of cutaneous melanoma is based largely on tumor thickness together with the presence of ulceration (for all lesions) or dermal mitotic figures (for pT1 lesions only), studies in urethral melanoma report conflicting information over its utility; however, the largest study to date shows thickness can be a prognostic factor [1–3, 27]. Improvement in survival has been noted for tumor thickness <2.0 mm, but these superficial tumors are rare in the urethra (mean thickness 7.1 mm) [2–4]. Nevertheless, we recommend application of the cutaneous staging system for the present time because of its superior ability to predict prognosis [10]. It is clear that a national registry of collected cases would be of tremendous value in determining the optimal staging method for this rare tumor (Table 12.2).

Treatment

With no established criteria on the surgical management of urethral melanoma, patients have undergone a wide variety of procedures with little data on their survival benefit. Margins of 2–2.5 cm are generally agreed upon in the literature to establish local control [3, 4]. Achieving adequate margins often requires extensive procedures in both males and females but remains an important step as failure to do so may result in up to 70 % rate of local recurrence [3]. While determining the presence of melanoma in situ at surgical resection margins is unreliable by frozen section, assessing the margin to rule out invasive melanoma is feasible and can allow the surgeon to remove additional tissue as needed.

Treatment of Primary Tumor

Surgical Management of the Primary Tumor in Males

Of the 50 procedures in males reported by El-Safadi et al. [1], 21 (42 %) underwent penectomy, 17 (34 %) partial penectomy, 7 (14 %) prostatectomy, and 6 (12 %) cystectomy with a median overall survival of 23.1 months. In a review by Papes et al. [9] among 14 patients with distal urethral melanoma who survived for 5 years, the median tumor thickness was 2 mm. These patients were treated with organ-sparing approaches including urethrectomy, partial urethrectomy, or partial penectomy with established local control; however, lesions >2 mm, which are more common, require more aggressive management [9, 23]. Although one study showed no survival benefit in radical procedures (i.e., anterior pelvic exenteration) versus less radical (local excision, partial or total urethrectomy), achieving adequate margins often requires a

Table 12.2 Cutaneous melanoma TNM classification system [12, 34]

T classification		
	Thickness	Ulceration status
T1	≤1.0 mm	(a) Without ulceration and level II/III
		(b) With ulceration or level IV/V
T2	1.01–2.0 mm	(a) Without ulceration
		(b) With ulceration
T3	2. 01–4.0 mm	(a) Without ulceration
		(b) With ulceration
T4	>4.0 mm	(a) Without ulceration
		(b) With ulceration

N classification		
	No. of metastatic nodes	Nodal metastatic mass
N1	One node	(a) Micrometastasis
		(b) Macrometastasis
N2	Two to three nodes	(a) Micrometastasis
		(b) Macrometastasis
N3	Four or more metastatic nodes or matted nodes or in-transit metastases/satellite(s) with metastatic node(s)	(a) Micrometastasis
		(b) Macrometastasis
		(c) In-transit metastases/satellite(s) without metastatic nodes

M classification		
	Site	Serum LDH
M1a	Distant skin, subcutaneous tissue, or nodal metastases	Normal
M1b	Lung metastases	Normal
M1c	All other visceral metastases	Normal
	Any distant metastasis	Elevated

more radical approach as in the case of melanomas located in the proximal penile, bulbar, or prostatic urethra [9, 23]. Figure 12.2 outlines a suggested surgical management of melanoma involving the male urethra. In the latter scenarios where debilitating surgery is considered to achieve negative margins, systemic therapy should also be considered as an initial approach. This is especially true where clinical trial participation is available (see discussion on systemic therapy).

Surgical Management of the Primary Tumor in Females

Among the 56 procedures in females reported by El-Safadi et al., 27 (48 %) underwent excision and total urethrectomy and 21 (38 %) received partial urethrectomy, 14 (25 %) cystectomy, and 12 (21 %) vulvectomy with median overall of 28.6 months [1]. In general, wide local excisions have shown similar results as more radical approaches while having decreased morbidities [3]. One study found that none of

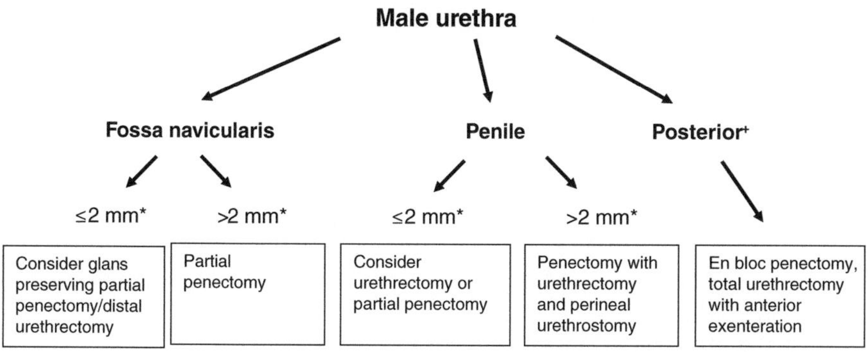

Fig. 12.2 Surgical management of male urethral melanoma (Adapted from Sanchez-Ortiz et al.) * Tumor thickness. + Includes bulbar, prostatomembranous urethra. For lesions <2mm, total urethrectomy with en bloc prostatectomy sparing the bladder and penis may be considered

the female patients who underwent partial urethrectomy experienced recurrence in the bladder, suggesting cystectomy may not be necessary [2, 4]. Rather than cystectomy, when indicated, DiMarco et al. proposed radical urethrectomy with bladder preservation and a continent catheterizable stoma as a more appropriate option [4]. The proposed procedure would include excision of the bladder neck, periurethral tissues, anterior vagina, and labia to achieve a negative surgical margin [4].

In some women, depending on the location within the urethra, cystourethrectomy and lymph node dissection or pelvic exenteration may be necessary to achieve adequate margins. However, if initial bladder neck biopsies performed at the time of disease assessment are free of tumor, we prefer to attempt to preserve the bladder and will assess the bladder neck margin at surgery using frozen section. In this setting, the margin is assessed for invasive melanoma only since melanoma in situ is not efficaciously addressed at frozen section (see tumor characteristics and pathologic features). If the findings at frozen section are not suspicious for invasive melanoma, the bladder will be spared. If the margin is suspicious at surgery, we will remove the bladder or take a second wide margin if feasible. Radical procedures are contraindicated when inguinal metastases are present or with large tumors found be to invading adjacent organs given the poor prognosis for such patients [3]. In this setting (as in male patients with advanced melanoma), we recommend neoadjuvant systemic therapy preferably in the context of a clinical trial as an initial approach. Figure 12.3 is a suggested approach for surgical management of the primary tumor.

Radiation Management of Primary Tumor

The role of radiation-based treatments is unknown as its use is limited to a few isolated cases with little known about the tumor thickness or stage of disease prior to treatment [2]. The data available so far has found radiation to be an ineffective primary treatment method [3, 4]. Although postoperative adjuvant radiation has been found to reduce local recurrence in desmoplastic subtype of cutaneous melanoma, its benefit in urethral melanoma has yet to be shown [2, 28].

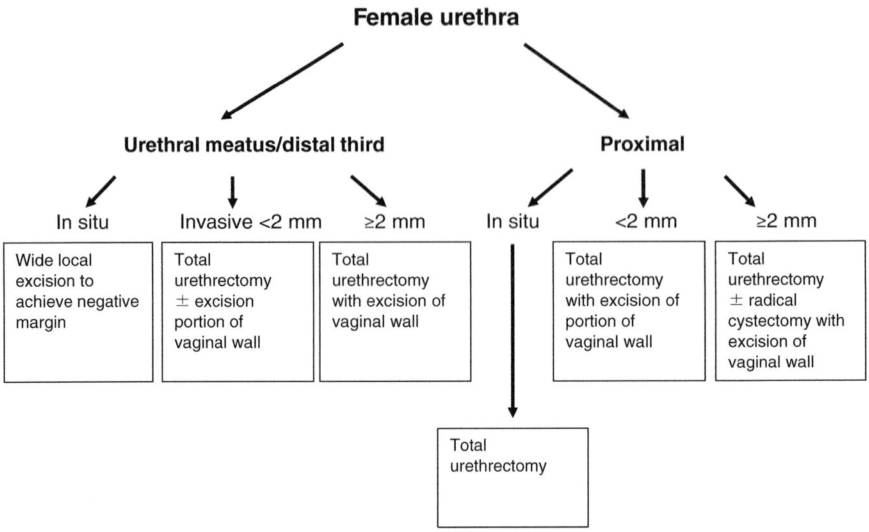

Fig. 12.3 Surgical management of female urethral melanoma

Treatment of the Inguinal Nodes

Surgical Management

Prophylactic lymph node dissection is not recommended in patients with clinically negative nodes [29]. DSNB has significantly affected the management of clinically node-negative patients with cutaneous melanoma where the survival among patients with microscopic lymph node metastases found subsequent to DSNB is superior to patients with clinically discovered lymph node metastases [10]. In addition, DSNB in clinically node-negative penile cancer has been shown to have a disease-specific 3-year survival advantage of 91 % over 79 % for surveillance [22]. Some authors have suggested that such a benefit could also be realized in urethral melanoma and have recommended DSNB as a procedure to stage the inguinal region in all patients with invasive urethral melanoma [4, 11].

In patients with palpable inguinal nodes, the decision to perform inguinal versus ilioinguinal lymph node dissection is a common dilemma. For cutaneous melanoma patients with suspected inguinal metastases, guidelines from the United Kingdom (UK) recommend inguinal dissection if there is a single clinically involved inguinal or femoral triangle node or a single positive superficial inguinal sentinel node [30]. According to the same guidelines, ilioinguinal dissection is recommended if there is more than one palpable metastatic inguinal node, radiological evidence of more than one metastatic inguinal node or at least one pelvic node metastasis, a conglomerate of inguinal metastatic nodes, or involvement of Cloquet's node [30].

Some have argued palpable inguinal nodes are commonly associated with pelvic nodal metastasis. Therefore, given the poor prediction of nodal involvement by CT, ilioinguinal dissection should be offered to these patients [31]. One study found the

5-year overall survival to be just 12 % in patients with palpable inguinal nodes that underwent ilioinguinal dissection, making the case that these dissections should be reserved for patients with radiologic evidence of pelvic involvement [32]. Routine ilioinguinal dissections would also lead to a substantial number of patients with no pelvic nodal involvement undergoing this more invasive procedure, which carries a higher morbidity versus inguinal dissection alone [32].

More recently, another study from the United Kingdom found that among patients presenting with palpable adenopathy, the 5-year survival in patients with cutaneous melanoma metastasis in the inguinal nodes alone was 51 and 28 % when both inguinal and pelvic nodes were involved [33]. Of note, the sensitivity of CT scan was only 57 %. Thus, this study provides evidence that prophylactic pelvic dissection may be worthwhile in patients with palpable inguinal adenopathy. Pelvic dissection provides important prognostic information, and with recent advances in systemic therapy, survival in the future may improve. Given these findings, we suggest that it is reasonable to offer pelvic dissection in patients with palpable inguinal adenopathy from urethral melanoma.

Treatment of Advanced Disease

The rarity of urethral and/or mucosal melanoma makes the performance of prospective randomized trials to assess treatment effects in patients with these melanoma subtypes challenging. Guidelines directing the decision to offer systemic treatment to patients with advanced mucosal melanoma are mostly extrapolated from the experience of the management of cutaneous melanoma, factoring in the limited data from a few retrospective or non-randomized studies in small groups of patients with mucosal histology.

Resected High-Risk Disease

The standard-of-care adjuvant options in patients with resected high-risk cutaneous melanoma included high-dose interferon alfa-2b (HDI) or pegylated interferon alfa-2b (PEG-IFN). Recently, adjuvant ipilimumab, an anti-cytotoxic T-lymphocyte antigen 4 (CTLA-4) monoclonal antibody, has demonstrated a relapse-free survival (RFS) advantage when compared with observation [35]. However, none of these adjuvant trials enrolled patients with mucosal melanoma [35–37].

At present, information on the efficacy of adjuvant therapy in patients with mucosal melanoma is confined to a randomized phase II study comparing HDI with cisplatin plus temozolomide chemotherapy. A total of 189 Asian patients with resected high-risk mucosal melanoma were randomly assigned into three groups: observation (group A), HDI for a year (group B), and cisplatin-temozolomide combination for six cycles (group C). At a median follow-up of 26.8 months, the median RFS were 5.4, 9.4, and 20.8 months in groups A, B, and C, respectively. Both adjuvant treatment options were superior to observation in terms of RFS ($p<0.001$ for both comparisons). When evaluating groups B and C, chemotherapy significantly improved RFS as compared with HDI ($p<0.001$). The median overall survival (OS) was 21.2 months in group A, 40.4 months in group B, and 48.7 months in group C. Comparison between groups B and C also revealed an OS advantage favoring chemotherapy ($p=0.009$). However, subgroup analyses suggested that the survival impact associated with chemotherapy appeared less prominent in patients with anorectal or genitourinary primary as compared with those with head and neck primary [38]. Despite the positive result of this phase II randomized study, the role of adjuvant chemotherapy in patients with resected high-risk mucosal melanoma requires larger phase III confirmatory study.

Unresectable or Metastatic Disease

Much progress in the development of systemic therapies for patients with unresectable or metastatic melanoma of cutaneous origin has recently been achieved with the advent of novel immunotherapies, e.g., the anti-CTLA4 and anti-programmed cell death-1 (PD-1) monoclonal antibodies, and targeted therapies targeting the mutation-driven constitutive activation of the mitogen-activated protein kinase (MAPK) pathway.

Immune Checkpoint Blockade Therapy

Since its approval by regulatory agencies worldwide, ipilimumab has become a standard treatment option for patients with unresectable or metastatic cutaneous melanoma, demonstrating a response rate of 10–15 % and a median OS of 10–11 months in both frontline and second-line settings [39, 40]. However, the only data on the efficacy of ipilimumab in patients with advanced mucosal melanoma were from retrospective analyses. Three reports of ipilimumab experience in the United States, Italian expanded access program, and Australia indicated clinical activity of this agent in advanced mucosal melanoma, with a response rate of 7–11 % per immune-related response criteria and a median OS of approximately 6 months [41–43]. Although these results are numerically inferior to those achieved in cutaneous melanoma, single-agent ipilimumab appears active against advanced mucosal melanoma, thus warrants further investigations.

The anti-PD-1 monoclonal antibodies, e.g., pembrolizumab and nivolumab, with more robust clinical activity and favorable safety profile compared with ipilimumab, have emerged as the standard front- and second-line therapy for patients with advanced melanoma of cutaneous origin [44]. Although the clinical trials evaluating the anti-PD-1 antibodies did not provide any specific efficacy and safety data in patients with mucosal melanoma, the study investigating nivolumab against investigators' choice of chemotherapy in patients with advanced melanoma whose disease progressed after ipilimumab, and if BRAF V600 mutation positive, a BRAF inhibitor, did include 11 % patients with mucosal melanoma [45]. At present, little is known regarding the efficacy of these novel immunotherapies in advanced mucosal melanoma except for a few case reports [46, 47] demonstrating anti-melanoma activity. The efficacy and safety profiles of the anti-PD-1 antibodies will need to be prospectively evaluated in patients with advanced mucosal melanoma.

Small-Molecule Targeted Therapy

For patients with advanced mutated *BRAF* V600 melanoma (approximately 45–50 % cutaneous melanoma), dual MAPK pathway blockade with combined BRAF and MEK inhibitors has been shown superior to BRAF inhibitor monotherapy in terms of response rate, progression-free survival (PFS), and OS [48, 49]. Adverse events secondary to paradoxical MAPK pathway activation by BRAF inhibitor are also reduced with combination therapy. Thus, the combination of BRAF and MEK inhibitors is an effective therapeutic option for patients with advanced mutated *BRAF* V600 melanoma, especially those who have rapidly progressing disease. However, the infrequent occurrence of *BRAF* mutations in mucosal melanoma limits the utility of this active regimen.

In contrast to *BRAF V600* mutation, *KIT* gene aberrations, i.e., mutations or amplifications, are more prevalent in mucosal melanoma. Therefore, targeting KIT kinase using small-molecule inhibitors is a sound therapeutic strategy. Three phase II studies have examined the efficacy and safety of imatinib, an inhibitor of KIT kinase, in patients with advanced melanoma harboring *KIT* mutations and/or amplifications [50].

In the study by Carvajal et al., imatinib 400 mg orally twice a day produced a durable response rate of 16 % (95 % CI, 2–30 %), with a median time to progression of 12 weeks (95 % CI, 11–18 weeks) and a median OS of 46.3 weeks (95 % CI, 28 weeks-not reached), in 25 evaluable patients with advanced *KIT*-mutated or *KIT*-amplified melanoma of mucosal, acral, or chronically sun-damaged cutaneous origin. Of note, objective responses seemed to cluster in tumors with L576P or K642E mutations or those with a mutant to wild-type allelic ratio of greater than 1 [51].

Two other studies evaluating imatinib 400 mg orally daily, with provision for dose increase to 600–800 mg per day at disease progression, reached similar clinical findings in comparable patient populations. Overall response rates ranged 23–29 %, with median time to progression of 3.5–3.7 months and median OS of 12.5–14.0 months [52, 53]. Mutations in *KIT* exons 11 or 13 appeared to predict clinical response to imatinib in one study, whereas *KIT* amplifications were correlated with low likelihood of response to imatinib in the other trial.

Combination Chemotherapy and Biochemotherapy

Evidence of the antitumor activity of chemo- and biochemotherapy in patients with advanced mucosal melanoma mostly originated from small retrospective studies. In the frontline and second-line settings, dacarbazine-containing combinations generated an overall response rate of 26.3 % and a median OS of 12.1 months in 95 patients with advanced melanoma of non-cutaneous origin, 22.1 % of whom had mucosal primaries in the gastrointestinal or genitourinary tracts [54]. Likewise, biochemotherapy (a combination of dacarbazine, vinblastine, cisplatin, interferon alfa-2b, interleukin-2) demonstrated robust clinical activity as both first- and second-line therapies in patients with advanced mucosal melanoma arising from the head and neck, vulvovaginal, or anorectal area, with response rates in the range of 30–40 % and median OS durations of 10–22 months [55–57].

In the salvage setting after a median of three prior systemic chemotherapeutic regimens, carboplatin-paclitaxel was shown effective in a retrospective study involving 32 patients, among whom ten had advanced mucosal melanoma. This heavily pretreated group of patients achieved an overall response rate of 21.9 % and a median OS of 5.2 months with the combination [58]. There were no statistically significant differences in response rates, PFS, and OS between patients with cutaneous and non-cutaneous melanoma.

Collectively, the aforementioned systemic treatments represent a valuable addition to the therapeutic arsenal for advanced mucosal melanoma; nevertheless, the survival impact of current systemic options remains limited in this patient subset. Thus, if appropriate, patients should be encouraged to participate in clinical trials evaluating new treatment strategies. For those who cannot take part in clinical trials, systemic therapy should be individualized according to patient- and disease-specific factors, such as mutation status, symptomatology, and disease tempo. Without sufficient evidence, it is difficult to determine with certainty the best therapeutic sequence.

Conclusion

Treatment decision for patients with advanced mucosal melanoma, specifically those with urethral melanoma, should be individualized by a multidisciplinary team of health-care professionals with skills and expertise in treating mucosal melanoma.

References

1. El-Safadi S, Estel R, Mayser P, Muenstedt K. Primary malignant melanoma of the urethra: a systematic analysis of the current literature. Arch Gynecol Obstet. 2014;289(5):935–43.
2. Oliva E, Quinn TR, Amin MB, Eble JN, Epstein JI, Srigley JR, et al. Primary malignant melanoma of the urethra: a clinicopathologic analysis of 15 cases. Am J Surg Pathol. 2000;24(6):785–96.
3. Papes D, Altarac S. Melanoma of the female urethra. Med Oncol. 2013;30(1):329-012-0329-2. Epub 2012 Dec 18.
4. DiMarco DS, DiMarco CS, Zincke H, Webb MJ, Keeney GL, Bass S, et al. Outcome of surgical treatment for primary malignant melanoma of the female urethra. J Urol. 2004;171(2 Pt 1):765–7.
5. Nguyen AT, Kavolius JP, Russo P, Grimaldi G, Katz J, Brady MS. Primary genitourinary melanoma. Urology. 2001;57(4):633–8.
6. Chang AE, et al. The National Cancer Data Base report on cutaneous and noncutaneous melanoma: a summary of 84,836 cases from the past decade. The American College of Surgeons Commission on Cancer and the American Cancer Society. Cancer. 1998;83(8):1664–78.
7. Seetharamu N, Ott PA, Pavlick AC. Mucosal melanomas: a case-based review of the literature. Oncologist. 2010;15(7):772–81.
8. Davies H, Bignell GR, Cox C, Stephens P, Edkins S, Clegg S, et al. Mutations of the BRAF gene in human cancer. Nature. 2002;417(6892):949–54.

9. Papes D, Altarac S, Arslani N, Rajkovic Z, Antabak A, Cacic M. Melanoma of the glans penis and urethra. Urology. 2014;83(1):6–11.
10. Balch CM, Soong SJ, Atkins MB, Buzaid AC, Cascinelli N, Coit DG, et al. An evidence-based staging system for cutaneous melanoma. CA Cancer J Clin. 2004;54(3):131–49. quiz 182–4.
11. van Geel AN, den Bakker MA, Kirkels W, Horenblas S, Kroon BB, de Wilt JH, et al. Prognosis of primary mucosal penile melanoma: a series of 19 Dutch patients and 47 patients from the literature. Urology. 2007;70(1):143–7.
12. Elder DE, Jucovy PM, Tuthill RJ, Clark Jr WH. The classification of malignant melanoma. Am J Dermatopathol. 1980;2(4):315–20.
13. Paladugu RR, Winberg CD, Yonemoto RH. Acral lentiginous melanoma. A clinicopathologic study of 36 patients. Cancer. 1983;52(1):161–8.
14. Oldbring J, Mikulowski P. Malignant melanoma of the penis and male urethra. Report of nine cases and review of the literature. Cancer. 1987;59(3):581–7.
15. Morita T, Suzuki H, Goto K, Hirota N, Tokue A. Primary malignant melanoma of male urethra with fistula formation. Urol Int. 1991;46(1):114–5.
16. Bostwick DG, Eble JN. Neoplasms of the prostate. Urol Surg Pathol. 1 ed. St. Louis: Mosby-Yearbook Inc. 1997;373–5.
17. Tetzlaff MT, Torres-Cabala CA, Pattanaprichakul P, Rapini RP, Prieto VG, Curry JL. Emerging clinical applications of selected biomarkers in melanoma. Clin Cosmet Investig Dermatol. 2015;8:35–46.
18. Dayyani F, Hoffman K, Eifel P, Guo C, Vikram R, Pagliaro LC, et al. Management of advanced primary urethral carcinomas. BJU Int. 2014;114(1):25–31.
19. Wood HM, Angermeier KW. Anatomic considerations of the penis, lymphatic drainage, and biopsy of the sentinel node. Urol Clin North Am. 2010;37(3):327–34.
20. McAninch JW, Lue TF. Smith & Tanagho's general urology. 18th ed. New York: McGraw-Hill; 2013. p. 14–5.
21. Bichakjian CK, Halpern AC, Johnson TM, Foote Hood A, Grichnik JM, Swetter SM, et al. Guidelines of care for the management of primary cutaneous melanoma. American Academy of Dermatology. J Am Acad Dermatol. 2011;65(5):1032–47.
22. Johnson TM, Bradford CR, Gruber SB, Sondak VK, Schwartz JL. Staging workup, sentinel node biopsy, and follow-up tests for melanoma: update of current concepts. Arch Dermatol. 2004;140(1):107–13.
23. Sanchez-Ortiz R, Huang SF, Tamboli P, Prieto VG, Hester G, Pettaway CA. Melanoma of the penis, scrotum and male urethra: a 40-year single institution experience. J Urol. 2005;173(6):1958–65.
24. Lont AP, Horenblas S, Tanis PJ, Gallee MP, van Tinteren H, Nieweg OE. Management of clinically node negative penile carcinoma: improved survival after the introduction of dynamic sentinel node biopsy. J Urol. 2003;170(3):783–6.
25. Sibon C, Chagnon S, Tchakerian A, Bafounta ML, Longvert C, Clerici T, et al. The contribution of high-resolution ultrasonography in preoperatively detecting sentinel-node metastases in melanoma patients. Melanoma Res. 2007;17(4):233–7.
26. van Rijk MC, Teertstra HJ, Peterse JL, Nieweg OE, Olmos RA, Hoefnagel CA, et al. Ultrasonography and fine-needle aspiration cytology in the preoperative evaluation of melanoma patients eligible for sentinel node biopsy. Ann Surg Oncol. 2006;13(11):1511–6.
27. Breslow A. Thickness, cross-sectional areas and depth of invasion in the prognosis of cutaneous melanoma. Ann Surg. 1970;172(5):902–8.
28. Stevens G, Thompson JF, Firth I, O'Brien CJ, McCarthy WH, Quinn MJ. Locally advanced melanoma: results of postoperative hypofractionated radiation therapy. Cancer. 2000;88(1):88–94.
29. Oxley JD, Corbishley C, Down L, Watkin N, Dickerson D, Wong NA. Clinicopathological and molecular study of penile melanoma. J Clin Pathol. 2012;65(3):228–31.
30. Marsden JR, Newton-Bishop JA, Burrows L, Cook M, Corrie PG, Cox NH, et al. Revised U.K. guidelines for the management of cutaneous melanoma 2010. Br J Dermatol. 2010;163(2):238–56.

31. Allan CP, Hayes AJ, Thomas JM. Ilioinguinal lymph node dissection for palpable metastatic melanoma to the groin. ANZ J Surg. 2008;78(11):982–6.
32. van der Ploeg AP, van Akkooi AC, Schmitz PI, van Geel AN, de Wilt JH, Eggermont AM, et al. Therapeutic surgical management of palpable melanoma groin metastases: superficial or combined superficial and deep groin lymph node dissection. Ann Surg Oncol. 2011;18(12):3300–8.
33. Glover AR, Allan CP, Wilkinson MJ, Strauss DC, Thomas JM, Hayes AJ. Outcomes of routine ilioinguinal lymph node dissection for palpable inguinal melanoma nodal metastasis. Br J Surg. 2014;101(7):811–9.
34. American Joint Committee on Cancer. AJCC cancer staging manual. 7th ed. New York: Springer; 2010.
35. Eggermont AM, et al. Adjuvant ipilimumab versus placebo after complete resection of high-risk stage III melanoma (EORTC 18071): a randomized, double-blind, phase 3 trial. Lancet Oncol. 2015;16(5):522–30.
36. Kirkwood JM, et al. Interferon alfa-2b adjuvant therapy of high-risk resected cutaneous melanoma: the Eastern Cooperation Oncology Group Trial EST 1684. J Clin Oncol. 1996;14(1):7–17.
37. Eggermont AM, et al. Adjuvant therapy with pegylated interferon alfa-2b versus observation alone in resected stage III melanoma: final results of EORTC 18991, a randomised phase III trial. Lancet. 2008;372(9633):117–26.
38. Lian B, et al. Phase II randomized trial comparing high-dose IFN-α2b with temozolomide plus cisplatin as systemic adjuvant therapy for resected mucosal melanoma. Clin Cancer Res. 2013;19(16):4488–98.
39. Hodi FS, et al. Improved survival with ipilimumab in patients with metastatic melanoma. N Engl J Med. 2010;363(8):711–23.
40. Robert C, et al. Ipilimumab plus dacarbazine for previously untreated metastatic melanoma. N Engl J Med. 2011;364(26):2517–256.
41. Postow MA, et al. Ipilimumab for patients with advanced mucosal melanoma. Oncologist. 2013;18(6):726–32.
42. Del Vecchio M, et al. Efficacy and safety of ipilimumab 3mg/kg in patients with pre-treated, metastatic, mucosal melanoma. Eur J Cancer. 2014;50(1):121–7.
43. Alexander M, et al. Ipilimumab in pretreated patients with unresectable cutaneous, uveal, and mucosal melanoma. Med J Aust. 2014;201(1):49–53.
44. National Comprehensive Cancer Network. NCCN guidelines—melanoma. V3.2015. http://www.nccn.org/professionals/physician_gls/pdf/melanoma.pdf. Accessed 16 Jul 2015.
45. Opdivo® (Nivolumab) US prescribing information 2015. Bristol-Myers Squibb. Princeton. http://packageinserts.bms.com/pi/pi_opdivo.pdf. Accessed 16 July 2015.
46. Min L, et al. Anti-PD1 following ipilimumab for mucosal melanoma: durable tumor response associated with severe hypothyroidism and rhabdomyolysis. Cancer Immunol Res. 2013;2(1):15–8.
47. Ohtsuka M, et al. Occurrence of psoriasiform eruption during nivolumab therapy for primary oral mucosal melanoma. JAMA Dermatol. 2015; Published online 15 Apr 2015.
48. Long GV, et al. Dabrafenib and trametinib versus dabrafenib and placebo for Val600 BRAF-mutant melanoma: a multicentre, double-blind, phase 3 randomised controlled trial. Lancet. 2015; Published online 29 May 2015.
49. Robert C, et al. Improved overall survival in melanoma with combined dabrafenib and trametinib. N Engl J Med. 2015;372(1):30–9.
50. Larkin J, et al. Combined vemurafenib and cobimetinib in BRAF-mutated melanoma. N Engl J Med. 2014;371(20):1867–76.
51. Carvajal RD, et al. KIT as a therapeutic target in metastatic melanoma. JAMA. 2011;305(22):2327–34.
52. Hodi FS, et al. Imatinib for melanomas harboring mutationally activated or amplified *KIT* arising on mucosal, acral, and chronically sun-damaged skin. J Clin Oncol. 2013;31(26):3182–90.
53. Guo J, et al. Phase II, open-label, single-arm trial of imatinib mesylate in patients with metastatic melanoma harboring *c-kit* mutation or amplification. J Clin Oncol. 2011;29(21):2904–9.

54. Yi JH, et al. Dacarbazine-based chemotherapy as first-line treatment in non-cutaneous metastatic melanoma: multicenter, retrospective analysis in Asia. Melanoma Res. 2011;21(3):223–7.
55. Bartell HL, et al. Biochemotherapy in patients with advanced head and neck mucosal melanoma. Head Neck. 2008;30(12):1592–8.
56. Harting MS, Kim KB. Biochemotherapy in patients with advanced vulvovaginal mucosal melanoma. Melanoma Res. 2004;14(6):517–20.
57. Kim KB, et al. Biochemotherapy in patients with metastatic anorectal mucosal melanoma. Cancer. 2004;100(7):1478–83.
58. Chang W, et al. Effect of paclitaxel/carboplatin salvage chemotherapy in non-cutaneous versus cutaneous metastatic melanoma. Melanoma Res. 2013;23(2):147–51.

Neuroendocrine and Small Cell Carcinomas of the Prostate: Sentinels of Lethal Evolution

13

John Paul Flores and Paul Mathew

Introduction

Neuroendocrine carcinomas and small cell carcinomas [NE/SCCs] encompass a broad range of neoplasms that arise from pulmonary and extra-pulmonary sites. Although pulmonary small cell carcinomas in smokers and the functional carcinoid tumors of the foregut associated with paraneoplastic endocrine syndromes are perhaps the best recognized of these diverse tumors, various organs can generate well-differentiated and poorly differentiated tumors from different cells of origin and with different genetic associations [1, 2]. In the prostate gland specifically, histopathological features distinguish high-grade poorly differentiated NE/SCCs from adenocarcinomas with Paneth cell differentiation and truly rare large cell neuroendocrine carcinomas and well-differentiated carcinoid tumors [3] from other histological variants of prostatic neoplasms [4, 5]. For the diagnostic pathologist, immunohistochemical stains for neuroendocrine markers including chromogranin, neuron-specific enolase, CD56, and synaptophysin are useful and important adjuncts to light microscopic findings but are not strictly required for the diagnosis [1]. For the clinician, the essential consideration is the awareness of the unique behavior and lethal potential of this entity which has major implications for management strategies. For the

J.P. Flores
Division of Hematology-Oncology, Tufts Medical Center, 800 Washington St, Boston, MA 02111, USA

P. Mathew, MD (✉)
Division of Hematology-Oncology, Department of Medicine, Tufts University School of Medicine, Boston, MA 02111, USA
e-mail: pmathew@tuftsmedicalcenter.org

L. Pagliaro (ed.), *Rare Genitourinary Tumors*,
DOI 10.1007/978-3-319-30046-7_13

translational research scientist, the clonal origins and genetic traits associated with this tumor provide an essential window into the evolutionary biology of the disease through which integrated strategies toward prevention and therapy may be conceived [6, 7].

Pathological Classification of Neuroendocrine Carcinomas of the Prostate

A recent consensus conference has suggested that there are six histological subtypes of neuroendocrine prostate cancer for consideration [3]:

1. Usual prostate adenocarcinoma with neuroendocrine (NE) differentiation

   This is defined as a morphologically typical acinar or ductal adenocarcinoma in which NE differentiation is demonstrated by immunohistochemistry (IHC), but would not otherwise be suspected. It is estimated that perhaps all prostatic adenocarcinomas will have at least some degree of NE differentiation, but this has no established clinical significance.
2. Adenocarcinoma with Paneth cell-like neuroendocrine differentiation

   This is defined as typical adenocarcinoma containing a proportion of cells expressing Paneth cell-like change – which is characterized by prominent eosinophilic cytoplasmic granules visible on routine light microscopy, positivity for chromogranin, and neurosecretory granules as seen by electron microscopy. Though it is a distinct pathologic entity with features of NE differentiation, usually marked after androgen deprivation therapy, its natural history is felt to be favorable [1]. Interestingly *AURKA* amplification has been recently associated with this entity [8].
3. Carcinoid tumor

   This is defined as a well-differentiated NE tumor occurring in the prostate showing classic morphology of carcinoid found in other sites, but is not associated with usual prostate carcinoma and does not arise from the urethra or extend from the bladder. This entity is extremely rare, with only five cases in the literature meeting the strict definition, with IHC showing positivity for NE markers and negative for PSA. Because of its rarity, clinical implications are unknown though it has been seen in young patients and in those with multiple endocrine neoplasia IIB syndrome and is thought to have a favorable prognosis.
4. Small cell carcinoma (SCC)

   This is a high-grade tumor featuring lack of prominent nucleoli, nuclear molding, fragility, and crush artifact. There is a high nuclear to cytoplasmic ratio, indistinct cell borders, and high apoptotic rate. These morphologic features are identical to small cell carcinomas of other sites such as the lung. NE markers are positive in the vast majority of cases, but PSA or other prostatic markers can be positive as well, though only in the minority of cases and often with less robust positivity. TTF-1 can be positive in small cell carcinoma of the prostate over 50 % of the time, limiting the use of this marker in differentiating from metastatic primary lung disease. CD44 expression overlaps significantly with adenocarcinoma reducing its utility [9].

5. Mixed neuroendocrine carcinoma – acinar adenocarcinoma

   This entity is defined by distinct NE components and conventional adenocarcinoma. Most commonly the mixture is small cell carcinoma with acinar carcinoma, though the NE component can be large cell NE and the adenocarcinoma component can be ductal or another variant. The transition between the two components is usually distinct and usually dominated by the NE component. Only the adenocarcinoma component is assigned a Gleason score and it is typically high grade. Uncommonly, the distinction among the neuroendocrine component and adenocarcinoma component is not clear, and the tumor appears to have features consistent with both morphologies.

6. Large cell neuroendocrine carcinoma

   This subtype is characterized as a high-grade tumor showing neuroendocrine differentiation and morphology consisting of large nests with peripheral palisading and often geographic necrosis. Cytology is characterized as non-small cell carcinoma with prominent nucleoli, vesicular clumpy chromatin, and/or large cell size with abundant cytoplasm. There is also a high mitotic rate. Immunohistochemistry is consistent with neuroendocrine differentiation. This subtype is also exceedingly rare. It has been reported to arise after typical prostate adenocarcinoma in the setting of hormonal therapy and can be seen in association with adenocarcinoma or small cell carcinoma. The limited clinical literature is suggestive of this being an aggressive malignancy with rapid dissemination [10].

The focus of this chapter will refer to the common subset of neuroendocrine prostate cancers, specifically high-grade neuroendocrine and small cell carcinomas [NE/SCCs]. Clinical syndromes in prostate cancer that mirror the natural history and chemotherapy responsiveness of these entities without containing histological evidence of NE/SCCs point to the diversity of aggressive prostate cancers [11, 12].

Clinical Management Considerations

Localized and Locally Advanced Disease

The frequency of incidental discovery of high-grade NE/SCCs coexistent with adenocarcinoma in needle biopsies of the prostate gland, performed in a general population as a result of screening or symptom-directed diagnostic efforts, is well under 0.1 % of all tumors. This attests to the rarity of the entity in this disease state. When detected, the tumor can comprise a minor or dominant component of the neoplastic volume, admixed with high-grade acinar [13] or less commonly ductal variant of adenocarcinoma. Very occasionally it can be found with low-grade Gleason 6 tumors with a sharp topographical demarcation. Given the rarity of this presentation, an evidence-based approach to management is undefined. Given the lethality of this disease, however, a *multidisciplinary approach* integrating systemic chemotherapy and local control measures is strongly recommended toward curative intent [14–16].

Given the proclivity for early hematogenous dissemination of these high-grade tumors analogous to the pulmonary counterpart, staging with computed tomography of the chest, abdomen, and pelvis, bone scan, and magnetic resonance imaging of the brain should be considered. It is uncertain if positron emission tomography (PET) scanning offers specific advantages over these studies [17].

Four to six cycles of etoposide and platinum adjuvant or neoadjuvant therapy may be integrated with local control enforced by surgery or radiotherapy as has been accomplished successfully in small cell bladder carcinoma [18]. There are no rules outside of the usual considerations in this setting including age and comorbidities, to choose one local control modality over another. However, as NE/SCCs are typically androgen-receptor (AR) negative, adjunctive hormonal therapy if given with radiation therapy is assumed to target only the PSA-expressing AR-positive component of the tumor which is usually present as well and theoretically cannot synergize with radiation therapy for control of the NE/SCC component. Toward optimal local control therefore, a combination of surgery and radiotherapy may be optimal, particularly in bulky tumors. Brain metastases are particular complications of NE/SCCs, but the use of prophylactic cranial irradiation in clinical settings of localized or locally advanced disease following definitive therapy is unsettled given the variable but low incidence of these events [19, 20].

A patient who presents with a bulky locally advanced high-grade adenocarcinoma associated with a disproportionately low PSA should be suspected of harboring elements of NE/SCC. Although this may not be present on initial diagnostic needle biopsies, rebiopsy after initial therapy with hormonal ablative therapy may disclose the presence of this tumor, particularly if there is a persistent bulky mass or regrowth of tumor following the first 8–12 weeks of initial castration therapy. For bulky tumors with NE/SCC elements, in a young otherwise fit man with minimal evidence of threatening distant disease, local control with radical surgery should be considered after initial efforts with etoposide-cisplatin-based chemotherapy, followed by postoperative radiotherapy. Such efforts toward local control may forestall invasion by the progressive tumor into the bladder, rectum, or pelvic sidewall with dire consequential morbidity that may prove more debilitating and life-threatening than distant disease.

Metastatic Disease

It is far more common to harbor suspicion of NE/SCC evolution in patients with metastatic castration-resistant prostate cancer as compared to primary castration-naïve presentations. Clinical features that suggest NE/SCC elements in this context include a PSA that is disproportionately low [21] compared to the systemic burden of the illness, the emergence of a bulky asymmetric mass in a nodal station or the prostate itself, lytic bone metastases with exophytic soft-tissue components, multiple liver metastases, or brain metastases [22]. Paraneoplastic syndromes such as ectopic ACTH production, hypercalcemia, inappropriate secretion of antidiuretic hormone, and the Lambert-Eaton myasthenia have been described and are uncommon.

Soluble blood markers including carcinoembryonic antigen, chromogranin, and neuron-specific enolase may be elevated, but no single marker is suitably diagnostic nor specific for the NE/SCC component. Of these, serum and tissue expression of chromogranin may be the best marker of neuroendocrine differentiation [23]. Nevertheless elevated values at baseline allow for selection of a panel of markers as adjunctive monitoring of therapy outcomes over time. A rising PSA or prostatic acid phosphatase testifies to progression in coexisting adenocarcinoma.

Histological evidence is essential to secure the diagnosis and biopsy of metastatic sites deemed suspect should be performed in a timely fashion. Morphological assessment of circulating tumor cells (CTCs) is a current research focus toward a liquid biopsy definition of NE/SCC. Etoposide and platin-based combination therapy is preferred over a secondary hormonal or a standard docetaxel strategy when a significant component of NE/SCC is histologically defined. When NE/SCC is the dominant disease, the role of continued hormonal ablation is questionable. Sequential docetaxel-carboplatin and etoposide-cisplatin regimens have been employed in syndromes of aggressive disease, and sequential responses were seen with the second regimen when reserved for disease progression after the first [24]. Median time to progression was short, 5.1 months and 3.0 months, respectively. Other chemotherapy agents such as doxorubicin [25] or topotecan have not been demonstrated to be active. Given the challenging outcomes with this disease state and rarity of durable control with chemotherapy with median survival of 9–16 months [24, 26–28], participation in a clinical trial that seeks to link the cellular and molecular phenotype of the disease with therapy outcome is strongly encouraged. In practical terms, initial systemic therapy with etoposide and platinum combination therapy may be conceived of as a bridge toward an effort with experimental therapeutics. Additional care should be taken in this context to monitor the CNS with periodic surveillance as preferential progression of disease in the brain has been observed.

As stated earlier, it is not uncommon to encounter mixed NE/SCC and high-grade adenocarcinoma in histological specimens with intermediate entities being increasingly discerned [29]. Following etoposide-cisplatin therapy, complete regression of the NE/SCC phenotype may be observed with persistence of the PSA-expressing disease which may subsequently dominate the progressive phenotype. Secondary hormonal strategies will continue to be relevant and appropriate in this context. Parenthetically, a theoretical concern is that the efforts toward more comprehensive ablation of AR signaling will perpetuate a microenvironment that fosters the reemergence or progression of the NE/SCC clone.

Current data suggests that NE/SCCs represent as much as 25 % of the lethal phenotype of the disease [6]. The apparent rise in incidence of NE/SCCs without discernible changes in mortality outcomes may relate to increased diagnostic awareness of this entity [30]. Although NE/SCCs have been defined as a histological entity associated with particular clinical presentations as described above, high-grade adenocarcinomas without histologically identifiable NE/SCC components can present with clinical features similar to that of NE/SCCs with short-lived hormonal control or bulky rapidly progressive disease, with or without robust PSA expression. Some of these aggressive tumors share molecular features of NE/SCCs [11]. This points to the broader spectrum of aggressive prostate cancer that requires elucidation in terms of genotype-phenotype linkage [12]. Other tumors may be driven by ligand-independent splice variants, amplified or mutant ARs, other steroid hormone receptors, and others by alternate stem progenitor phenotypes [31]. Until recently [32], there were no molecular narratives defined to allow demarcation of these advanced tumors with personalized therapy. This is the leading edge of the challenge toward the control of advanced prostate cancer given the limited control exerted by existing chemohormonal strategies.

In this sense, NE/SCCs represent a sentinel at the evolutionary front of the disease, but only one of several which may coexist and present distinctive challenges toward molecular solutions [33]. High-resolution data sets from the integrated genomic [34, 35] and proteomic landscape of prostate tumors when linked to carefully curated clinical and histological phenotypes may allow for a progressive insight into this heterogeneity and a clinically applicable reclassification of the disease.

Current Cellular and Molecular Themes in NE/SCCs of the Prostate

Translational Implications

A fusion between the *TMPRSS2* and *ETS* family of genes is observed in up to 70 % of primary adenocarcinomas of the prostate [36] and also in preinvasive PIN (prostatic intraepithelial neoplasia) lesions [37]. The *TMPRSS2-ERG* fusion gene is present in 50–70 % of NE/SCCs usually associated with interstitial deletion of *ERG* and concordant with the usual acinar component suggestive of shared clonal origins [38, 39], similar to that described with p53 mutation [40]. In mixed NE/SCCs and adenocarcinomas, perfect concordance in *TMPRSS2-ERG* status by FISH was seen in both components with loss of AR and AR-regulated *ERG* expression in the NE/SCC component [41], with sharp demarcation between these components. From an applied perspective, determination of the presence of the *TMPRSS2-ERG* fusion in a NE/SCC lesion may be useful to distinguish between bladder and prostatic origin of a locally advanced pelvic NE/SCC [39, 42]. There is no good evidence in humans to suggest that high-grade NE/SCCs arise from the supportive neuroendocrine cells in the basal layer of the normal prostate gland. A similar evolutionary pedigree of clonal origins is suggested in pulmonary small cell carcinomas that arise from the background of EGFR-mutant non-small cell lung cancers treated with EGFR inhibitors; these SCCs display the EGFR mutation defined in the primary non-small cell carcinoma [43]. Concordant patterns of allelic loss of heterozygosity and nonrandom X chromosome inactivation between urothelial and small cell bladder carcinomas also support linked clonal origins in these tumors [44].

A suite of additional genomic anomalies have been described in association with NE/SCCs. *PTEN* losses with dysregulated PI3-kinase and Akt expression are observed in the majority of high-grade prostate cancers. *PTEN* loss functions as a cooperative oncogene with *ERG* [45] but does not occur in discernibly higher frequency in NE/SCCs. In significant contrast, Rb protein loss is seen in 90 % of SCCs compared to 43 % of concurrent acinar carcinomas, 7 % of primary acinar carcinomas, and 15 % of metastatic castration-resistant acinar carcinomas. The *RB* pathway may be an essential gatekeeper of SCC transition [46]. Furthermore, loss of cyclin D1 expression in 88 % of small cell carcinomas (compared with only 2 % of acinar carcinomas) with a high p16 to cyclin D1 ratio reflecting functional Rb inactivation was recently described [47]. Rare adenocarcinomas that demonstrated loss of cyclin D1 were associated with clinical features of SCC. High-frequency nuclear p53 expression in NE/SCCs secondary to mutation is associated with inactivation of the IL8-CXCR2-p53 inhibitory pathway which regulates neuroendocrine differentiation [48]. However, combined inactivation of the *RB* and *TP53* tumor suppressor pathways may be the most potent explanatory factor in the pathogenesis of NE/SCCs across organ sites. Conditional inactivation of both p53 and Rb targeted to the murine prostatic epithelium generates carcinomas with luminal epithelial and neuroendocrine differentiation [49]. Overexpression and gene amplification of *AURKA* and *MYCN* in 40 % of NE/SCCs contrasted with only 5 % of adenocarcinomas. Experimental evidence of the cooperativity between *AURKA* and *MYCN* in the induction of neuroendocrine phenotype in prostate cancers with sensitivity to Aurora kinase inhibitor therapy has led to ongoing clinical trials in NE/SCCs [41]. *REST*, a transcriptional complex that functions as a master repressor of neuroendocrine differentiation, was found to be downregulated in a significant proportion of tumors [50]. Taken together, the consequences of these genetic alterations include activation of neural pathways, cell cycle, and mitotic programs, which are a hallmark of NE/SCCs.

A gene signature specific for human prostatic basal cells is differentially enriched in varying phenotypes of late-stage castration-resistant prostate cancers. Metastatic samples with a NE/SCC phenotype were found to be more stemlike [51] than either adenocarcinoma or a recently described atypical carcinoma which is intermediate to small cell carcinoma and adenocarcinoma [29]. The NE/SCC tumors had higher CD49f Hi Scores with enrichment of E2F and SOX2 targets implicated in self-renewal capacities [51]. Lentiviral transduction of *NMYC* and myristoylated *AKT* into benign human prostate CD49f Hi cells can initiate biphenotypic tumors with adenocarcinoma and NE/SCC components, supporting the idea that a tissue stem cell is the source of these tumor populations when faced with specific genomic challenges [51]. A castrate microenvironment may interact with these genomic challenges to accelerate the evolution of these biphenotypic histological entities to explain their rarity in castration-naïve primary tumors versus advanced castration-resistant tumors. Emergence from a common stem precursor under these conditions may therefore represent the source of these NE/SCC tumors rather than dedifferentiation or transdifferentiation. The molecular programs that regulate the stem component of NE/SCCs may therefore represent targets for therapy.

In this regard, several decades previously, experiments in the Shionogi model of AR-positive rat mammary carcinoma with androgen cycling, i.e., castration therapy alternated with acute testosterone replacement therapy, had demonstrated the delayed emergence of castration resistance when compared to chronic castration therapy, as a result of inhibition of stem population expansion. The related clinical trials of intermittent hormonal therapy which failed to demonstrate a clinical advantage have not reproduced the cycling procedures employed in this model [52]. It remains to be determined whether such modified androgen therapy could slow the emergence of NE/SCCs in prostate cancers.

Given the multiplicity of losses of major tumor suppressor genes with attendant genomic complexity and the emergence of stem transcriptional programs, it is unlikely that single-pathway inhibitors will have a discernible impact on the illness. Induction of synthetic lethality with combinatorial therapeutics will require additional insight into the wiring of survival pathways in NE/SCCs. Mutational inactivation of the p53 and Rb tumor suppressors may contribute to the acquisition of additional genetic damage including loss of homologous DNA damage repair capacity and vulnerability to inhibitors of DNA damage repair such as that recently demonstrated with olaparib in heavily pretreated metastatic castration-resistant disease [32]. A higher incidence of triple-negative breast carcinomas is seen in patients with germline BRCA-mutant backgrounds, but it is as yet undetermined if a higher risk of AR-negative prostatic NE/SCCs emerges in men with *BRCA* germline mutations who develop prostate cancer. Acquisition of diverse genetic lesions in *BRCA*-mutant tumors may spur the development of tumor neoantigens which may serve as targets for derepressed immunosurveillance with immune checkpoint inhibitors. Durable responses with PD-1 inhibitors in pulmonary small cell carcinomas in the second-line setting suggest a potential for this strategy in NE/SCCs of the prostate [53, 54].

Refinements in therapeutic concepts such as these may emerge from increasingly diversified experimental models of NE/SCCs. It has been suggested that the commonly employed bone-derived AR-PSA- PC-3 cell line is more accurately a representative of small cell carcinoma [55]. Investigators are now moving to immune-competent murine models, patient-derived xenografts [42, 56–58], tumor organoids [59], and biobanks [60] toward a more accurate and representative set of resources for translational studies.

Case Presentation 1

A 62-year-old South Asian male presented with a screening PSA of 10.6 ng/ml. Digital rectal examination revealed a palpable nodule in the left lobe of the prostate. Transrectal ultrasound-directed biopsy showing Gleason 5 + 5 = 10 adenocarcinoma in 9/12 scores. Staging studies were negative for metastases. He was treated with oral bicalutamide and external beam radiation for his localized high-risk prostate cancer to a PSA nadir to 0.46 ng/ml, 5 months after diagnosis. His PSA thereafter increased to 2.1 ng/ml in 6 months. He initiated GnRH agonist therapy 6 months later. Eighteen months later, pelvic lymphadenopathy was noted on a PET scan and his PSA rose to 8.6 ng/ml. With progressive disease in the lung and nodes identified on repeat imaging, he sought another opinion. A strong family history of ovarian

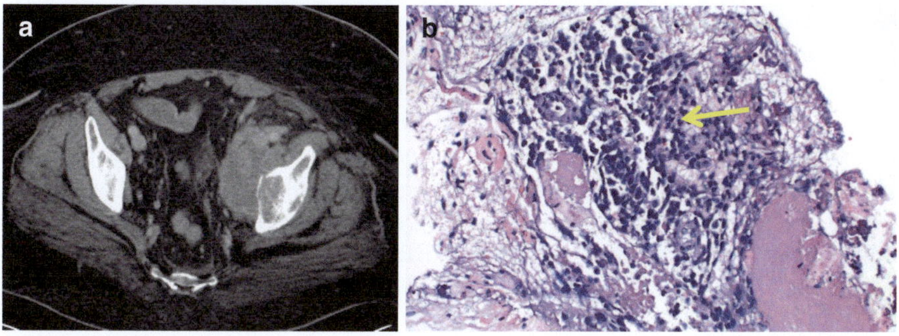

Fig. 13.1 (**a**) Bulky left external iliac node with direct lytic erosion into the left hemipelvis. (**b**) The arrow shows small blue cells positive for cytokeratin consistent with high-grade neuroendocrine carcinoma

and breast carcinoma among first-degree relatives led to a diagnosis of a germline *BRCA-2* mutation. He received sequential nilutamide, abiraterone and prednisone, and enzalutamide with initial response but presented with left hip pain and lower extremity swelling within 14 months. Restaging studies demonstrated multiple new liver metastases, progressive sclerotic bone metastases, and a bulky left external iliac node with lytic erosion of tumor directly into the ipsilateral hemipelvis abutting the acetabulum (Fig. 13.1a). Despite the apparent heavy burden of disease, PSA was 15 ng/ml. CT-guided needle biopsy of the bulky left external iliac node showed metastatic high-grade neuroendocrine carcinoma (Fig. 13.1b). Immunohistochemistry demonstrated that the tumor was pancytokeratin, CAM 5.2, CD56, chromogranin, and synaptophysin positive; Ki-67 was >90 % and PSA and PSAP were negative. Serum CEA and neuron-specific enolase were elevated, but chromogranin was normal. He was treated with four cycles of carboplatin with etoposide with complete resolution of his liver metastases and partial response in the bulky nodal mass, which was consolidated with involved-field radiation therapy. His leg swelling and pain resolved. He was started on an oral polyadenosine-ribose polymerase-1 (PARP-1) inhibitor on a clinical trial and remained on this for 8 months at which time his PSA rose to 30 ng/ml with increasing sclerotic bone metastases and mediastinal adenopathy. His CEA remained at a stable nadir and his neuron-specific enolase normalized without recurrence of liver metastases and no evidence of brain metastases. His PARP-1 inhibitor was discontinued and docetaxel therapy initiated for control of the acinar component of his disease.

Case 1 Discussion: The disproportionately low PSA, asymmetric bulky nodal mass, and multiple liver metastases together lent suspicion for the existence of a NE/SCC component to his disease that was confirmed on biopsy. Etoposide and platinum-based systemic therapy resulted in a complete resolution of disease in the liver, and the control of the solitary bulky mass was consolidated with radiation therapy. This effectively allowed for a bridge to PARP-1 inhibitor therapy which likely contributed significantly toward maintenance of remission of the NE/SCC component until the adenocarcinoma component progressed, requiring conventional taxane chemotherapy. The discordant pattern of progression influenced by the PARP-1 inhibitor is intriguing. Whether germline BRCA-2 mutation or somatic biallelic inactivation of BRCA-2 or other forms of homologous DNA repair deficiency [32, 34] also influences the emergence of the NE/SCC phenotype in advanced castration-resistant disease has not been reported. Tumors with germline BRCA mutations may harbor neoantigens in higher frequency and PD-1 expressing immune infiltrates, which may predict for response to immune checkpoint inhibitors, as have been suggested in BRCA-mutant ovarian tumors [61].

Case Presentation 2

A 59-year-old Caucasian male presented with new-onset obstructive urinary symptoms and a PSA of 10.1 ng/ml. Digital rectal examination revealed a very bulky nodular tumor involving both lobes extending to bilateral sulci and seminal vesicles. Staging studies revealed pelvic and retroperitoneal adenopathy but no bone metastases or other visceral disease. On MRI imaging, the tumor involved the bladder neck and abutted the rectal wall without clear invasion. There was no elevation in serum CEA, chromogranin, or neuron-specific enolase. Initial hormonal ablative therapy was accompanied by improvement in voiding symptoms and decline in PSA to a nadir of 0.7 ng/ml with regression yet persistence of the bulky mass in the prostate in the left lobe. Rebiopsy of the gland indicated high-grade carcinoma and neuroendocrine differentiation with immunohistochemical staining but no frank histological features of NE/SCC. He was treated with six cycles of docetaxel and carboplatin. After the completion of the sixth cycle, an impression of tumor regrowth in the left lobe of his prostate was suggested by digital rectal examination, and restaging CT scans indicated regrowth of disease in a single pelvic node. Retroperitoneal and other pelvic nodes remained stable and there was no evidence of bone or visceral metastases. Radical prostatectomy and bilateral pelvic lymph node dissection were performed, and pathology revealed mixed high-grade and neuroendocrine carcinoma with areas suggestive of small cell carcinoma (Fig. 13.2a). Immunohistochemical stains showed focal positivity for PSA and PAP but also synaptophysin (Fig. 13.2b) and chromogranin. One of nine lymph nodes harbored

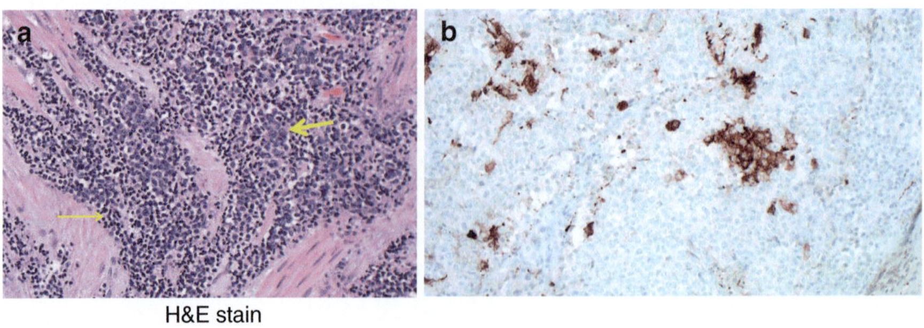

Fig. 13.2 (**a**) *Thick arrow* indicates larger tumor cells and *thin arrow* shows crushed tumor cells with lymphocytes imparting a small cell appearance. (**b**) Tumor cells staining for synaptophysin

metastatic carcinoma, and multiple surgical margins were positive. Postoperative radiation therapy followed by consideration of etoposide-cisplatin chemotherapy was recommended. A screen for a germline *BRCA* mutation prompted by a history of multiple first-degree relatives with breast and prostate carcinoma was negative.

Case 2 Discussion: Although several features of his initial presentation suggested the possibility of a NE/SCC component, histological and biochemical evidence supportive of this entity was difficult to obtain. Nevertheless the phenotype of the illness with its unusual bulk, local aggressiveness, low PSA phenotype, and unimpressive regression with castration therapy pointed to a highly aggressive or "anaplastic" phenotype. A multimodality regimen of neoadjuvant docetaxel-carboplatin followed by surgery and postoperative radiotherapy was planned. In shared decision-making, the patient was counseled that this multidisciplinary effort would not be curative, given the presence of extra-pelvic nodal metastases at diagnosis, but might contribute toward reduced morbidity from uncontrolled locally invasive tumor and prolong his survival.

Conclusion

These highly aggressive phenotypes of illness, like the NE/SCC counterparts, represent sentinels of disease evolution that may be explained by the cellular and molecular themes summarized in this chapter. Additional measures for tumor control would require specific insights into the biology of this disease and linked therapeutics. These frontiers of prostate cancer biology will continue to be explored.

Acknowledgements The authors would like to acknowledge Elizabeth Genega, MD for assistance with photography of representative pathology.

References

1. Klimstra DS, Beltran H, Lilenbaum R, Bergsland E. The spectrum of neuroendocrine tumors: histologic classification, unique features and areas of overlap. Am Soc Clin Oncol Educ Book. 2015;35:92–103.
2. Zheng X, Liu D, Fallon JT, Zhong M. Distinct genetic alterations in small cell carcinoma from different anatomic sites. Exp Hematol Oncol. 2015;4:2.
3. Epstein JI, Amin MB, Beltran H, et al. Proposed morphologic classification of prostate cancer with neuroendocrine differentiation. Am J Surg Pathol. 2014;38:756–67.
4. Humphrey PA. Histological variants of prostatic carcinoma and their significance. Histopathology. 2012;60:59–74.
5. Randolph TL, Amin MB, Ro JY, Ayala AG. Histologic variants of adenocarcinoma and other carcinomas of prostate: pathologic criteria and clinical significance. Mod Pathol Off J U S Can Acad Pathol. 1997;10:612–29.
6. Terry S, Beltran H. The many faces of neuroendocrine differentiation in prostate cancer progression. Front Oncol. 2014;4:60.
7. Vlachostergios PJ, Papandreou CN. Targeting neuroendocrine prostate cancer: molecular and clinical perspectives. Front Oncol. 2015;5:6.
8. Park K, Chen Z, MacDonald TY, et al. Prostate cancer with Paneth cell-like neuroendocrine differentiation has recognizable histomorphology and harbors AURKA gene amplification. Hum Pathol. 2014;45:2136–43.

9. Wang CC, De Marzo AM, Lotan TL, Epstein JI. Overlap of CD44 expression between prostatic small cell carcinoma and acinar adenocarcinoma. Hum Pathol. 2015;46:554–7.
10. Evans AJ, Humphrey PA, Belani J, van der Kwast TH, Srigley JR. Large cell neuroendocrine carcinoma of prostate: a clinicopathologic summary of 7 cases of a rare manifestation of advanced prostate cancer. Am J Surg Pathol. 2006;30:684–93.
11. Aparicio A, Tzelepi V. Neuroendocrine (small-cell) carcinomas: why they teach us essential lessons about prostate cancer. Oncology (Williston Park, NY). 2014;28:831–8.
12. Beltran H, Tomlins S, Aparicio A, et al. Aggressive variants of castration-resistant prostate cancer. Clin Cancer Res Off J Am Assoc Cancer Res. 2014;20:2846–50.
13. Wang W, Epstein JI. Small cell carcinoma of the prostate. A morphologic and immunohistochemical study of 95 cases. Am J Surg Pathol. 2008;32:65–71.
14. Bolton DM, Chiu ST, Clarke S, Angus D. Primary small cell carcinoma of the prostate: unusual modes of presentation. Aust N Z J Surg. 1994;64:91–4.
15. Deorah S, Rao MB, Raman R, Gaitonde K, Donovan JF. Survival of patients with small cell carcinoma of the prostate during 1973–2003: a population-based study. BJU Int. 2012;109:824–30.
16. Weiner AB, Patel SG, Richards KA, Szmulewitz RZ, Eggener SE. Population-based analysis of treatment modalities and survival for clinically localized small-cell carcinoma of the prostate. Prostate Cancer Prostatic Dis. 2014;17:286–91.
17. Sahiner I, Akkas BE, Ucmak Vural G. Clinical impact of 18F-fluorodeoxyglucose positron emission tomography/computed tomography in the evaluation of small cell carcinoma of the prostate. Rev Esp Med Nucl Imag Mol. 2013;32:193–5.
18. Siefker-Radtke AO, Dinney CP, Abrahams NA, et al. Evidence supporting preoperative chemotherapy for small cell carcinoma of the bladder: a retrospective review of the M. D. Anderson cancer experience. J Urol. 2004;172:481–4.
19. Naidoo J, Teo MY, Deady S, Comber H, Calvert P. Should patients with extrapulmonary small-cell carcinoma receive prophylactic cranial irradiation? J Thorac Oncol Off Publ Int Assoc Study Lung Cancer. 2013;8:1215–21.
20. Yazici O, Ozdemir NY, Sendur MA, Aksoy S, Zengin N. Current approaches for prophylactic cranial irradiation in extrapulmonary small cell carcinoma. Curr Med Res Opin. 2014;30:1327–36.
21. Leibovici D, Spiess PE, Agarwal PK, et al. Prostate cancer progression in the presence of undetectable or low serum prostate-specific antigen level. Cancer. 2007;109:198–204.
22. Erasmus CE, Verhagen WI, Wauters CA, van Lindert EJ. Brain metastasis from prostate small cell carcinoma: not to be neglected. Can J Neurol Sci J Can Sci Neurol. 2002;29:375–7.
23. di Sant' Agnese PA. Divergent neuroendocrine differentiation in prostatic carcinoma. Semin Diagn Pathol. 2000;17:149–61.
24. Aparicio AM, Harzstark AL, Corn PG, et al. Platinum-based chemotherapy for variant castrate-resistant prostate cancer. Clin Cancer Res Off J Am Assoc Cancer Res. 2013;19:3621–30.
25. Papandreou CN, Daliani DD, Thall PF, et al. Results of a phase II study with doxorubicin, etoposide, and cisplatin in patients with fully characterized small-cell carcinoma of the prostate. J Clin Oncol Off J Am Soc Clin Oncol. 2002;20:3072–80.
26. Amato RJ, Logothetis CJ, Hallinan R, Ro JY, Sella A, Dexeus FH. Chemotherapy for small cell carcinoma of prostatic origin. J Urol. 1992;147:935–7.
27. Cohen A, Richards KA, Patel S, Weiner A, Eggener SE, Szmulewitz RZ. Metastatic small cell carcinoma of the prostate: population-based analysis of patient characteristics and treatment paradigms. Urol Oncol. 2015;33:70.e1–7.
28. Marcus DM, Goodman M, Jani AB, Osunkoya AO, Rossi PJ. A comprehensive review of incidence and survival in patients with rare histological variants of prostate cancer in the United States from 1973 to 2008. Prostate Cancer Prostatic Dis. 2012;15:283–8.
29. Small EJ, Huang J, Youngren J, Sokolov A, Aggarwal RR, et al. Characterization of neuroendocrine prostate cancer (NEPC) in patients with metastatic castration resistant prostate cancer (mCRPC) resistant to abiraterone or enzalutamide: preliminary results from the SU2C/PCF/

AACR West Coast Prostate Cancer Dream Team (WCDT). J Clin Oncol Off J Am Soc Clin Oncol. 2015;33(suppl);abstr 5003.
30. Alanee S, Moore A, Nutt M, et al. Contemporary incidence and mortality rates of neuroendocrine prostate cancer. Anticancer Res. 2015;35:4145–50.
31. Watson PA, Arora VK, Sawyers CL. Emerging mechanisms of resistance to androgen receptor inhibitors in prostate cancer. Nat Rev Cancer. 2015.
32. Mateo J, Carreira S, Sandhu S, et al. DNA-repair defects and olaparib in metastatic prostate cancer. N Engl J Med. 2015;373:1697–708.
33. Prandi D, Baca SC, Romanel A, et al. Unraveling the clonal hierarchy of somatic genomic aberrations. Genome Biol. 2014;15:439.
34. Robinson D, Van Allen EM, Wu YM, et al. Integrative clinical genomics of advanced prostate cancer. Cell. 2015;161:1215–28.
35. Baca SC, Garraway LA. The genomic landscape of prostate cancer. Front Endocrinol. 2012;3:69.
36. Tomlins SA, Rhodes DR, Perner S, et al. Recurrent fusion of TMPRSS2 and ETS transcription factor genes in prostate cancer. Science (New York, NY). 2005;310:644–8.
37. Mosquera JM, Perner S, Genega EM, et al. Characterization of TMPRSS2-ERG fusion high-grade prostatic intraepithelial neoplasia and potential clinical implications. Clin Cancer Res Off J Am Assoc Cancer Res. 2008;14:3380–5.
38. Han B, Mehra R, Suleman K, et al. Characterization of ETS gene aberrations in select histologic variants of prostate carcinoma. Mod Pathol Off J U S Can Acad Pathol. 2009;22:1176–85.
39. Lotan TL, Gupta NS, Wang W, et al. ERG gene rearrangements are common in prostatic small cell carcinomas. Mod Pathol Off J U S Can Acad Pathol. 2011;24:820–8.
40. Hansel DE, Nakayama M, Luo J, et al. Shared TP53 gene mutation in morphologically and phenotypically distinct concurrent primary small cell neuroendocrine carcinoma and adenocarcinoma of the prostate. Prostate. 2009;69:603–9.
41. Beltran H, Rickman DS, Park K, et al. Molecular characterization of neuroendocrine prostate cancer and identification of new drug targets. Cancer Discov. 2011;1:487–95.
42. Aparicio A, Tzelepi V, Araujo JC, et al. Neuroendocrine prostate cancer xenografts with large-cell and small-cell features derived from a single patient's tumor: morphological, immunohistochemical, and gene expression profiles. Prostate. 2011;71:846–56.
43. Oser MG, Niederst MJ, Sequist LV, Engelman JA. Transformation from non-small-cell lung cancer to small-cell lung cancer: molecular drivers and cells of origin. Lancet Oncol. 2015;16:e165–72.
44. Cheng L, Jones TD, McCarthy RP, et al. Molecular genetic evidence for a common clonal origin of urinary bladder small cell carcinoma and coexisting urothelial carcinoma. Am J Pathol. 2005;166:1533–9.
45. Carver BS, Tran J, Gopalan A, et al. Aberrant ERG expression cooperates with loss of PTEN to promote cancer progression in the prostate. Nat Genet. 2009;41:619–24.
46. Tan HL, Sood A, Rahimi HA, et al. Rb loss is characteristic of prostatic small cell neuroendocrine carcinoma. Clin Cancer Res Off J Am Assoc Cancer Res. 2014;20:890–903.
47. Tsai H, Morais CL, Alshalalfa M, et al. Cyclin D1 loss distinguishes prostatic small-cell carcinoma from most prostatic adenocarcinomas. Clin Cancer Res Off J Am Assoc Cancer Res. 2015.
48. Chen H, Sun Y, Wu C, et al. Pathogenesis of prostatic small cell carcinoma involves the inactivation of the P53 pathway. Endocr Relat Cancer. 2012;19:321–31.
49. Zhou Z, Flesken-Nikitin A, Corney DC, et al. Synergy of p53 and Rb deficiency in a conditional mouse model for metastatic prostate cancer. Cancer Res. 2006;66:7889–98.
50. Lapuk AV, Wu C, Wyatt AW, et al. From sequence to molecular pathology, and a mechanism driving the neuroendocrine phenotype in prostate cancer. J Pathol. 2012;227:286–97.
51. Smith BA, Sokolov A, Uzunangelov V, et al. A basal stem cell signature identifies aggressive prostate cancer phenotypes. Proc Natl Acad Sci USA. 2015.

52. Mathew P. The bifunctional role of steroid hormones: implications for therapy in prostate cancer. Oncology (Williston Park, NY). 2014;28:397–404.
53. Ott PA, Fernandez MEE, Hiret S, Kim D-W, Moss RA, al. E. Pembrolizumab (MK-2475) in patients with extensive-stage small cell lung cancer: preliminary safety and efficacy results from KEYNOTE-028. J Clin Oncol Off J Am Soc Clin Oncol. 2015;33:abstr 7502.
54. Antonia SJ, Bendell JC, Taylor MH, et al. Phase I/II Study of nivolumab with or without ipilimumab for treatment of recurrent small cell lung cancer (SCLC): CA209-032. J Clin Oncol Off J Am Soc Clin Oncol. 1015;33:abstr 7503.
55. Tai S, Sun Y, Squires JM, et al. PC3 is a cell line characteristic of prostatic small cell carcinoma. Prostate. 2011;71:1668–79.
56. Berman-Booty LD, Knudsen KE. Models of neuroendocrine prostate cancer. Endocr Relat Cancer. 2015;22:R33–49.
57. Lopez-Barcons LA. Small-cell neuroendocrine carcinoma of the prostate: are heterotransplants a better experimental model? Asian J Androl. 2010;12:308–14.
58. True LD, Buhler K, Quinn J, et al. A neuroendocrine/small cell prostate carcinoma xenograft-LuCaP 49. Am J Pathol. 2002;161:705–15.
59. Vela I, Chen Y. Prostate cancer organoids: a potential new tool for testing drug sensitivity. Expert Rev Anticancer Ther. 2015;15:261–3.
60. Liu X, Ory V, Chapman S, et al. ROCK inhibitor and feeder cells induce the conditional reprogramming of epithelial cells. Am J Pathol. 2012;180:599–607.
61. McAlpine JN, Porter H, Kobel M, et al. BRCA1 and BRCA2 mutations correlate with TP53 abnormalities and presence of immune cell infiltrates in ovarian high-grade serous carcinoma. Mod Pathol Off J U S Can Acad Pathol. 2012;25:740–50.

Mucinous, Signet Ring, Ductal, and Sarcomatoid Variants of Prostate Cancer

14

Parminder Singh, Dan Albertson, Sumanta K. Pal, and Neeraj Agarwal

Prostate Cancer

Prostate cancer is the second most common malignancy in men after lung cancer [1]. In the USA alone, there will be an estimated 221,000 new cases and 27, 500 deaths due to prostate cancer in 2015 [2]. The most common type of prostate cancer is prostate adenocarcinoma. Conventional prostate adenocarcinoma is well studied both pathologically and clinically. There are standardized histological criteria for conventional prostate adenocarcinoma which demonstrates typical acinar morphology. The sum of the two most common patterns is combined to provide the *Gleason score*, which correlates well with the clinical course of the disease. National Comprehensive Cancer Network (NCCN) guidelines describe clinical and pathological parameters for assigning risk categories to the patient and provide a clear guidance on how to treat conventional prostate adenocarcinoma [3].

However, there are morphologic subtypes of prostate adenocarcinoma and other carcinomas which are rarely observed in prostate, either alone or in combination with conventional adenocarcinoma. Gleason grading and the clinical course of these

P. Singh, MD
Division of Hematology and Medical Oncology, University of Arizona Cancer Center, Banner University Medical Center, Tucson, AZ, USA

D. Albertson, MD
Department of Pathology, Huntsman Cancer Institute, University of Utah, Salt Lake City, UT, USA

S.K. Pal, MD
Department of Medical Oncology and Experimental Therapeutics, City of Hope, Comprehensive Cancer Center, Duarte, CA, USA

N. Agarwal, MD (✉)
Division of Medical Oncology, Huntsman Cancer Institute, University of Utah, Ste 2123, Salt Lake City, UT 84112, USA
e-mail: neeraj.agarwal@hci.utah.edu

L. Pagliaro (ed.), *Rare Genitourinary Tumors*,
DOI 10.1007/978-3-319-30046-7_14

subtypes is less well understood, and guidelines for treatment do not exist. A knowledge of appropriate pathological diagnosis and appropriate treatment is important for improved outcomes of these patients. The following sections describe some of these rare subtypes of prostate adenocarcinoma and suggest optimal treatment options based on the current literature.

Mucinous Adenocarcinoma

Epidemiology

Primary mucinous adenocarcinoma, also known as colloid adenocarcinoma of the prostate, is a rare histologic variant of prostate cancer. The incidence of mucinous prostate cancer varies in different reports but is considered to occur in the range of 0.21–0.43 % of all cases [4–7]. Boyd is credited with the first description of a case of mucinous prostate adenocarcinoma in 1882 [8]. Recently, in a large series of prostatectomies, the mean age at diagnosis of patients with this subtype was observed to be 56 years (range, 44–69) [9]. Elbadawi and colleagues proposed for the first time the diagnostic criteria for mucinous adenocarcinoma: (1) abundant secretion by tumor cells of histochemically proven acidic or neutral mucin, (2) sparing of or only secondary involvement of prostatic ducts and prostatic urethral urothelium, (3) nonpapillary growth with colloid carcinoma pattern, and (4) the absence of an extraprostatic mucinous carcinoma [10]. Epstein and colleagues further modified the diagnostic criterion to require the following: lakes of extracellular mucin to be present in ≥25 % of tumor resected during a single procedure [5]. Mucinous adenocarcinoma is generally considered to have a more aggressive clinical course; however, recent reports suggest that this may not be the case [11, 12].

Pathology

Grossly, the prostate in mucinous adenocarcinoma demonstrates a mucoid or gelatinous cut surface. Histologically, mucinous adenocarcinoma is characterized by extracellular pools of mucin containing free-floating tumor cells that demonstrate a variety of patterns including solid, cribriform, microacinar, or potentially signet ring like cells. The cells usually have an oval to round nuclei with clear or eosinophilic cytoplasm. Chromatin is finely dispersed with occasional prominent nucleoli. Mitoses are rarely observed in these specimens [13]. The proportion of mucinous component varies among patients. It is generally accepted that at least 25 % of the total tumor volume should be composed of mucin to establish the diagnosis [5, 10]. Previously, any mucinous component was graded as Gleason 4. More recently, primary emphasis is based on the underlying architectural pattern of the glands [9]. This reflects observations that the clinical course of pure mucinous adenocarcinoma may be more indolent and similar to conventional adenocarcinoma of the prostate. The International Society of Urological Pathologists has stated no consensus on

Gleason grading for this subtype leaving it to the evaluating pathologist to decide how to most appropriately grade the tumor [14]. Biopsies of metastatic sites in patients with advanced diseases have demonstrated both mucinous and non-mucinous components [15].

Primary prostatic mucinous adenocarcinoma is positive for PSA and prostatic acid phosphatase (PAP) and usually negative for CEA. The positivity observed can be both diffuse and focal [13]. ERG gene expression is observed in up to 50 % of these specimens [16]. MUC2 expression has been observed in nearly 100 % of the samples analyzed and reported in literature [17]. MUC2 expression is considered a key factor in morphogenesis of mucinous adenocarcinoma. In conventional prostate adenocarcinoma, MUC2 expression was observed focally in 24 % of cases and mainly in areas with extensive mucinous metaplasia [17].

Up to 70 % of prostate adenocarcinoma may demonstrate glandular areas with intraluminal mucin or focal mucin lakes. It is now believed that there is aberrant cellular secretion from the mucin-secreting epithelium normally found in the prostate. These tumors should not be labeled as mucinous adenocarcinoma [18]. It has been observed in histochemical studies that the mucin present in mucinous prostate adenocarcinoma is heavily O-acetylated as compared to mucin secreted in conventional prostate adenocarcinoma [19]. It is not clear if there is an association between the amount of mucin production and disease course.

Clinical Features and Management

Mucinous adenocarcinoma is very similar in its presentation to conventional adenocarcinoma of the prostate. In addition to the symptoms of urinary frequency, urgency, obstruction, hematuria, nocturia, suprapubic discomfort, and weight loss, some patients may have mucosuria after prostatic massage, and some rarely have hydronephrosis on presentation. The metastatic pattern of mucinous prostate carcinoma closely follows the conventional counterpart with bone being the most common site of metastases followed by lymph nodes and lung [9, 20]. Seventy-seven percent of the reported cases with mucinous adenocarcinoma of the prostate had PSA elevation [15]. The mean preoperative PSA level reported in a large series was 9.0 ng/ml (range, 1.9–34.3 ng/ml) [9]. Magnetic resonance (MR) images show bright signal intensity on long TR/TE images, and in comparison, a conventional adenocarcinoma nodule in the peripheral zone is of lower signal intensity than the surrounding glandular stroma [21–23]. MR spectroscopy may not be a good imaging modality for evaluating mucinous prostate carcinoma because large mucin lakes render a tumor metabolically less active [22].

Secondary involvement of the prostate with mucinous adenocarcinoma of the colon, bladder, or urethra may mimic primary mucinous prostate carcinoma. Hence, the initial work-up of men with prostatic mucinous adenocarcinoma on biopsy should include ruling out a primary mucinous adenocarcinoma in other organs. Primary prostatic adenocarcinoma can be differentiated easily by light microscopy and immunohistochemical techniques. A prostatic origin is characterized by positive PSA, PAP expression, and negative CK7, CK20, and 34betaE12 expression in the biopsy specimens [24]. Both ERG and MUC2 expression are observed in mucinous adenocarcinoma of prostate [16, 17]. ERG expression may suggest subtype of conventional prostate adenocarcinoma.

The majority of men (up to 77 %) with primary mucinous adenocarcinoma of the prostate respond to androgen deprivation therapy [15]. The prognosis and long-term outcomes for mucinous adenocarcinoma of the prostate are not clearly established because of the rare nature of this disease, with reports describing aggressive and indolent disease courses. The standardization of diagnostic criteria and exclusion of mixed mucinous and signet-type carcinoma from the exclusive mucinous group has helped to improve our understanding of the biology of this disease [5, 10]. In a series, 47 patients with localized mucinous prostate cancer managed with prostatectomy alone, the 5-year actuarial PSA progression-free survival was 97.2 %. A matched group of conventional prostatic adenocarcinoma, using Kattan nomogram, had 5-year actuarial PFS of 85.4 % [9]. The authors concluded that patients with localized disease should be treated with definitive surgery or radiation therapy as described for conventional prostatic adenocarcinoma, as their outcome may be similar to that in conventional prostate adenocarcinoma. The prognosis of patients with advanced mucinous adenocarcinoma is considered to be similar to high-grade conventional prostatic adenocarcinoma with survival of 50 % at 3 years [15]. The presence of signet ring cells confers a relatively worse prognosis [15].

Signet Ring Cell Carcinoma (SRCC) of the Prostate

Primary SRCC of the prostate is a rare disease with reported incidence being less than 0.5 % of all prostate cancers. It was first described in 1981 by Giltman [25]. The signet ring cell is described traditionally as a cell whose nucleus is displaced by a large intracytoplasmic vacuole composed of mucin, as seen in gastrointestinal, breast, and bladder cancer. Prostatic signet ring cells may be negative or minimally positive for mucin, but morphologically appear similar to signet ring carcinomas from other sites (Fig. 14.1). Considering the rarity of the disease, diagnostic criteria are not standardized. It is widely accepted that more than 25 % cells should demonstrate signet ring cell morphology for it to be designated as SRCC [26, 27].

Pathology

SRCC of the prostate is characterized by large number of signet ring cells without obvious gland formation. They are arranged in the pattern of sheets, small clusters, or as single cells. The presence of signet ring cells is considered Gleason grade 5. Traditional stains for mucin including alcian blue, PAS-D, and mucicarmine may be negative or only focally positive [27]. The cells are characterized by nuclear displacement with clear cytoplasm. Electron microscopic analysis demonstrates that signet ring morphology is a result of intracytoplasmic lumina or vacuoles. These

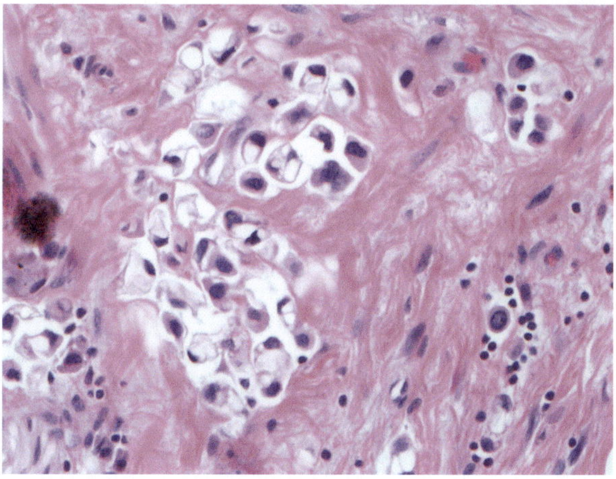

Fig. 14.1 Poorly differentiated prostate adenocarcinoma with signet ring cells (400×). Note the malignant cells with prominent intracytoplasmic inclusions

lumina contain rod-shaped crystalloids which do not possess limiting membrane and are devoid of substructure [28]. Most of the tumors described in literature are associated with other forms of high-grade prostatic adenocarcinoma [27, 29].

These tumors are strongly immunoreactive to PSA, PAP, and cytokeratin AE1/AE3 and are often negative for other mucin markers, CEA, CK7, and CK20. The proliferative fraction of the SRCC of the prostate, as measured by MIB-1, is generally lower than SRCC of other sites such as the bladder or stomach [27].

Clinical Features and Management

The clinical course described in literature for SRCC prostate cancer is variable and likely may reflect the retrospective nature of reports and the rarity of disease. Many investigators have reported this variant to follow an aggressive clinical course with inferior outcomes, compared to conventional prostatic adenocarcinomas [30–32]. Others have reported long-term survival especially for clinically localized disease which has undergone definitive treatment [33–35]. The mean age of reported cases in the literature is 68.2 years (range, 50–84 years). More than 40 % patients reported in the literature presented with advanced stages of disease [36].

As in conventional prostatic adenocarcinomas, the prognosis of primary SRCC of the prostate correlates with the stage of the disease, with higher stages being associated with poorer outcomes [32, 36]. The clinical presentation is similar to prostate adenocarcinoma with localized disease commonly presenting with obstructive urinary symptoms. Elevated serum PSA levels may not be seen in all patients. Metastatic SRCC from other sites, artifactual signet ring cells, and SRC lymphoma should be ruled out at the time of initial work-up. Artifactual SRC that are observed sometimes after TURP or transrectal biopsies are actually vacuolated lymphocytes or smooth muscle cells [37]. The patients with SRCC of the prostate may not respond to androgen deprivation therapy [15].

There are reports of patients with localized SRCC of the prostate treated with aggressive local therapy who had a good long-term outcome [30, 31, 35, 36]. For those patients who are identified at an early localized disease stage, we recommend definitive therapy including either radical prostatectomy or definitive radiation with androgen deprivation therapy.

Based on anecdotal reports of response to androgen deprivation therapy, although short lasting, we recommend that patients presenting with advanced SRCC of the prostate undergo surgical or medical castration [32, 38]. It should be noted, however, that in 1 case series of men with mucinous and signet ring features, none of the 11 patients who had advanced stage pure signet ring or mixed histology features demonstrated response to androgen deprivation therapy [15]. Clinical trials evaluating chemotherapy upfront with androgen deprivation for newly diagnosed metastatic or advanced prostate cancer have not included these subtypes of prostate cancer. In the absence of data from randomized controlled trials, clinical judgment should be used in considering combining docetaxel with androgen deprivation in patients with widely metastatic disease [39].

Ductal Carcinoma of the Prostate

Ductal carcinoma, also known as endometrioid carcinoma or papillary carcinoma of the prostate, was first described in 1967 by Melicow and Pachter. The initial description suggested its possible origin from prostatic utricle, which is considered to be the remnant of mullerian ducts in men [40]. This was based on the histopathological appearance and proximity to the utricle which had dysplasia present in its epithelium [18]. This misnomer led the initial investigators to not use androgen deprivation or estrogen for treatment [41]. Later reports showed positivity of these tumor cells for PSA, PAP, and androgen receptor, indicating a prostatic rather than mullerian origin [42].

Epidemiology

Pure ductal carcinoma of the prostate is rare with incidence varying from 0.2 to 1.3 % of all prostate cancers among large series. Prostatic adenocarcinoma with both acinar (convention prostatic adenocarcinoma) and ductal features is observed in up to 6 % of patients (Figs. 14.2 and 14.3) [43]. Immunohistochemical evidence showing ER receptor negativity and AR receptor positivity suggest that this disease may respond to androgen ablation. The patients who are diagnosed with ductal carcinoma on transurethral (TUR) biopsy should undergo transrectal biopsies to rule out concurrent conventional (acinar) tumors. The clinical presentation of this cell type resembles to that in conventional prostate adenocarcinoma. These tumors are now believed to arise from periurethral or prostatic ducts and grow into the urethra as papillary tumors lined with columnar epithelium. These papillary lesions may be responsible for hematuria commonly noticed in these patients [44]. The tumors

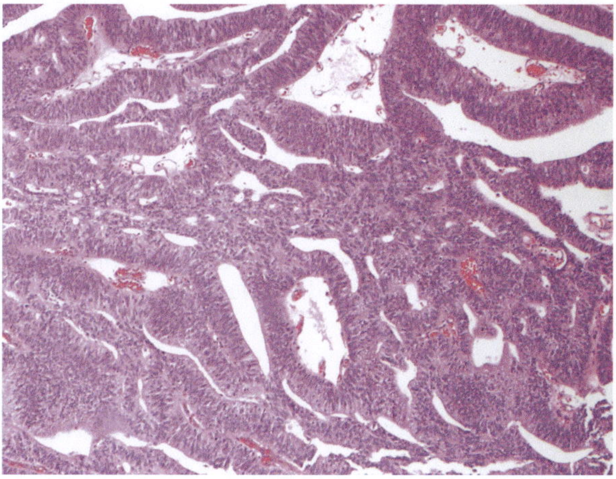

Fig. 14.2 Large duct prostate adenocarcinoma (100×)

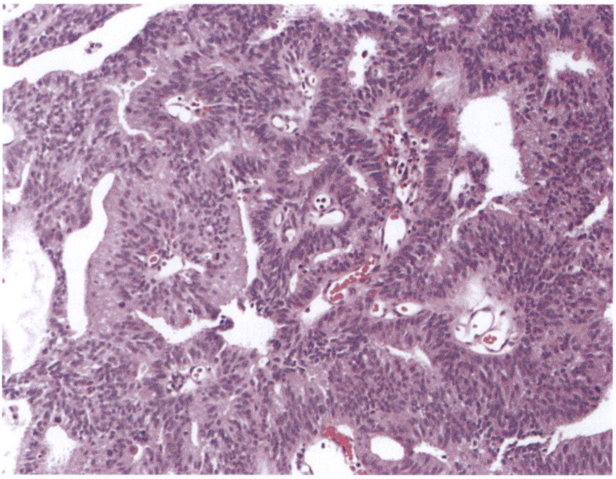

Fig. 14.3 Large duct prostate adenocarcinoma (200×)

arising from the secondary or peripheral ducts may not have urethral component. Ductal carcinoma should not be confused with intraductal carcinoma of the prostate observed in higher-grade cases of conventional acinar adenocarcinomas [45].

Pathology

Microscopically ductal carcinoma of the prostate has two distinct subtypes: cribriform subtype, which is characterized by solid tumor, and papillary subtype, characterized typical papillary areas [42]. These tumors are composed of papillary fronds supported by a complex, branching fibro-connective tissue core, usually lined with tall columnar epithelium. The epithelial cells have elongated nuclei with prominent nucleoli. Needle biopsies usually demonstrate tumor fragmentation and stromal reaction [46].

Ductal carcinoma can be confused with high-grade prostatic intraepithelial neoplasia (PIN). Several features can help distinguish these two lesions. Firstly, ductal carcinomas demonstrate true papillary fronds with a well-established fibrovascular core. Secondly, they are characterized by stromal fibrosis, hemosiderin deposition, and perineural invasion indicating the true invasiveness of the carcinoma [46]. These features are absent in high-grade PIN. Papillary urothelial carcinoma in the TUR specimen may also resemble papillary ductal carcinoma of the prostate. In urothelial carcinoma, the nuclei of the cancer cells are pleomorphic with angulated nuclear outlines and variable numbers and site of nucleoli. Ductal carcinoma on the other hand generally has more uniform nuclei [6]. Immunohistochemistry shows that ductal carcinomas are strongly positive for PSA, PAP [44], and AR and negative for ER [42]. Our experience has also shown negative staining for GATA-3, in comparison to urothelial carcinoma which is often GATA-3 positive.

Clinical Features and Management

Prostatic ductal carcinoma is clinically associated with elevated serum levels of PSA and PAP. Since these tumors are uniformly androgen receptor positive, these patients respond to androgen deprivation, albeit for shorter durations than those seen with conventional prostatic adenocarcinoma [42, 47]. In one of the largest retrospective reviews of 54 men with ductal carcinoma of the prostate, the actuarial risk of biochemical progression after radical prostatectomy was 34 %. A retrospective comparison with other large series of conventional carcinoma prostate showed a statistically significant shorter time to progression after definitive treatment ($p<0.00001$) [46]. The prognosis of prostatic ductal carcinoma is not well defined. Overall, these patients are considered to have aggressive disease since they progress quickly after initial response to androgen deprivation as compared to those seen in conventional prostatic adenocarcinoma. A retrospective study of 29 ductal carcinoma patients with matched 116 conventional prostate carcinoma patients, for age, clinical stage, margin status, PSA, and follow-up, showed poorer prognosis than the conventional group ($p=0.016$) [48].

Based on the reported data, we recommend stage and risk-based definitive treatment of localized ductal carcinoma of the prostate, as done for men with conventional prostatic adenocarcinomas. Patient with advanced stage should be offered medical or surgical castration, and subsequently novel androgen synthesis and AR inhibitors, and chemotherapeutic agents once they experience progression.

Sarcomatoid Carcinoma

Sarcomatoid carcinoma is another very rare variant of prostate adenocarcinoma which is characterized by spindled and/or pleomorphic sarcomatoid morphology admixed with conventional acinar adenocarcinoma or found in subsequent sections.

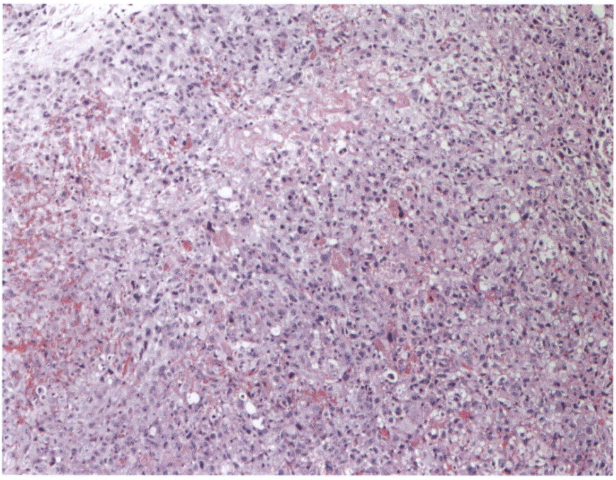

Fig. 14.4 Sarcomatoid prostate adenocarcinoma (100×)

Most of the patients have either prior history of conventional adenocarcinoma or are diagnosed concurrently. The presence of sarcomatoid component reflects the ability of high-grade prostate adenocarcinoma to dedifferentiate into a more primitive mesenchymal-like state. Some investigators have hypothesized that androgen deprivation and radiation may induce or facilitate epithelial to mesenchymal transformation [49, 50]. Patients with predominant sarcomatoid carcinoma may not have elevated PSA.

These patients should be differentiated from primary sarcoma of the prostate. Primary sarcoma of the prostate resembling rhabdomyosarcoma, leiomyosarcoma, angiosarcoma, fibrosarcoma, high grade pleomorphic sarcoma, osteogenic sarcoma, and neurogenic sarcoma had been described in the literature. Light microscopy and immunohistochemistry can easily help to differentiate these tumors from sarcomatoid differentiation [51].

Pathology

The sarcomatoid component of sarcomatoid prostate cancer can demonstrate a variety of morphologic appearances. The sarcomatoid areas most commonly demonstrate spindle cells with large, pleomorphic, hyperchromatic nuclei (Figs. 14.4 and 14.5). Occasionally, the cells appear more plump, with abundant eosinophilic cytoplasm and pleomorphic or vesicular nuclei – resembling high-grade pleomorphic sarcoma (malignant fibrous histiocytoma) [51, 52]. The sarcomatous component may also demonstrate focal or widespread resemblance to other types of sarcoma such as fibrosarcoma, chondroblastic osteosarcoma, and others [53]. The conventional adenocarcinoma component associated with this subtype shows typical patterns including glandular, cribriform, comedo, or papillary and usually demonstrates a higher Gleason score (Fig. 14.6). In a retrospective case series of 32 patients with

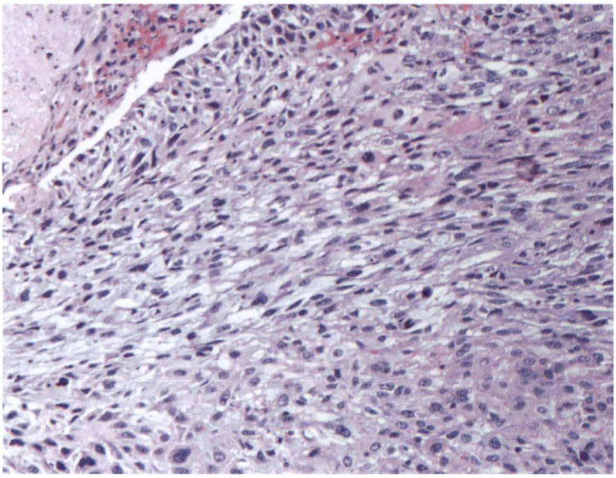

Fig. 14.5 Sarcomatoid prostate adenocarcinoma (200×)

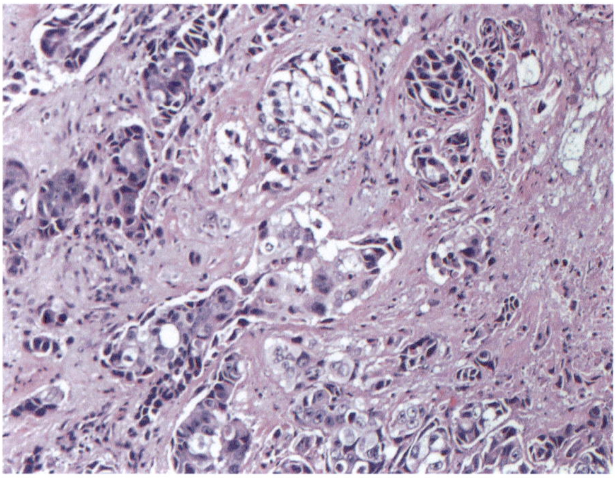

Fig. 14.6 Sarcomatoid prostate adenocarcinoma (same case as Figs. 14.5 and 14.6) with component of high-grade conventional adenocarcinoma (200×)

sarcomatoid carcinoma of the prostate, 93 % of the specimens showed 8 or higher-grade Gleason sum scores in the acinar component [54]. The sarcomatoid component in these specimens ranged from 5 to 99 %. Undifferentiated spindle cell appearances were observed in a majority of the cases.

The sarcomatoid component is observed to be positive for vimentin. Other markers like desmin, myoglobin, and S-100 staining are variable as described in the reported cases. These sarcomatous areas are PSA, PAP, and AR negative. A recent study using FISH for analyzing ERG deletion demonstrated that sarcomatoid component was positive for this deletion in the absence of positive ERG IHC [55]. This finding is supportive of an epithelial rather than mesenchymal origin. The adenocarcinoma component is classically positive for prostate cancer-specific immunostains like PSA and PAP.

Clinical Features and Management

It is generally considered that sarcomatoid carcinoma of the prostate is a very aggressive variant. The patients presenting with advanced disease have a very poor prognosis and die within months of their diagnosis. There are case reports of patients who were diagnosed in early stages, underwent surgery followed by radiation and androgen deprivation therapy, and had longer survival [56]. However, in a larger series of 21 patients from Mayo Clinic, including both localized (10/21) and advanced disease patients (11/21), 7-year survival was observed to be 14 % [53]. In another study of 42 patients with sarcomatoid carcinoma of the prostate, actuarial risk of death at 1 year was 20 %. No correlation was observed between patient survival and morphologic features, prior therapy, or coexistent high-grade acinar carcinoma. Treatment with single-agent chemotherapy agents, such as docetaxel, carboplatin, and cisplatin, has not been shown to improve outcomes in patients with advanced sarcomatoid carcinoma [54].

We recommend to treat these patients aggressively if diagnosed at an early stage with surgery, followed by definitive radiation, and concomitant androgen deprivation therapy. Patients with advanced stage should receive androgen deprivation therapy, especially if sarcomatoid carcinoma is admixed with conventional acinar adenocarcinoma. Chemotherapy may be considered early since the sarcomatous component may not respond to androgen deprivation.

Future Directions

The different histological subtypes noted herein have two common facets: (1) a lack of well-defined biology and (2) a lack of a well-defined treatment strategy. Recent genomic profiling studies of conventional prostatic adenocarcinoma suggests a high frequency of aberrations outside of the canonical androgen receptor signaling axes [57]. These studies point toward new potential treatment paradigms for advanced disease, targeting genes related to DNA repair (e.g., *ATM*, *BRCA1*, or *BRCA2*) or unique signal transduction cascades (e.g., *PIK3CA*, *BRAF*, etc.). The same approach should be taken to characterize rare histologies of prostate cancer. Only when the biological underpinnings of the disease are better understood that we will begin to define personalized treatment strategies for these orphan diseases.

References

1. Torre LA, Bray F, Siegel RL, Ferlay J, Lortet-Tieulent J, Jemal A. Global cancer statistics, 2012. CA Cancer J Clin. 2015;65:87–108.
2. Siegel RL, Miller KD, Jemal A. Cancer statistics, 2015. CA: Cancer J Clin. 2015;65:5–29.
3. Mohler JL, Kantoff PW, Armstrong AJ, et al. National comprehensive cancer network. J Natl Compr Canc Netw. 2014;12(5):686–718. PMID: 24812137.
4. Xie LP, Qin J, Zheng XY, et al. Age and pathological features of 481 prostate cancer patients. Zhonghua Nan Ke Xue. 2005;11:428–30.

5. Epstein JI, Lieberman PH. Mucinous adenocarcinoma of the prostate gland. Am J Surg Pathol. 1985;9:299–308.
6. Grignon DJ. Unusual subtypes of prostate cancer. Mod Pathol. 2004;17:316–27.
7. Bohman KD, Osunkoya AO. Mucin-producing tumors and tumor-like lesions involving the prostate: a comprehensive review. Adv Anat Pathol. 2012;19:374–87.
8. Boyd S. A case of colloid scirrhus of the prostate. Trans Pathol Soc Lond. 1882;33:200–3.
9. Osunkoya AO, Nielsen ME, Epstein JI. Prognosis of mucinous adenocarcinoma of the prostate treated by radical prostatectomy: a study of 47 cases. Am J Surg Pathol. 2008;32:468–72.
10. Elbadawi A, Craig W, Linke CA, Cooper Jr RA. Prostatic mucinous carcinoma. Urology. 1979;13:658–66.
11. Watarai Y, Demura T, Togashi M, et al. Mucinous adenocarcinoma of the prostate. A case report and analysis of the literature. Nihon Hinyokika Gakkai Zasshi. 1994;85:1276–9.
12. Kalaitzis C, Koukourakis M, Giannakopoulos S, et al. Metastatic mucinous adenocarcinoma of the prostate with PSA value of 8.6 ng/mL at 5-year-followup after prostatectomy, radiotherapy, and androgen deprivation. Case Rep Urol. 2014;2014:218628.
13. Ro JY, Grignon DJ, Ayala AG, Fernandez PL, Ordonez NG, Wishnow KI. Mucinous adenocarcinoma of the prostate: histochemical and immunohistochemical studies. Hum Pathol. 1990;21:593–600.
14. Epstein JI, Allsbrook Jr WC, Amin MB, Egevad LL, Committee IG. The 2005 International Society of Urological Pathology (ISUP) Consensus Conference on Gleason Grading of Prostatic Carcinoma. Am J Surg Pathol. 2005;29:1228–42.
15. Saito S, Iwaki H. Mucin-producing carcinoma of the prostate: review of 88 cases. Urology. 1999;54:141–4.
16. Johnson H, Zhou M, Osunkoya AO. ERG expression in mucinous prostatic adenocarcinoma and prostatic adenocarcinoma with mucinous features: comparison with conventional prostatic adenocarcinoma. Hum Pathol. 2013;44:2241–6.
17. Osunkoya AO, Adsay NV, Cohen C, Epstein JI, Smith SL. MUC2 expression in primary mucinous and nonmucinous adenocarcinoma of the prostate: an analysis of 50 cases on radical prostatectomy. Mod Pathol. 2008;21:789–94.
18. Ro JY, Ayala AG, Wishnow KI, Ordonez NG. Prostatic duct adenocarcinoma with endometrioid features: immunohistochemical and electron microscopic study. Semin Diagn Pathol. 1988;5:301–11.
19. Saez C, Japon MA, Conde AF, Poveda MA, Luna-More S, Segura DI. Sialomucins are characteristically O-acylated in poorly differentiated and colloid prostatic adenocarcinomas. Mod Pathol. 1998;11:1193–7.
20. Manne RK, Haddad FS. Mucinous adenocarcinoma of prostate. Urology. 1989;33:247–9.
21. Schiebler ML, Schnall MD, Outwater E. MR imaging of mucinous adenocarcinoma of the prostate. J Comput Assist Tomogr. 1992;16:493–4.
22. Westphalen AC, Coakley FV, Kurhanewicz J, Reed G, Wang ZJ, Simko JP. Mucinous adenocarcinoma of the prostate: MRI and MR spectroscopy features. AJR Am J Roentgenol. 2009;193:W238–43.
23. Outwater E, Schiebler ML, Tomaszewski JE, Schnall MD, Kressel HY. Mucinous carcinomas involving the prostate: atypical findings at MR imaging. J Magn Reson Imaging. 1992;2:597–600.
24. Curtis MW, Evans AJ, Srigley JR. Mucin-producing urothelial-type adenocarcinoma of prostate: report of two cases of a rare and diagnostically challenging entity. Mod Pathol. 2005;18:585–90.
25. Giltman L. Signet ring adenocarcinoma of the prostate. J Urol. 1981;126:134–5.
26. Randolph TL, Amin MB, Ro JY, Ayala AG. Histologic variants of adenocarcinoma and other carcinomas of prostate: pathologic criteria and clinical significance. Mod Pathol. 1997;10:612–29.
27. Torbenson M, Dhir R, Nangia A, Becich MJ, Kapadia SB. Prostatic carcinoma with signet ring cells: a clinicopathologic and immunohistochemical analysis of 12 cases, with review of the literature. Mod Pathol. 1998;11:552–9.

28. Ro JY, el-Naggar A, Ayala AG, Mody DR, Ordonez NG. Signet-ring-cell carcinoma of the prostate. Electron-microscopic and immunohistochemical studies of eight cases. Am J Surg Pathol. 1988;12:453–60.
29. Matsuoka Y, Arai G, Ishimaru H, Takagi K, Ito Y. Primary signet-ring cell carcinoma of the prostate. Can J Urol. 2007;14:3764–6.
30. Remmele W, Weber A, Harding P. Primary signet-ring cell carcinoma of the prostate. Hum Pathol. 1988;19:478–80.
31. Skodras G, Wang J, Kragel PJ. Primary prostatic signet-ring cell carcinoma. Urology. 1993;42:338–42.
32. Kwon WA, Oh TH, Ahn SH, Lee JW, Park SC. Primary signet ring cell carcinoma of the prostate. Can Urol Assoc J. 2013;7:E768–71.
33. Yoshimura K, Fukui I, Ishikawa Y, Maeda H, Yamauchi T, Kawai T. Locally-confined signet-ring cell carcinoma of the prostate: a case report of a long-term survivor. Int J Urol. 1996;3:406–7.
34. Lilleby W, Axcrona K, Alfsen GC, Urnes T, Hole KH. Diagnosis and treatment of primary signet-ring cell carcinoma of the prostate. Acta Oncol. 2007;46:1195–7.
35. Kanematsu A, Hiura M. Primary signet ring cell adenocarcinoma of the prostate treated by radical prostatectomy after preoperative androgen deprivation. Int J Urol. 1997;4:522–3.
36. Fujita K, Sugao H, Gotoh T, Yokomizo S, Itoh Y. Primary signet ring cell carcinoma of the prostate: report and review of 42 cases. Int J Urol. 2004;11:178–81.
37. Alguacil-Garcia A. Artifactual changes mimicking signet ring cell carcinoma in transurethral prostatectomy specimens. Am J Surg Pathol. 1986;10:795–800.
38. Celik O, Budak S, Ekin G, Akarken I, Ilbey YO. A case with primary signet ring cell adenocarcinoma of the prostate and review of the literature. Arch Ital Urol Androl. 2014;86:148–9.
39. Gravis G, Fizazi K, Joly F, et al. Androgen-deprivation therapy alone or with docetaxel in non-castrate metastatic prostate cancer (GETUG-AFU 15): a randomised, open-label, phase 3 trial. Lancet Oncol. 2013;14:149–58.
40. Melicow MM, Pachter MR. Endometrial carcinoma of proxtatic utricle (uterus masculinus). Cancer. 1967;20:1715–22.
41. Merchant Jr RF, Graham AR, Bucher Jr WC, Parker DA. Endometrial carcinoma of prostatic utricle with osseous metastases. Urology. 1976;8:169–73.
42. Oxley JD, Abbott CD, Gillatt DA, MacIver AG. Ductal carcinomas of the prostate: a clinico-pathological and immunohistochemical study. Br J Urol. 1998;81:109–15.
43. Dube VE, Farrow GM, Greene LF. Prostatic adenocarcinoma of ductal origin. Cancer. 1973;32:402–9.
44. Epstein JI, Woodruff JM. Adenocarcinoma of the prostate with endometrioid features. A light microscopic and immunohistochemical study of ten cases. Cancer. 1986;57:111–9.
45. Dawkins HJ, Sellner LN, Turbett GR, et al. Distinction between intraductal carcinoma of the prostate (IDC-P), high-grade dysplasia (PIN), and invasive prostatic adenocarcinoma, using molecular markers of cancer progression. Prostate. 2000;44:265–70.
46. Brinker DA, Potter SR, Epstein JI. Ductal adenocarcinoma of the prostate diagnosed on needle biopsy: correlation with clinical and radical prostatectomy findings and progression. Am J Surg Pathol. 1999;23:1471–9.
47. Young BW, Lagios MD. Endometrial (papillary) carcinoma of the prostatic utricle – response to orchiectomy. A case report. Cancer. 1973;32:1293–300.
48. Kim A, Kwon T, You D, et al. Clinicopathological features of prostate ductal carcinoma: matching analysis and comparison with prostate acinar carcinoma. J Korean Med Sci. 2015;30:385–9.
49. Locke JR, Soloway MS, Evans J, Murphy WM. Osteogenic differentiation associated with x-ray therapy for adenocarcinoma of the prostate gland. Am J Clin Pathol. 1986;85:375–8.
50. Meeter UL, Richards JN. Osteogenic sarcoma of the prostate. J Urol. 1960;84:654–7.
51. Shannon RL, Ro JY, Grignon DJ, et al. Sarcomatoid carcinoma of the prostate. A clinicopathologic study of 12 patients. Cancer. 1992;69:2676–82.

52. Fyfe G, Fisher RI, Rosenberg SA, Sznol M, Parkinson DR, Louie AC. Results of treatment of 255 patients with metastatic renal cell carcinoma who received high-dose recombinant interleukin-2 therapy. J Clin Oncol. 1995;13:688–96.
53. Dundore PA, Cheville JC, Nascimento AG, Farrow GM, Bostwick DG. Carcinosarcoma of the prostate. Report of 21 cases. Cancer. 1995;76:1035–42.
54. Hansel DE, Epstein JI. Sarcomatoid carcinoma of the prostate: a study of 42 cases. Am J Surg Pathol. 2006;30:1316–21.
55. Rodrigues DN, Hazell S, Miranda S, et al. Sarcomatoid carcinoma of the prostate: ERG fluorescence in-situ hybridization confirms epithelial origin. Histopathology. 2015;66:898–901.
56. Lauwers GY, Schevchuk M, Armenakas N, Reuter VE. Carcinosarcoma of the prostate. Am J Surg Pathol. 1993;17:342–9.
57. Robinson D, Van Allen EM, Wu YM, et al. Integrative clinical genomics of advanced prostate cancer. Cell. 2015;161:1215–28.

Prostate Sarcomas and Squamous Cell Carcinomas

15

Louis L. Pisters

Introduction

Primary prostate sarcomas are rare tumors arising from nonepithelial mesenchymal components of the prostate stroma. These tumors account for less than 0.1 % of prostate malignancy in adults [1]. Leiomyosarcomas are the most common histological subtype in adults, whereas rhabdomyosarcoma is more common in pediatric patients. Surgery remains the mainstay in treatment and the surgical approach varies depending on tumor extent. Radical prostatectomy is appropriate for those patients whose tumors are confined to the prostate. Cystoprostatectomy or total pelvic exenteration is the preferred approach for those patients with significant bladder or rectal invasion. Systemic chemotherapy and preoperative radiation therapy may be considered preoperatively in locally advanced cases or as definite treatment in those patients with metastatic disease. Although the overall prognosis for patients with prostate sarcomas remains poor, surgical resection with or without preoperative chemotherapy and radiation can cure select patients without metastatic disease.

Squamous cell carcinoma of the prostate is very rare also constituting less than 0.1 % of all prostate cancers in a pure form. Patients typically present with obstructive urinary symptoms. Prostate squamous cell carcinoma has a tendency to recur locally (after initial treatment with surgery or radiation therapy) and also spreads distantly to the bones (osteolytic metastasis), liver, and lungs. The cancer is very aggressive with a median survival time of only 14 months. A multimodality treatment approach with systemic therapy combined with local treatment with surgery and/or radiation therapy should be considered.

L.L. Pisters, MD
Department of Urology, The University of Texas MD Anderson Cancer Center, 1515 Holcombe Blvd., Houston, TX, USA
e-mail: lpisters@mdanderson.org

L. Pagliaro (ed.), *Rare Genitourinary Tumors*,
DOI 10.1007/978-3-319-30046-7_15

This chapter focuses on pure prostate sarcomas and squamous cell carcinomas including patient evaluation and management. High-grade prostate adenocarcinoma can rarely differentiate into sarcomatoid or squamous cell carcinoma phenotypes, and an extensive discussion of these mixed histology prostate cancers is beyond the scope of this chapter.

Sarcoma: Patient Presentation and Evaluation

Most patients with leiomyosarcoma present in the fifth to eighth decade of life, whereas most adults with rhabdomyosarcoma of the prostate present in their late teens or twenties [2]. The most common symptoms are urinary obstruction in 76 % of patients followed by pelvic or perineal pain in almost 50 % [2]. Other less common symptoms include urinary frequency, rectal pain, constipation, and hematuria or pain with ejaculation [2]. Physical examination may reveal an enlarged prostate or prostate mass on digital rectal examination or palpable lower abdominal mass in the context of a large prostate sarcoma. Many prostate sarcomas have a relatively smooth posterior surface and may be difficult to distinguish from enlargement of the prostate with benign prostatic hypertrophy (BPH) on digital rectal examination. Rhabdomyosarcoma of the prostate should be suspected in any young adult with urinary obstruction and an enlarged prostate or pelvic mass on digital rectal examination. PSA values are not elevated in patients with prostate sarcoma. Ultrasonography (either transrectal or transabdominal) or cross-sectional imaging with CT or MRI will demonstrate a prostate mass that may be either relatively homogeneous or heterogeneous (Fig. 15.1). Cross-sectional imaging of the lungs and liver is an important component of initial staging, since these are the most common metastatic sites. Pelvic or retroperitoneal lymph node metastases are less common but occasionally occur, particularly with rhabdomyosarcomas. Other less common metastatic sites are the brain, kidney, and abdominal wall. A biopsy is helpful in establishing a pathologic diagnosis and distinguishing sarcoma from other atypical prostate lesions such as benign leiomyoma or stromal tumor of uncertain malignant potential (STUMP). An image-guided needle biopsy using transrectal ultrasound or CT may be optimal as different regions of a heterogeneous tumor may be sampled. Transurethral resection of the prostate is sometimes performed on a patient with obstructive symptoms and suspected BPH with final pathology demonstrating sarcoma. Once a diagnosis of prostate sarcoma is made, consideration should be given to referring the patient to a tertiary center specializing in sarcoma treatment.

Specific Types of Prostate Sarcoma

Leiomyosarcoma

Although leiomyosarcoma is the most common subtype of prostate sarcoma, there are less than 250 cases in the literature [3–7]. Leiomyosarcomas vary in size from 1 to 25 cm, with the majority of lesions between 5 and 10 cm [3–7].The majority of

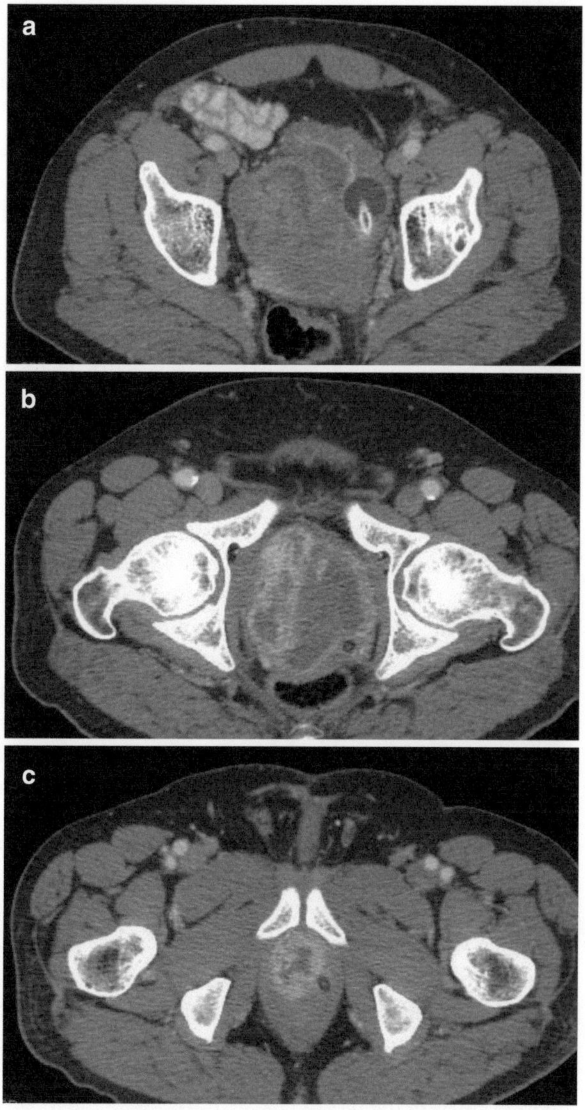

Fig. 15.1 A 61-year-old male presented with urinary retention and was found to have a 10 cm sclerosing epithelioid fibrosarcoma of the prostate. (**a–c**) Axial computed tomography images of the tumor at presentation. Note the position and deviation of the urethral catheter by the tumor. He was treated with 5,000 cGy preoperative radiation therapy followed by radical prostatectomy with negative margins and was cancer-free with 6 months of follow-up

prostate leiomyosarcomas have been high grade with frequent mitosis and necrosis. Rare cases of low-grade leiomyosarcoma have been reported. Smooth muscle markers such as actin, desmin, and calponin are typically positive on immunohistochemical studies [2]. Focal keratin positivity can be seen in epithelioid cases. Positivity for estrogen receptor has been reported for both prostate leiomyosarcoma and STUMPs [2].

Prostate leiomyosarcomas often have aggressive behavior similar to high-grade leiomyosarcomas arising in other sites. Approximately one quarter of patients have metastatic disease at presentation, and many develop metastatic disease in spite of local and systemic treatments. The overall prognosis for prostate leiomyosarcoma is poor with 50–75 % of patients dying within 2–5 years. All ten patients in a recent Chinese report of prostate leiomyosarcoma died, in spite of six of them having no metastatic disease at presentation [3]. However, many of the patients in the Chinese report had locally advanced tumors with most being greater than 10 cm in size [3]. The completeness of surgical resection is important, and negative surgical margins have been associated with improved survival [4].

Rhabdomyosarcoma

Embryonal rhabdomyosarcoma involving the prostate is far more common in children than in adults. The other two types of rhabdomyosarcoma, pleomorphic and alveolar, are exceedingly rare in the prostate [2]. There are 52 cases of adult prostate rhabdomyosarcoma in the literature [3–11]. Most patients with prostate rhabdomyosarcoma present with urinary obstruction. Tumors are often advanced and a significant number of patients have metastatic disease at presentation. Patients typically have a large mass; most rhabdomyosarcomas are greater than 7 cm in diameter. The presence of anaplasia may indicate a more aggressive rhabdomyosarcoma [2]. Sarcoma botryoides is a rare subtype of embryonal rhabdomyosarcoma with rare prostate cases reported [12, 13]. Pathologists should confirm the diagnosis of rhabdomyosarcoma with immunostaining for markers of skeletal muscle differentiation including Myo-D1 and myogenin [2]. Unfortunately, adults with rhabdomyosarcoma do not respond as well as children to either systemic chemotherapy or radiation. In spite of this, neoadjuvant systemic chemotherapy and radiation should be considered prior to surgical intervention for those patients who do not have metastatic disease at presentation, due to the aggressive nature of these malignancies. In the report by Musser, patients with rhabdomyosarcomas had significantly worse survival than those with leiomyosarcoma (hazard ratio, 3.00; 95 % confidence interval 1.13–7.92, $p=0.27$) [5].

Prostate Angiosarcoma

Angiosarcoma is an exceptionally rare prostate sarcoma that is remarkably aggressive and often leads to mortality within a year of diagnosis. Patients with angiosarcoma often present with hematuria and dysuria. Other presenting symptoms include abdominal or pelvic pain, urinary frequency, or constipation. There are about 10 reported cases in the world [14–20]. Although the mean age at diagnosis is 40 years, angiosarcoma has been reported in a wide range of ages from 2 to 80 years [14–20]. Three of the ten cases reported in the literature had received prior radiation therapy for prostate adenocarcinoma, leading to the hypothesis that radiation therapy may have been causal in the development of the angiosarcoma. Although some patients have initially presented with locally advanced disease, metastatic progression is predictable. Common metastatic sites include the lymph nodes, spleen, lung, and liver.

From a pathologic perspective, immunostaining for endothelial markers CD31, CD34, and ERG can confirm endothelial cell differentiation [2]. Factor VIII-related antigen is a less sensitive marker for angiosarcoma since it may be lost in some cases [2]. Importantly, some angiosarcomas may be keratin positive on immunohistochemistry which is especially true for the epithelioid variant of angiosarcoma [2]. The keratin positivity of some angiosarcomas may lead to a misdiagnosis of carcinoma [2].

Prostate angiosarcoma is a challenging malignancy to treat because it has been resistant to all systemic chemotherapy, radiation, and surgery. Since this sarcoma type has been resistant to all standard sarcoma treatment regimens, consideration should be given to going directly to an experimental approach. Patients could participate in a phase I study or consider a personalized medicine approach based on the molecular profile of a patient's malignancy.

Stromal Tumor of Uncertain Malignant Potential (STUMP)

In 1998, a proposal was made to unify a wide variety of prostate stromal lesions under the term stromal tumors of uncertain malignant potential (STUMP) [21]. The stromal lesions encompassed under the STUMP category were previously known as atypical stromal hyperplasia, atypical spindle cell proliferation, prostatic stromal hyperplasia, phyllodes tumor, and cystic epithelial-stromal tumors [21–26]. Although most of the STUMPs have a benign clinical course, some are believed to progress into prostate stromal sarcoma, and hence the term "uncertain malignant potential" should be included according to Herawi and Epstein [26]. However, it should be noted that in general it is exceedingly rare for a benign mesenchymal tumor to become a sarcoma. Although sarcomatous transformation of a neurofibroma into a neurofibrosarcoma has been described, benign mesenchymal tumors almost never transform into malignant counterparts, such as lipoma transforming into liposarcoma or hemangioma developing into hemangiosarcoma. There are four different histologic patterns of STUMP [2]. The most common histologic pattern is normal to hypercellular stroma with spindle cells showing degenerative atypia admixed with benign prostate glands [2]. The second pattern also occurs with an admixture of normal prostate glands and consists of hypercellular bland fusiform stromal cells with eosinophilic cytoplasm [2]. The third pattern consists of hypercellular stroma with or without atypia associated with prostate glands in a pattern that bears a resemblance to phyllodes tumor of the breast (these tumors were previously referred to as phyllodes hyperplasia or phyllodes tumor) [2]. The fourth pattern of STUMP consists to sheets of myxoid stroma with bland stromal cells, typically lacking admixed prostate glands [2]. In general, STUMP cases have few or no mitotic figures and no necrosis. If a significant number of mitotic figures or necrosis is present, then prostate stromal sarcoma should be considered [2].

Although there is a wide variation in age of presentation, many patients with STUMP are 60 years or older [21–26]. Symptoms associated with STUMP include bladder outlet obstruction, hematuria, or palpable rectal mass [21–26]. Some patients have presented with an elevated PSA level [21–26], but this may be due to the presence of a separate cause for the elevated PSA such as benign prostatic hyperplasia, prostate inflammation, or prostate adenocarcinoma. The stromal component of STUMPs does not produce PSA, but the elevated PSA in these patients may lead to a transrectal ultrasound examination that reveals the STUMP. In general

STUMPs do not metastasize and radical prostatectomy with negative surgical margins is curative. In Herawi's report, 7 of 14 stromal sarcomas were associated with STUMP, raising the possibility that STUMPs may dedifferentiate into sarcomas in rare cases [26]. As a result, patients with STUMP should either undergo radical prostatectomy or be closely observed if they are not good surgical candidates or decline surgery.

Prostate Stromal Sarcoma

Stromal sarcomas may arise de novo or may rarely develop from a pre-existing STUMP and can occur in any zone of the prostate [26]. These sarcomas were previously known as malignant phyllodes tumors. Although there is a wide and overlapping range of age at diagnosis for prostate sarcoma and STUMP, most patients with prostate stromal sarcoma are less than 50 years old and tend to be younger than patients with STUMP [21, 27–31]. Symptoms of prostate stromal sarcoma include urinary retention, hematuria, and hematospermia [21, 30–32]. Prostate stromal sarcomas frequently extend directly into the seminal vesicles and occasionally involve the bladder (Fig. 15.2) and rectum. Size does not seem to correlate well with metastatic potential, and the reported dimensions range from small microscopic tumors to tumors as large as 18 cm [21, 26, 31, 33]. Prostate stromal sarcomas can metastasize to the liver and lung [26, 29, 31]. Prostate stromal sarcoma in general appears to be less aggressive than rhabdomyosarcoma and angiosarcoma with better survival. The principal treatment for prostate stromal sarcoma is surgical extirpation with less data supporting radiation therapy or chemotherapy [26, 30–33].

Pathologically prostate stromal sarcoma resembles STUMPs morphologically but has increased cellularity, stromal cellular atypia, mitosis, and necrosis. Leaflike structure, resembling breast phyllodes tumor, is the most common pattern. Prostate stromal sarcomas are progesterone receptor positive and most cases are diffusely positive for CD34 and vimentin. Prostate stromal sarcomas may express estrogen receptor and cases are occasionally focally positive for desmin. High-grade prostate stromal sarcomas frequently express beta-catenin, high Ki-67 labeling index, and p53 expression [2].

Treatment of Adult Prostate Sarcoma

Surgery remains a mainstay in the treatment of adult prostate sarcoma. Surgery must be individualized based on the extent of disease and may include radical prostatectomy, cystoprostatectomy, or total pelvic exenteration. The goals of surgical treatment are to obtain local control and potentially cure those patients that do not have metastatic disease. The surgeon should make every effort to obtain negative surgical margins, since positive margins are associated with worse survival [4]. Consideration should be given to preoperative chemotherapy or radiation therapy in those patients who present with locally advanced lesions in whom negative surgical margins may be difficult to obtain [4]. Neoadjuvant therapy may improve the likelihood of negative surgical margins and may improve local control, but there is no clear data to show a survival advantage for any specific neoadjuvant therapy. Patients with metastatic disease, including those with limited regional lymph node

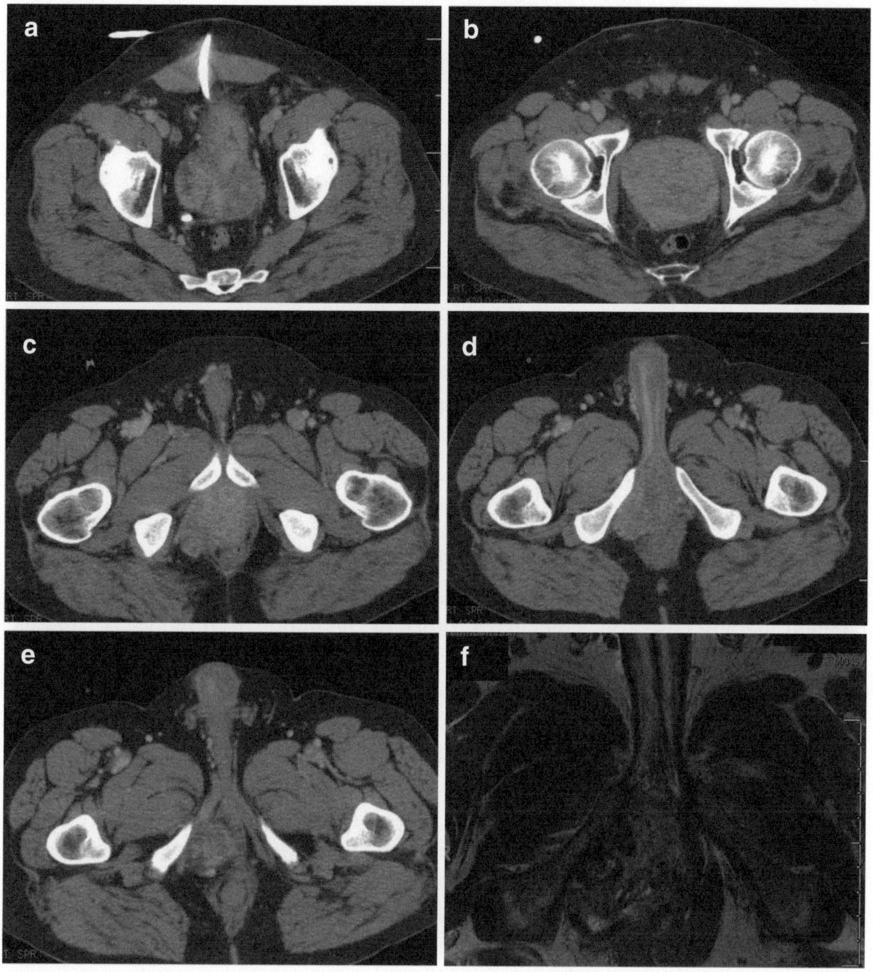

Fig. 15.2 A 45-year-old male presented with urinary obstruction and was found to have a large prostate stromal sarcoma. (**a–e**) Axial computed tomography images. Note suprapubic tube and involvement of bladder and right pelvic sidewall structures. (**f**) Axial T2 magnetic resonance images demonstrating right pelvic sidewall involvement. The patient was treated with preoperative doxorubicin and ifosfamide, prior to a planned radical cystoprostatectomy

involvement, often die of progressive disease. Local treatment may be considered for palliation of select symptomatic patients with metastatic disease, but patients should have a clear understanding of the palliative nature of such treatment.

Since the prognosis for many patients with prostate sarcoma is adverse, it seems reasonable to extrapolate data from extremity sarcoma literature and apply it to those with prostate sarcoma. Radiation therapy may improve local control [34], but cannot compensate well for large-volume or grossly positive margins [35]. A meta-analysis of adjuvant chemotherapy for localized soft tissue sarcoma demonstrated improved progression-free survival but unchanged overall survival [36]. For those patients with locally advanced prostate sarcoma and significant bladder or rectal wall invasion, it seems reasonable to consider neoadjuvant radiation and/or systemic chemotherapy prior to surgery to try to improve local control and delay or prevent systemic progression. Although adjuvant radiation can be given after cystoprostatectomy or pelvic exenteration, small bowel often falls down into the local field making it harder to deliver a meaningful dose of radiation. For this reason, it seems reasonable to consider preoperative radiation for locally advanced cases. Although there are no strong data to support the routine use of intraoperative radiation, this modality may be helpful in select patients. Intraoperative radiation can be used to treat focal regions where the surgical margins may be compromised at surgery. Since the overall dose of radiation delivered intraoperatively is too low to be effective as a stand-alone modality, patients who have received preoperative radiation may be the best candidates for this approach.

For those patients who develop a local recurrence following initial surgery, salvage surgery may rarely be curative and can be considered in select patients, especially those with a prolonged initial disease-free interval [4].

Patients with metastatic disease and those with angiosarcoma have an adverse prognosis and should be considered for experimental trials. Existing targeted therapies such as imatinib might be beneficial in select patients [37]. However, personal targeted therapy based on molecular profiles of the tumor from biopsy or surgical resected specimens may be the future for such patients.

Prostate Squamous Cell Carcinoma (PSCC)

PSCC is extremely rare in pure form and represents less than 0.1 % of all prostate malignancies. Kanthan conducted a review of the Saskatchewan Cancer Agency records over the past 30 years and found a total of six pure PSSS among 13,497 cases of prostate malignancies (0.004 %) [38]. PSCC is most frequently seen as a mixed tumor following treatment with radiation or hormonal therapy for prostate adenocarcinoma. In these mixed cases, it has been hypothesized that the SCC component may be derived from squamous metaplasia which undergoes malignant transformation in response to the radiation or hormonal therapy [39]. There are rare cases of pure PSCC that occur in the setting of chronic inflammation with urinary tract infection or prostatitis [40, 41]. The cell of origin of PSCC is uncertain – basal or reserve cells of the prostatic acini as proposed by Sieracki [42] or the transitional epithelium lining the urethra or major ducts as proposed by Kahler [43] and Thompson [44].

Presentation and Evaluation

Most patients with pure PSCC present with urinary obstructive symptoms and are 60 years or older. Digital rectal examination may show a mass involving the prostate with or without involvement of the seminal vesicles and bladder base. Pure PSCC does not express PSA and the serum PSA level is usually normal. An elevated PSA may indicate a mixed tumor with adenocarcinoma component. Cystoscopy may reveal irregular friable mucosa. An extensive prostate biopsy with sampling of multiple regions is essential in making the diagnosis. Mott has suggested five criteria for the diagnosis of pure PSCC: (1) a clearly malignant neoplasm as judged by disordered growth and cellular anaplasia; (2) definite squamous features of keratinization, squamous pearls, and/or numerous distinct intercellular bridges; (3) a lack of any glandular or acinar pattern (indicative of adenocarcinoma with squamous transformation); (4) no prior estrogen therapy; and (5) the absence of primary SCC elsewhere, particularly within the bladder [41]. Patients with mixed tumors with both adenocarcinoma and PSCC have high-grade adenocarcinoma elements [45]. Therefore, if a patient has a prior history of low-to-intermediate-grade prostate adenocarcinoma and is found to have PSCC, it is important to extensively re-biopsy the patient to evaluate for focal high-grade adenocarcinoma elements. PSCC can involve the rectum resulting in a rectal mass for which the differential diagnosis includes SCC of anal origin. Any patient with a prior history of prostate adenocarcinoma who develops SCC of the rectum or anus should be evaluated for a mixed tumor. Many patients with PSCC with rectal invasion have mixed tumors; extensive biopsies with immunostaining for PSA usually help make the correct diagnosis and exclude SCC of anal origin [45]. Cross-sectional imaging is essential to evaluate local tumor extent and evaluate the patient for metastatic disease. The possible metastatic sites for PSCC include the pelvic and retroperitoneal lymph nodes, liver, lungs, and bone. Some patients present with bone pain and a bone metastases are lytic lesions on imaging.

Once the diagnosis of PSCC is made, consideration should be given to referring the patient to a tertiary medical center due to the poor prognosis.

Treatment of PSCC

PSCC has an adverse prognosis with a median overall survival of only 14 months. PSCC is prone to both local recurrence after initial local therapy and distant metastasis. Both surgery and radiation therapy can be used as local treatments. Since PSCC occurs in patients who are typically greater than 60 years, treatment selection must take into account the patient's overall health. In a healthy patient with a negative metastatic evaluation, the current optimal therapy may be neoadjuvant chemoradiation prior to surgical extirpation with consideration of intraoperative radiation therapy in select cases if there is concern regarding a focal positive margin. In an older patient who may not tolerate extirpative surgery, chemoradiation alone may be best. Rare cases of long-term disease-free survival have been reported with either surgery [46] or radiation [42]; however, combining these treatments may improve local control. Pure PSCC does not respond to hormonal therapy [41], but a mixed prostate adenocarcinoma/SCC might have a slight response. A variety of single and multi-agent chemotherapy regimens have been employed with none showing clear superiority [47–51]. Several possible advantages to using preoperative chemotherapy include possible shrinking of the tumor mass, possible treatment of subclinical metastatic disease, and the added benefit of giving the patient a 3-month or so window of time to allow the biology of their disease to be determined. Although PSCC is a potentially aggressive cancer, the literature is replete with case reports of patients with either pure PSCC or mixed PSCC that have died within a few weeks or months of diagnosis. Patients with these "super" aggressive pure or mixed PSCCs are unlikely to benefit from surgical extirpation, and these patients could be spared surgery. Patients who experience disease progression during a period of initial systemic chemotherapy could be considered for alternative chemotherapy or experimental therapy. Similar to other aggressive malignancies, personal targeted therapy based on molecular profiles of the tumor from biopsy or surgical resected specimens may be the future for such patients.

Conclusion

Both adult prostate sarcoma and PSCC are potentially aggressive malignancies that are best managed in a tertiary care center. Accurate pathology for both malignancies may be challenging and extensive biopsy is likely to render the correct diagnosis. Multimodality therapy including surgery, radiation therapy, and systemic treatment is currently the best approach. Future therapy may include targeted treatments based on the molecular profile of a patient's tumor.

References

1. Tetu B, Srigley JR, Bostwich DG. Soft tissue tumors. In: Bostwick DG, editor. Pathology of the prostate. New York: Churchill-Livingston; 1990. p. 117.
2. Tavora F. Mesenchymal tumors of the bladder and prostate: an update. Pathology. 2013;45(2):104–15.
3. Wang X. Twenty-five cases of adult prostate sarcoma: treated at a high volume institution from 1989 to 2009. Urology. 2013;82:160–5.
4. Sexton WJ. Adult prostate sarcoma: the M.D. Anderson cancer center experience. J Urol. 2001;166:521–5.
5. Musser JE. Adult prostate sarcoma: the memorial sloan kettering experience. Urology. 2014;84:624–8.
6. Mondaini N. Clinical characteristics and overall survival in genitourinary sarcomas. Treated with curative intent. A multicenter study. Eur Urol. 2005;47:468–73.
7. Cheville JC. Leiomyosarcoma of the prostate. Cancer. 1995;76:1422–7.
8. Waring PM, Newland RC. Prostatic embryonal rhabdomyosarcoma in adults. A clinic pathologic review. Cancer. 1992;69:755–62.
9. Nabi G, Dinda AK, Dogra PN. Primary embryonal rhabdomyosarcoma of prostate in adults. Diagnosis and management. Int Urol Nephrol. 2002;34:531–4.
10. Biscelia M, Magro G, Carosi I, et al. Primary embryonal rhabdomyosarcoma of the prostate in adults. Report of a case with review of the literature. Int J Surg Pathol. 2012;19(83):1–7.
11. Ren FY, Lu JP, Wang JJ, et al. Adult prostate sarcoma: radiological – clinical correlation. Clin Radiol. 2009;64(17):1–7.
12. Treetipastit J, Kittikowit W, Zielenska M, et al. Mixed embryonal/alveolar rhabdomyosarcoma of the prostate. Report of a case with molecular genetic studies and literature review. Pediatr Dev Pathol. 2009;12(38):3–9.

13. Miller HC, Benjamin JA, McEnvoy RK. Sarcoma botryoides: a 7 year survival. J Urol. 1969;101:567–9.
14. Humphrey PA. Angiosarcoma for the prostate. J Urol. 2012;187:684–5.
15. Kaliq W, Meyer CF, Uzoaru I, Wolf RM, Antonararkis ES. Prostate angiosarcoma: a case report and literature review. Med Oncol. 2012;29:2901–3.
16. Kaliq W, Meyer CF, Uzoaru I, Wolf RM, Antonararkis ES. Prostate angiosarcoma: is there any association with previous radiation therapy? BJU Int. 2012;110:E819–25.
17. Chandan VS, Wolsh L. Postirradition angiosarcoma of the prostate. Arch Pathol Lab Med. 2013;127:876–8.
18. Oliva Encina J, Gil Martinez P, Allepuz Losa C, et al. Prostatic angiosarcoma: report of a new case. (Spanish). Actas Urol Exp. 2001;25:78–80.
19. Chan KW. Angiosarcoma of the prostate. An immunohistochemical study of a case. Pathology. 1990;22:108–10.
20. Nanus DM, Kelsen D, Clark DG. Radiation – induced angiosarcoma. Cancer. 1987;60:777–9.
21. Gaudin PB, Rosai J, Epstein JI. Sarcomas and related proliferative lesions of specialized prostatic stroma. A clinic pathologic stud of 22 cases. Am J Surg Pathol. 1998;22:148–62.
22. Vassilakis GB. Pure leiomyoma of prostate. Urology. 1978;11:93–4.
23. Bostwick DG, Hossain D, Wian J, et al. Phyllodes tumor of the prostate. Long-term follow-up study of 23 cases. J Urol. 2004;172:894–9.
24. Attah EB, NKposong EO. Phyllodes type of atypical prostatic hyperplasia. J Urol. 1976;115:762–4.
25. Hossain D, Meier I, Wian J, et al. Prostatic stromal hyperplasia with atypia: follow-up study for 18 cases. Arch Pathol Lab Med. 2008;132:1729–33.
26. Herawi M, Epstein JI. Specialized stromal tumors of the prostate: a clinic pathologic study of 50 cases. Am J Surg Pathol. 2006;30:694–704.
27. Hansel DE, Herawi M, Montgomery E, Epstein JI. Spindle cell lesions of the adult prostate. Mod Pathol. 2007;20:148–50.
28. Herawi M, Montgomery EA, Epstein JI. Gastrointestinal stromal tumors (GIST) on prostate needle biopsy: a clinicopathologic study of 8 cases. Am J Surg Pathol. 2006;30:1389–95.
29. Rammeh Rommani S, Zermani R, Sfaxi M, et al. Prostatic stromal sarcoma. (French). Prog Urol. 2006;16:381–2.
30. Aguilar B, Villalobos M, Sotomayor M. Phyllodes tumor of the prostate. Urology. 2009;73:271.
31. Fraggetta F, Pepe P, Giunta ML, Aragona F. Primary high grade sarcoma of the specialized prostatic stroma: a case report with clinic-pathologic considerations. Pathological. 2008;100:482–4.
32. Morikawa T, Nagata M, Tomita K, et al. Phyllodes tumor of the prostate with exuberant glandular hyperplasia. Pathol Int. 2006;56:158–61.
33. Bostwick DG, Hossain D, Qian J, et al. Phyllodes tumor of the prostate: long-term follow-up study of 23 cases. J Urol. 2004;172:894–9.
34. Strander H, Turesson I, Cavallin-Stahl E. A systematic overview of radiation therapy effects in soft tissue sarcomas. Acta Oncol. 2003;42:516–31.
35. Schwartz DL, Einck J, Bellon J, et al. Fast neutron radiotherapy for soft tissue and cartilaginous sarcomas at high risk for local recurrence. Int J Radiat Oncol Boils Phys. 2001;50:449–56.
36. Adjuvant chemotherapy for localized respectable soft tissue sarcoma of adults: meta-analysis of individual data. Sarcoma Meta-analysis Collaboration. Lancet. 1997;350:1647–54.
37. Heinrich MC, Corless CL, Demetri GD, et al. Kinase mutations and imatinib response in patients with metastatic gastrointestinal stromal tumor. J Clin Oncol. 2003;21:4342–9.
38. Kanthan R. Squamous cell carcinoma of the prostate. A report of 6 cases. Urol Int. 2004;72(1):28–31.
39. Moyana TN. Adenosquamous cell carcinoma of the prostate. Am J Surg Pathol. 1987;11:403–7.

40. Sarma DP, Weilbaecher TG, Moon TD. Squamous cell carcinoma of prostate. Urology. 1991;37(3):260–2.
41. Mott LJ. Squamous cell carcinoma of the prostate. Report of 2 cases and review of the literature. J Urol. 1979;121:833–5.
42. Sieracki JC. Epidermoid carcinoma of the human prostate: report of three cases. Lab Invest. 1955;4:232–40.
43. Kahler JE. Carcinoma of the prostate gland: a pathologic study. J Urol. 1939;41:557–4.
44. Thompson GJ, Albers DD, Broders AC. Unusual carcinomas involving the prostate gland. J Urol. 1953;69:416–25.
45. Parwani AV. Prostate carcinoma with squamous differentiation. Am J Surg Pathol. 2004;28:5.
46. Masuda H, Yamada T, Nagahama K, Nagamutu H, Negishi T. Primary squamous cell carcinoma of the prostate: a case report. Jpn J Urol Surg. 1992;5:519–21.
47. Majeed F. Primary squamous cell carcinoma of the prostate: a novel chemotherapy regimen. J Urol. 2002;168:640.
48. Kuwahara M, Matsushita K, Yoshinga H, Aki M, Fujisaki N, Furihata M, Ohtsuki Y. Primary squamous cell carcinoma of the prostate: a case report. Hinyokika Kiyo. 1993;39:77–80.
49. Uchibayashi T, Hisazumi H, Hasegawa M, Shiba N, Muraishi Y, Tanaka T, Nonomura A. Squamous cell carcinoma of the prostate. Scand J Urol Nephrol. 1997;31:223–4.
50. Okada E, Kamizaki H. Primary squamous cell carcinoma of the prostate. Int J Urol. 2000;7:347–50.
51. Munoz F, Pierfracesco F. Squamous cell carcinoma of the prostate: long-term survival after combined chemo-radiation. Radiat Oncol. 2007;2:15.

Sex Cord-Stromal Tumors of the Testis

16

Marc Barry, Arpit Rao, and Richard Lauer

Leydig Cell Tumor of the Testis

Background

Leydig cells are an essential component of normal testicular stroma and are responsible for the development of male phenotype of the fetus and secretion of testosterone throughout life under the influence of the luteinizing hormone. The pathogenesis of Leydig cell tumors is poorly understood. The most common presentation is as a unilateral testicular mass, and metastatic disease is uncommon. Surgical resection is the mainstay of treatment as this tumor type is not sensitive to chemotherapy or radiotherapy. The prognosis is excellent for surgically resectable disease.

Incidence

Leydig cell tumors of the testis (LCT) are the commonest sex cord-stromal tumors, constituting about 3 % of testicular neoplasms overall and up to 9 % of all testicular neoplasms in prepubertal males [1, 2]. Although these can occur at any age, a bimodal distribution has been reported, with most cases occurring between 5–10 and 30–60 years of age. Approximately 10 % are bilateral, and 10 % are malignant. Malignant LCT has not been described in prepubertal males.

M. Barry, MD (✉)
Department of Pathology, University of New Mexico School of Medicine, Albuquerque, NM, USA
e-mail: MarcBarry@salud.unm.edu

A. Rao, MD • R. Lauer, MD
Division of Hematology/Oncology, Department of Internal Medicine, University of New Mexico School of Medicine,
MSC10-5550, 1 University of New Mexico, Albuquerque, NM 87131, USA

L. Pagliaro (ed.), *Rare Genitourinary Tumors*,
DOI 10.1007/978-3-319-30046-7_16

Historically, about 10 % of patients were thought to have metastatic disease at presentation, as defined by distant spread beyond the testis. This is suggested to be a significant overestimate in the current era due to increasingly earlier incidental detection of LCT because of wider use of scrotal ultrasound [3].

Presentation

The commonest initial manifestation is unilateral painless testicular mass, occurring in about 50 % of patients. Most patients are asymptomatic at diagnosis.

Because of the pivotal role of Leydig cells in the androgen axis, these tumors frequently elaborate androgens, and the majority of prepubertal patients present with precocious puberty manifested as pubic hair growth, accelerated skeletal and muscle development, and mature masculine voice. Adults with excessive androgen production are usually asymptomatic.

In about 8–15 % of patients, secretion of excessive estrogens may lead to feminization with gynecomastia, infertility, and genital underdevelopment. In adults, loss of libido, erectile dysfunction, and infertility may result. Older patients are more likely to present with metastatic disease with symptoms of a shorter duration, and without any endocrine manifestations [1].

Workup

Laboratory Workup

In pure Leydig cell tumors, testicular tumor markers including serum alpha-fetoprotein (AFP), beta subunit of human chorionic gonadotropin (β-HCG), and lactate dehydrogenase (LDH) should be within the reference range [3–5]. Serum testosterone levels are usually elevated. Serum estradiol levels may be increased when clinical feminization is evident [4, 5].

Imaging Workup [6]

Historically, the majority of patients with LCT underwent diagnostic imaging for a unilateral testicular mass/swelling. However, LCT are being increasingly detected in asymptomatic patients who undergo evaluation for infertility. Scrotal ultrasound is usually the initial imaging test. LCT are commonly hypo-echoic peripheral well-defined masses, but may also be iso- or hyper-echoic. Color Doppler most often has decreased central signal and increased peripheral signal. Ultrasound is unable to reliably distinguish between LCT and other tumors of the testis.

MRI of the testis is a useful diagnostic modality for LCT, which are nonenhancing on non-contrast T1-weighted sequences. These demonstrate a distinctive strong homogenous enhancement on T1 with contrast sequences, supposedly due to increased vascularity and myxoid-fibrous stroma. T1 delayed post-contrast sequences show a central washout of the contrast. T2 sequences commonly show a well-defined peripheral rim.

Staging workup for suspected malignancy includes a CT scan of the abdomen for the evaluation of retroperitoneal spread and chest radiography.

Pathology

Grossly, Leydig cell tumors are usually well circumscribed and have a solid or lobulated appearance on sectioning. They are usually yellow-tan to brown-gray in color. About 25 % have foci of necrosis and/or hemorrhage. Most are less than 4 cm in diameter, and tumors less than 1 cm are more common in the pediatric population. LCT are generally confined to the testis, but local extratesticular spread may be seen in 10–15 % of cases [1].

Microscopically, LCT may show a variety of patterns of growth: most commonly solid/diffuse (Fig. 16.1) or nodular, but trabecular or cord-like, pseudoglandular, tubular, nested, and microcystic patterns of growth may also be seen [21]. Sometimes multiple patterns may be seen in one tumor (Fig. 16.1). Fibrous septa and myxoid or edematous stroma (Fig. 16.1) have been described. Rarely, there may be associated calcification or ossification [22]. The cells of LCT generally resemble nonneoplastic Leydig cells: they are large and polygonal with abundant eosinophilic cytoplasm and have round nuclei containing a single prominent nucleolus (Fig. 16.2). Occasionally, due to lipid accumulation, LCT may have vacuolated or clear cytoplasm [22], and rarely the cells may be spindled or appear small, with scant cytoplasm. In up to 40 % of LCT, crystalloids of Reinke may be seen: these are strongly eosinophilic needle-shaped or rhomboid crystals present focally within the cytoplasm (Fig. 16.2).

About 90 % of LCT are immunoreactive for alpha-inhibin, melan-A, and calretinin. CD99 is positive in two thirds. Tumors are negative or focally positive for cytokeratins and S-100 and are negative for various markers of germ cell tumors such as OCT3/4, CD30, and CD117.

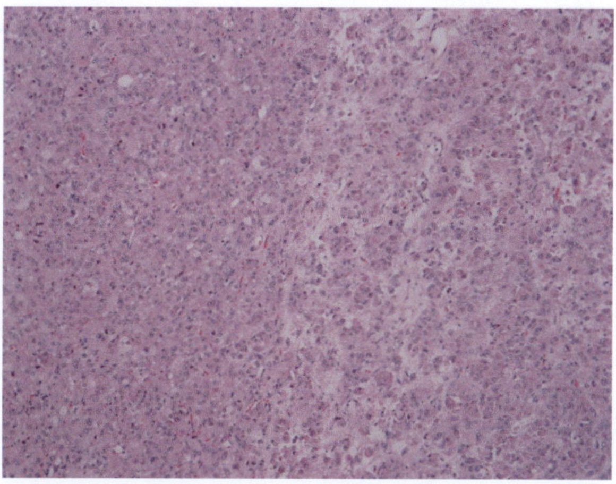

Fig. 16.1 Leydig cell tumor: tumor is present as eosinophilic cells with a diffuse sheetlike architecture and also focally as small nests embedded within some edematous stroma (100× magnification)

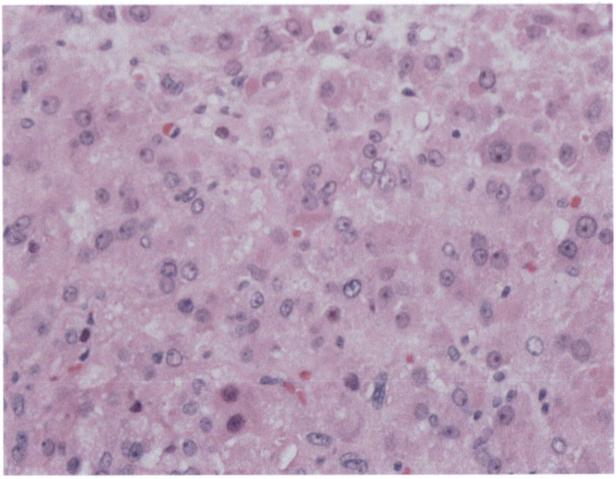

Fig. 16.2 Leydig cell tumor: tumor cells are large polygonal cells with abundant eosinophilic cytoplasm, round nuclei with prominent nucleoli. This case shows minimal nuclear atypia. A crystalloid of Reinke is present as a eosinophilic rhomboid structure centrally in the slide (400× magnification)

The pathologic differential diagnosis for LCT is wide, especially if the LCT shows variant architecture or cytology. It includes Leydig cell hyperplasia, the "tumors" that occur with adrenogenital syndrome and Nelson syndrome, other sex cord-stromal tumors, including large cell calcifying Sertoli cell tumor, yolk sac tumor (vs. microcystic LCT), seminoma (vs. LCT with clear cytoplasm), malakoplakia, and various non-testicular malignancies such as lymphoma, sarcoma, melanoma, and carcinoma such as prostatic adenocarcinoma [21].

Up to 10 % of LCT behave malignantly, and the only definitive criterion for malignancy in LCT is the presence of metastatic disease. Malignancy is not seen in prepubertal cases and is rare in adult patients with endocrine manifestations. In a study of the largest series of LCT [1], Kim et al. describe a number of clinicopathologic features, that, when taken together, may be useful in predicting subsequent malignant behavior: older age at tumor presentation, tumor size larger than 5 cm, infiltrative tumor margins, lymph-vascular space invasion, significant nuclear atypia, and increased mitotic rate (>3 per 10 high-power fields). All malignant LCT in this series had four or more of these findings, whereas 12 of 14 benign LCT had none. A more recent study by Cheville et al. [2] confirmed these findings in general, but recommended a cutoff of >5 mitoses per 10 high-power fields. This study also found that 7 out of 7 malignant LCT had aneuploidy as compared with 7 out of 18 benign LCT and that the proliferation index as measured by MIB-1 immunohistochemistry is 18.6 % in malignant LCT versus 1.2 % in benign LCT. They noted, however, that the results of aneuploidy and MIB-1 staining did not add additional information to the conventional clinicopathologic variables. In another smaller study [23], McCluggage et al. also find support for the clinicopathologic criteria of Kim, but in addition found MIB-1 staining helpful, in that all of the benign tumors had MIB-1 index of 0–2 %, whereas three of four malignant tumors had staining of 20–50 % of cells (one malignant tumor had 1 % staining). They also describe more than 50 % of cells with nuclear staining for p53 in two of the four malignant tumors as compared to 1–2 % staining in all benign (and two of the malignant) LCT.

None of the clinicopathologic features outlined above (apart from metastasis) is definitive for malignancy; however, as outlined, the presence of multiple of these features in patient/tumor allows some risk stratification for subsequent malignant behavior and helps identify which patients require extended follow-up.

Treatment

Type of Surgery

Surgical management is the mainstay of treatment for LCT. Two approaches have been described in the literature: radical inguinal orchiectomy (RIO) and testis-sparing surgery (TSS). The former has been the most commonly performed surgical procedure and remains the standard of care for patients with LCT. If performed, careful attention should be paid to early control of the spermatic cord and without violation of the scrotal skin to prevent hematogenous and cutaneous dissemination, respectively.

TSS warrants a multidisciplinary approach and preferably should be performed at specialized centers. An intraoperative ultrasound may be used to locate the mass, which is then enucleated with a rim of normal testicular parenchyma using an inguinal approach. A frozen section analysis can then be performed [7–10], and if features worrisome for malignancy are detected, a RIO is then performed. If the mass is benign, the testis is irrigated and returned to the scrotal sac.

Retroperitoneal Lymph Node Dissection (RPLND)

Studies evaluating the role of RPLND in LCT are limited. In one series, among the six patients who underwent RPLND for malignant phenotype LCT, three with stage I disease remained disease-free at follow-up (range, 25–135 months), and three with stage II disease subsequently died (range, 11–52 months) despite further treatment (including surgery, chemotherapy, or radiotherapy). The patients with stage II disease had initially presented with stage I disease and were being managed by surveillance [11].

In another series with younger patients (median age, 36 years), three patients with stage I and two patients with stage II disease had no disease recurrence at follow-up (range, 24–214 months) [12]. A series evaluating utility of minimally invasive RPLND in young patients (median age, 41 years) with stage I malignant phenotype LCT had no disease recurrence at follow-up (range, 3–29 months). Unfortunately, two intraoperative vascular complications required an open conversion [13].

Finally, a recent series evaluated the outcomes of RPLND in four patients with stage I and two patients with stage II malignant phenotype LCT. The number of adverse pathological features was the dominant determinant for disease recurrence and survival. Two patients with stage I disease, both of which had five adverse pathological features, developed early relapse and died of metastatic disease within 24 months of surgery. Two other patients with stage I LCT remained disease-free at follow-up. One patient with stage II LCT had disease recurrence, but was alive at 49 months after surgery.

In summary, RPLND with or following RIO should be considered for patients with LCT irrespective of clinical stage if having a malignant pathological phenotype, as the risk of metastatic disease increases significantly with increasing number of high-risk features.

Surveillance

Most recurrences occur within 2 years of the initial diagnosis, but late recurrences occurring as far as 8 years after surgery have been reported. Recurrent disease shares the original tumor's histopathological features, and metastasis may occur in the retroperitoneal lymph nodes (70 %), liver (45 %), lung (40 %), and bone (25 %) [14]. The frequency of surveillance imaging remains undefined. The suggested follow-up for tumors with malignant features is similar to that for non-seminomatous germ cell tumors with chest imaging and abdominal CT every 4 months during the first year, every 6 months during the second year, and yearly thereafter. Patients should be adequately monitored for at least 10–15 years after surgery due to the possibility of late recurrences.

Chemotherapy and Radiotherapy

LCT are chemo- and radiotherapy-resistant tumors. Combination chemotherapy with the bleomycin-etoposide-platinum used for germ cell malignancies is not particularly effective in LCT, resulting in only transient responses [11, 15–18]. Combination of mitotane and doxorubicin has been ineffective as well [14]. The tyrosine kinase inhibitor imatinib failed to demonstrate efficacy in human trials after showing promising results in animal models [19, 20]. The efficacy of taxanes, gemcitabine, and anti-angiogenic agents remains undetermined. Radiation therapy has not been shown to be beneficial in any setting in malignant LCT.

Prognosis

Benign LCT have an excellent prognosis after definitive treatment. Median survival for malignant phenotype LCT is variable and is worse for patients with advanced stage disease with more high-risk features.

Sertoli Cell Tumor of the Testis

Background

Sertoli cells play a critical role in spermatogenesis and regulation of testicular homeostasis. Inhibin and activin hormones produced by Sertoli cells modulate the secretion of follicle-stimulating hormone by the hypothalamus. Sertoli cell tumor (SCT) of the testis is an exceedingly rare entity. The majority of cases are sporadic, but the association of Sertoli cell neoplasms and hamartomatous proliferations with genetic syndromes, such as Peutz-Jeghers syndrome [24–26], androgen insensitivity syndrome (testicular feminization syndrome) [27], and Carney complex [26, 28], has been well described. The World Health Organization classifies these tumors into Sertoli cell tumor "not otherwise specified" (NOS), large cell calcifying SCT, and sclerosing SCT subtypes [29]. SCTs are mostly benign neoplasms, but malignancy does occur.

Incidence

Sertoli cell tumors of the testis constitute around 1 % of testicular neoplasms in the reported literature. Patients can present at any age with no known peak incidence [30]. Malignant cases form a small proportion (10 %) of cases [31–33].

Presentation

The commonest manifestation is as a slowly enlarging unilateral painless testicular mass. In younger patients, these may be discovered as testicular masses on ultrasonography done for workup of gynecomastia [25].

As compared to their malignant counterparts, benign SCTs are more likely to occur in younger patients (mean age, 17 versus 39 years old), be small (mean, 1.4 cm versus 5.4 cm), and multifocal or bilateral (28 % vs. 0 % of malignant tumors). Retroperitoneal lymph nodes are the commonest metastatic site, but hematogenous spread to the lungs, liver, and bone has been described in the literature [32].

Workup

Laboratory Workup

In pure Sertoli cell tumors, testicular tumor markers including serum alpha-fetoprotein (AFP), beta subunit of human chorionic gonadotropin (β-HCG), and lactate dehydrogenase (LDH) should be within the reference range. In young patients with clinical syndromes such as Peutz-Jeghers, Sertoli cell neoplasia has been associated with gynecomastia. This is thought to be a direct result of elevated levels of aromatase – an enzyme that converts testosterone and androstenedione to estradiol – within neoplastic cells [25].

Imaging Workup

Scrotal ultrasound is usually the initial imaging performed and shows a hypo- to hyper-echoic inhomogeneous lesion containing cystic areas. Large cell calcifying SCT tends to present as a well-circumscribed diffusely hyper-echoic intratesticular mass with heavy acoustic shadowing due to the presence of calcifications and moderate hypervascularity [34, 35]. MRI findings are varied and nondiagnostic. T1-weighted images show homogenous intermediate signal intensity with markedly enhanced well-defined thin walls. T2-weighted images show high signal intensity of the lesion [36].

Imaging of contralateral testis should be considered because a substantial proportion of Sertoli cell tumors are multifocal and bilateral (although multifocal and/or bilateral SCTs tend to be benign). In addition, CT of the chest and abdomen should be performed after a diagnosis has been established, because some SCTs are metastatic at the time of initial diagnosis.

Pathology

Sertoli cell tumors of the usual type (not otherwise specified (NOS)) are generally unilateral well-circumscribed yellow-white or tan masses, usually less than 4 cm in diameter and confined to the testis at initial presentation. Cystic change may be seen. There may be foci of hemorrhage, but necrosis is rare [21]. Microscopically, the characteristic finding is that of tubule formation (Figs. 16.3 and 16.4). These tubules may be hollow or solid. Cords, solid nests and sheets, trabeculae (Fig. 16.3), and rarely a retiform pattern may also be seen [21]. The tumor cells show a moderate amount of pale to eosinophilic cytoplasm (Fig. 16.4) and may appear clear or vacuolated if intracellular lipid is prominent. The nuclei tend to be bland, with small nucleoli, and generally there are few mitoses (Fig. 16.4). Occasional tumors may show significant cellular pleomorphism and mitotic activity. By immunohistochemistry, SCTs show staining for vimentin and variable staining for inhibin, calretinin, and cytokeratins. The pathologic differential diagnosis includes the nonneoplastic Sertoli cell nodules ("Pick adenomas") commonly seen in cryptorchid testes, the

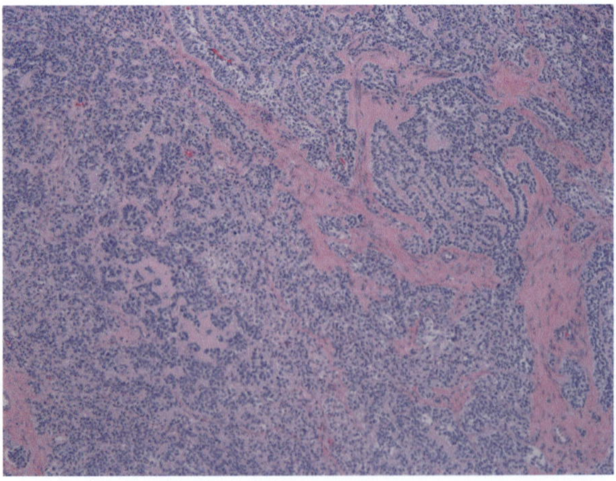

Fig. 16.3 Sertoli cell tumor: the tumor in this case shows a variety of architectural patterns, including hollow and solid tubular, nested, and solid patterns (100× magnification)

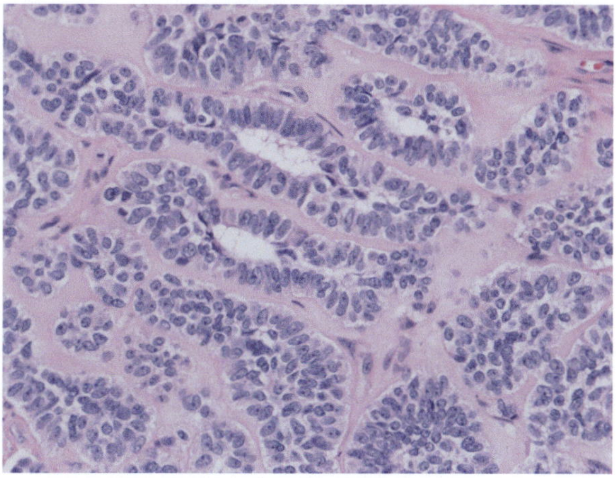

Fig. 16.4 Sertoli cell tumor: characteristic tubular architecture is present, with tumor cells showing pale cytoplasm and quite uniform bland nuclei with small nucleoli. Nuclear grooves are not seen (400× magnification)

benign hamartomatous and adenomatous Sertoli cell lesions of androgen insensitivity syndrome, Leydig cell tumor, undifferentiated sex cord-stromal tumor, and even occasionally seminoma. SCTs (NOS) are usually benign, but about 10 % show malignant behavior [30–44]. Malignant behavior in SCT (NOS) may also be seen in children. Metastases are generally to retroperitoneal or inguinal lymph nodes, but may also be to lung and skin. As with Leydig cell tumor, the best criterion for malignancy in SCT is metastasis, but malignant behavior is associated with a number of pathologic features: tumor size of 5 cm or greater, mitotic rate of greater than 5 per 10 high-power fields, significant nuclear atypia, necrosis, and lymph-vascular space invasion [21, 30, 31, 47]. Young and colleagues diagnose SCT as malignant if it has two or more of these features, and if there is one of the features they diagnose "uncertain malignant potential" [21]. Otherwise, they note that the SCT has a very low risk of malignant behavior. Two other features that correlate with malignancy are a MIB-1 proliferation index of >30 % [48] and a predominance of a diffuse growth pattern [31].

Large cell calcifying SCT is a variant with an unusual clinical association: 30–40 % of cases are associated with Carney complex, an inherited condition that is associated with mucocutaneous pigmentation, cardiac myxomas, myxomas of other sites, pituitary adenoma, and bilateral adrenal cortical hyperplasia. About half of cases are associated with germline mutation in the *PRKAR1A* gene. The association with large cell calcifying SCT is important to remember when diagnosing this tumor, because patients with Carney syndrome are at risk for sudden death secondary to cardiac myxomas. Large cell calcifying SCTs are generally well-circumscribed yellow-tan masses, usually less than 4 cm in diameter. Some have a gritty texture on sectioning, due to calcification. Microscopically, there are nests, cords, and sheets of cells with abundant eosinophilic cytoplasm in a fibrocollagenous or myxoid stroma [32, 45, 46]. Usually there is associated stromal microcalcification, and there may be a characteristic stromal neutrophilic infiltrate. Intratubular tumor is frequently present. Nuclei appear round, with prominent nucleoli. Mitoses are usually scant. The main morphological differential diagnosis is with Leydig cell tumor. Malignant behavior is seen in up to 20 % of cases, typically in older patients and typically not associated with Carney complex [31, 47]. Pathological features that have been associated with malignancy include tumor size >4 cm, extratesticular spread, mitotic count >3 per 10 high-power fields, significant nuclear atypia, lymphovascular invasion, and necrosis [32]. Kratzer and colleagues found that malignant tumors had two or more of these features [32].

Sclerosing SCT is an uncommon variant that usually presents as a testicular mass alone. Microscopically, the characteristic finding is of cells that are similar to SCT (NOS) set in a densely fibro-sclerotic stroma [42, 43]. About 40 cases have been reported in the literature, and only 1 showed malignant behavior [43].

Intratubular large cell hyalinizing Sertoli cell neoplasia is a form of Sertoli cell proliferation that is associated with, and very characteristic of, Peutz-Jeghers syndrome (thus associated with *STK11/LKB1* gene mutations) [25]. Clinically, it is usually associated with gynecomastia. Microscopically, this lesion comprises an intratubular Sertoli cell proliferation that is multifocal and bilateral, with large eosinophilic cells and associated intratubular incorporation of globules of basement membrane material [25], (Fig. 16.5). Intratubular large cell hyalinizing Sertoli cell neoplasia is itself benign, but in about 30 % of cases, an invasive tumor develops, that is morphologically reminiscent of large cell calcifying SCT [25].

Androgen insensitivity syndrome (testicular feminization syndrome) is associated with hamartomatous and adenomatous Sertoli cell proliferations. These may be multifocal and bilateral, but are clinically benign [27, 49].

Treatment

Type of Surgery

There are several commonalities between the management of Leydig cell tumors and Sertoli cell tumors, with surgical resection being the mainstay of treatment for both. Radical inguinal orchiectomy (RIO) and testis-sparing surgery (TSS) have been performed with the former being the standard of care.

While RIO has the advantage of familiarity for the surgeons, TSS may offer fertility and sexual function preservation. TSS warrants a greater multidisciplinary approach and preferably should be performed at specialized centers. It involves localization of testicular mass using intraoperative ultrasound followed by enucleation with a rim of normal testicular parenchyma using an inguinal approach. If malignant features are detected on a frozen section, a RIO is then performed. If the mass lacks adverse pathologic features, the testis is irrigated and returned to the scrotal sac. A series of 55 patients with Leydig cell tumors and 11 with Sertoli cell tumors evaluated outcomes of TSS versus RIO [38]. Patients undergoing TSS had

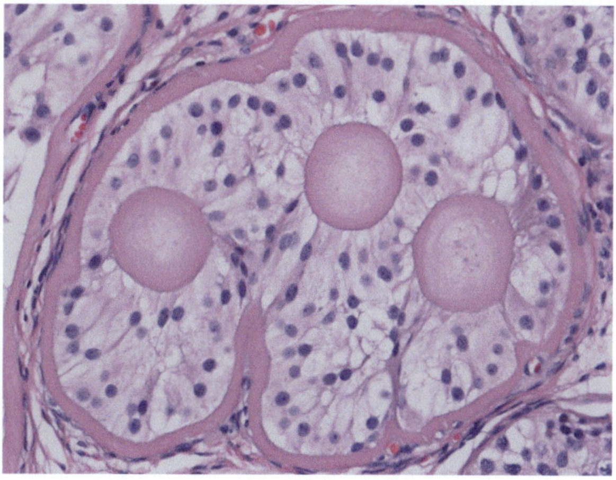

Fig. 16.5 Intratubular large cell hyalinizing Sertoli cell tumor: the microscopic section shows a seminiferous tubule that is completely replaced by large eosinophilic Sertoli cells and prominent globular eosinophilic basement membrane material. This entity is very characteristic of Peutz-Jeghers syndrome (400× magnification)

100 % relapse-free and overall survival at 5 years, but none had two or more adverse pathological features, and the median tumor size was only 0.7 cm (range, 0.6–1.3). One patient treated with TSS initially developed a local recurrence 26 months later and required orchiectomy.

Retroperitoneal Lymph Node Dissection (RPLND)

Studies evaluating the role of RPLND in SCT are limited. In one series, among the four patients who underwent RPLND for Sertoli cell tumors, two patients with stage I disease remained disease-free at follow-up (range, 9–63 months). One patient with stage II-B having three adverse histological features and one with III-A disease and having two adverse histological features died of the disease after 9 and 69 months, respectively [14].

Immediate RPLND for stage I disease is controversial as a low proportion of these patients have nodal metastasis. However, immediate RPLND is recommended for all clinical stage II-A or higher (due to the lack of effective subsequent therapies and inadequate data about optimal surveillance strategies), and if tumor size is large and three or more risk factors are present [14, 37, 38].

Chemotherapy

Chemotherapy and radiation therapy are not consistently effective, although occasional tumors have responded [32].

Additional Workup

Because of the known association of SCT and other Sertoli cell proliferations with genetic syndromes, careful attention should be paid to the presenting features, especially in younger patients with large cell calcifying Sertoli cell tumors and with intratubular large cell hyalinizing Sertoli cell neoplasia. Depending on the specifics of the pathologic findings, these patients should be evaluated for Carney complex, Peutz-Jeghers syndrome, or androgen insensitivity syndrome. Carney complex is particularly concerning because of association with cardiac myxoma, which may result in sudden death if undiagnosed.

Surveillance

Patients undergoing TSS must be carefully followed for local recurrence with testicular ultrasound. Additionally, in one series, on a mean of 3.8 years of follow-up of 16 patients with Sertoli cell tumors after radical orchiectomy, 3 of 12 patients who had no metastasis at presentation developed late metastasis. Retrospectively, histologic findings of these three patients showed adverse features: lymph-vascular space invasion in 2, nuclear atypia in 2, and necrosis in one patient [30].

For some young patients with small multifocal and bilateral large cell calcifying SCT, conservative treatment may be considered, with testicular surveillance and antiestrogenic therapy if there are estrogenic symptoms [21, 50]. Similarly, when on clinical and radiologic grounds the lesions associated with Peutz-Jeghers syndrome are regarded to be confined to the tubules (intratubular large cell hyalinizing Sertoli cell neoplasia), careful surveillance in combination with aromatase inhibitors could be considered [21, 25, 51, 52]. Evidence for invasion should prompt orchiectomy.

Owing to the rarity of these tumors, the frequency of surveillance imaging remains undefined. Suggested follow-up is similar to non-seminomatous germ cell tumors with chest imaging and abdominal CT every 4 months during the first year, every 6 months during the second year, and yearly thereafter. There has been only one late metastasis beyond 5 years after diagnosis, and hence, a minimal of 5 years of follow-up is recommended [39].

Prognosis

Malignant Sertoli cell tumors have a median survival of around 2 years [40, 41].

Granulosa Cell Tumor of the Testis

Background

Granulosa cell tumors of the testis (GRCT) are exceedingly rare neoplasms, occurring much more commonly in the ovary than in the testis. Granulosa cell tumors of the testis have been classified into adult and juvenile subtypes based on their histopathological characteristics. Malignant forms of adult-type GRCT have been reported, and these are resistant to the radiotherapy and chemotherapy regimens used in germ cell tumors. Surgical resection is the mainstay of treatment and results in excellent cure rates in localized disease.

Incidence

Adult-type GRCT is exceedingly uncommon, with total number of cases between 50 and 100 in the literature. Peak incidence of adult GRCT is around 40 years of age with a range of 12–87 years, and with more than half of the cases occurring in patients in fifth and sixth decades of life [55, 56]. Juvenile GRCT is the commonest testicular tumor in males younger than 6 months of age, with most reported cases diagnosed under 2 years of age [53, 54]. They may occur in undescended testes of infants with disorders of sex development and anomalies of sex chromosomes [70].

Presentation

The commonest manifestation is as a unilateral painless testicular mass. Some adult GRCT may present with endocrine symptoms: gynecomastia (up to 20 %) and loss of libido and potency. Hormonal features are not seen in patients with juvenile GRCT. There is considerable heterogeneity in clinical presentation in adult GRCT, with time from symptom onset to clinical evaluation ranging between few months to as long as a decade [55].

Metastasis has not been reported in juvenile GRCT, and only a small proportion of adult GRCT metastasize, with retroperitoneal lymph nodes being the commonest site [57].

Workup

Laboratory Workup

Elevations of tumor markers including alpha-fetoprotein, lactate dehydrogenase, and inhibin-B have been reported, but their prognostic value is unclear [58, 59].

Imaging Workup

Scrotal ultrasound is usually the initial imaging performed and shows a well-circumscribed hypo-echoic lesion possibly containing cystic areas [60]. A "Swiss cheese" pattern with effacement of normal testicular parenchyma by tumor mass containing multiple septated cysts and color Doppler showing a hypervascular rim has been described [58]. CT may show a hypo-echoic lesion with rim enhancement on T1 contrast weighted images [61].

Pathology

Adult-type granulosa cell tumors are usually well-circumscribed, solid, and/or cystic yellow-to-tan-to-gray masses. They usually measure 3–5 cm but may measure up to 18 cm. Microscopically, the most common pattern is microfollicular, with

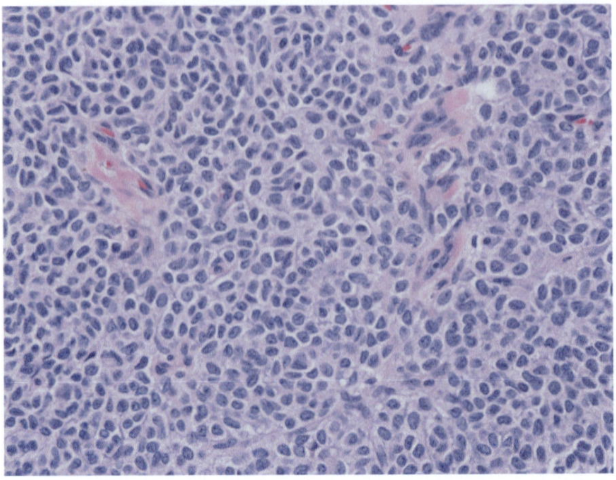

Fig. 16.6 Granulosa cell tumor: tumor cells are present in a diffuse architectural pattern in this case, and the cells show a scant amount of pale cytoplasm, and fairly uniform round-to-oval "coffee bean" nuclei with visible longitudinal nuclear groove (400× magnification)

Call-Exner bodies, but other patterns may be seen, including macrofollicular, trabecular, insular, gyriform, and diffuse (Fig. 16.6). The tumor cells have scant pale cytoplasm, and pale round-to-oval nuclei, often with nuclear grooves, thus resembling a "coffee bean" (Fig. 16.6). Mitoses are generally infrequent, but occasionally a high mitotic rate may be seen [67]. Tumor cells are usually positive by immunohistochemistry for alpha-inhibin, vimentin, estrogen, and progesterone receptors and may show variable positivity for cytokeratins [67]. Typical germ cell tumor markers, including OCT3/4 and alpha-fetoprotein (AFP), are negative. The pathologic differential diagnosis may include unclassified sex cord-stromal tumor, Sertoli cell tumor, or mixed germ cell-sex cord-stromal tumor [21]: careful attention to morphology and the use of selective immunostains (to exclude a germ cell component) will aid in the correct diagnosis.

Most adult-type GRCT are benign, but malignancy has been described. The small number of malignant cases limits the prognostic power of features other than metastasis, but the following have been described as indicating a greater risk for malignant behavior: large tumor size (>7 cm), lymph-vascular space invasion, tumor hemorrhage, and tumor necrosis [67, 69]. In a review of the literature, one group of authors suggests that tumor size >5 cm is the only feature statistically associated with malignancy [66].

Juvenile-type GRCT are solid and/or cystic yellow-to-gray nodules. The corresponding microscopic appearance shows a variably sized follicular and/or solid appearance. The tumor cells have a moderate amount of cytoplasm and round-to-oval hyperchromatic nuclei without grooves [21]. The mitotic index may be high. By immunohistochemistry, the tumor cells usually stain for alpha-inhibin and are negative for AFP. Because of the young age of presentation of juvenile-type GRCT, an important differential diagnosis is yolk sac tumor: careful examination for follicular architecture, positive immunostaining for alpha-inhibin, and negative staining for AFP should aid in the diagnosis of GRCT.

Juvenile GRCT are benign, without reported metastatic disease, despite the finding that occasional tumors may have a high mitotic index.

Treatment

Type of Surgery

The majority of reported cases of juvenile GRCT underwent radical inguinal orchiectomy (RIO), and all had excellent outcomes with no local or distant recurrences on prolonged follow-up [53, 54, 58, 62–64]. Orchiectomy using a prescrotal approach has also been described, but careful attention must be paid to avoid tumor spillage [59]. Testis-sparing surgery (TSS) may be feasible for small tumors with normal preoperative tumor markers (in particular, a normal alpha-fetoprotein level), and intraoperative frozen section that is consistent with this entity [64, 65].

RIO has been the procedure of choice for adult GRCT as well. The role of preoperative and/or intraoperative staging using RPLND is unknown. Treatment decisions must be individualized, and risks of retroperitoneal exploration balanced against the lack of good surveillance strategy and treatment options for patients with recurrent disease.

Retroperitoneal Lymph Node Dissection (RPLND)

Owing to the benign nature of juvenile GRCT, routine RPLND is not recommended. Routine RPLND has not been shown to improve outcomes in adult GRCT, and decision to perform the procedure must be individualized. As noted above, the following features are regarded as indicating a greater risk for malignancy: large tumor size (>7 cm), lymph-vascular space invasion, tumor hemorrhage, and tumor necrosis [67, 69].

Chemotherapy

Chemotherapy is not of proven value in patients with GRCT.

Surveillance

Surgical resection of tumor is thought to be curative for patients with juvenile GRCT, and no further follow-up is suggested.

Adult GRCT tend to recur mostly within the first 3 years of resection, but there are several important caveats. Patients with slow-growing tumors (longer time from symptom onset to clinical diagnosis) may develop late recurrence and need longer surveillance duration, although such an association is not well established. We suggest a frequency of clinical evaluation of every 3 months for the first 2 years and every 6 months thereafter. If transition to a primary care provider is considered at the 5-year mark, the patient and receiving provider must be made aware about the possibility of recurrences as late as 10 years from initial diagnosis.

Prognosis

Juvenile GRCT and stage I adult GRCT without high-risk features have a cure rate approaching 100 %. Survival drops significantly for adult GRCT presenting at stages higher than II-A, and recurrence and/or widespread metastasis are not uncommon.

Tumors of the Fibrothecoma Group

Background

Fibrothecomas of the testis are exceedingly rare neoplasms. Most reported testicular fibrothecomas are actually fibromas of gonadal stromal origin. Thecomas are vanishingly rare, with only two possible cases reported [29, 71, 72]. Establishing an accurate diagnosis is critical because of the overlap with testicular sarcomas and undifferentiated sex cord-stromal tumors. No malignant cases of fibrothecoma have been reported and these tumors carry an excellent prognosis.

Incidence

No incidence data is available due to the rarity of these tumors. In one review, median age at diagnosis was 31 years (range, 5–67 years) [73].

Presentation

The commonest presentation is painless unilateral scrotal swelling, but scrotal pain can be the presenting symptom. No hormonal symptoms have been described in cases of fibrothecoma; unlike ovarian thecomas, testicular fibrothecomas have not been associated with feminizing symptoms or elevation of serum levels of estrogen. Metastatic spread or recurrences have not been reported with testicular fibrothecomas [73]. Ovarian fibrothecomas occur in about 25 % of patients with nevoid basal cell carcinoma syndrome (Gorlin syndrome), which is caused by mutations in the *Protein patched homolog 1* (*PTCH*) gene. One of the cases of testicular thecoma occurred in a young male with this syndrome, which may point toward an association [72]. Evaluation for this syndrome might be considered for young patients with testicular thecoma.

Workup

Laboratory Workup

No cases have been associated with elevation of tumor markers including alpha-fetoprotein, lactate dehydrogenase, and inhibin-B. Perioperative assessment of estradiol, testosterone, luteinizing hormone, and follicle-stimulating hormone is likely not useful even in cases of testicular thecomas because surgery is considered curative.

Imaging Workup

Scrotal ultrasound in cases of pure fibromas may show heterogeneous echotexture, and larger masses may have abundant free fluid. Fibrothecomas are usually well circumscribed, but these may abut the tunica albuginea [75]. Average tumor size is around 2 cm.

Pathology

Grossly, testicular fibrothecomas are usually solid, well-circumscribed, tan-to-yellow/white masses. They generally lack necrosis and hemorrhage. Occasional tumors may show infiltration into the surrounding testicular parenchyma [75]. Microscopically, these tumors resemble their ovarian equivalents: most resembling typical or cellular variants of ovarian fibromas [21]. Fibrothecomas are composed of spindled-to-ovoid uniform cells in short fascicular and/or storiform arrangements, with variable amounts of collagen deposition. The degree of cellularity may be moderate to very cellular. Mitotic activity may be seen: most tumors have less than five mitoses per 10 high-power fields, but some tumors show nine to ten mitoses per 10 high-power fields [21, 75, 76]. Fibrothecomas show variable immunohistochemical staining, with frequent positivity for inhibin, calretinin, vimentin, pan keratin, Melan-A, S-100, muscle-specific actin, BCL2, CD34, and desmin [75]. An important pathologic differential diagnosis is between fibrothecoma and unclassified sex cord-stromal tumor, as the latter may behave malignantly. Although unclassified sex cord-stromal tumors may have areas that resemble fibrothecoma, areas of transition to epithelial areas should be seen [21].

Treatment

Type of Surgery

The majority of patients with fibrothecoma undergo radical inguinal orchiectomy (RIO) and they have had excellent outcomes with no local or remote recurrences on prolonged follow-ups of up to several years [74–76]. Testis-sparing surgery (TSS) has been described in one case of pure fibroma, and excisional biopsy in a case of fibrothecoma, and may be considered for small tumors that allow sparing of sufficient testicular parenchyma [76].

Retroperitoneal Lymph Node Dissection (RPLND)

RPLND is not routinely recommended for pure fibroma or pure fibrothecomas as no malignant spread has been demonstrated in reported literature.

Chemotherapy

Testicular fibrothecomas are benign tumors and no chemotherapy is indicated.

Surveillance

In a recent study, 16 cases of testicular fibrothecoma were followed for an average of 71.8 months (range, 3–144 months), and no recurrences or metastasis were detected. Follow-up beyond 5 years is not recommended and can be abbreviated further based on the patient's preference.

Prognosis

Testicular fibrothecomas have uniformly excellent prognosis with no documented recurrences or disease-specific mortality.

References

1. Kim I, Young RH, Scully RE. Leydig cell tumors of the testis. A clinicopathological analysis of 40 cases and review of the literature. Am J Surg Pathol. 1985;9(3):177–92.
2. Cheville JC, Sebo TJ, Lager DJ, Bostwick DG, Farrow GM. Leydig cell tumor of the testis: a clinicopathologic, DNA content, and MIB-1 comparison of nonmetastasizing and metastasizing tumors. Am J Surg Pathol. 1998;22(11):1361–7.
3. Hendry J, Fraser S, White J, Rajan P, Hendry DS. Retroperitoneal lymph node dissection (RPLND) for malignant phenotype Leydig cell tumours of the testis: a 10-year experience. SpringerPlus. 2015;4:20.
4. Heer R, Jackson MJ, El-Sherif A, Thomas DJ. Twenty-nine Leydig cell tumors: histological features, outcomes and implications for management. Int J Urol Off J Jpn Urol Assoc. 2010;17(10):886–9.
5. Suardi N, Strada E, Colombo R, Freschi M, Salonia A, Lania C, Cestari A, Carmignani L, Guazzoni G, Rigatti P, Montorsi F. Leydig cell tumour of the testis: presentation, therapy, long-term follow-up and the role of organ-sparing surgery in a single-institution experience. BJU Int. 2009;103(2):197–200.
6. Tsitouridis I, Maskalidis C, Panagiotidou D, Kariki EP. Eleven patients with testicular Leydig cell tumors: clinical, imaging, and pathologic correlation. J Ultrasound Med Off J Am Inst Ultrasound Med. 2014;33(10):1855–64.
7. Connolly SS, D'Arcy FT, Bredin HC, Callaghan J, Corcoran MO. Value of frozen section analysis with suspected testicular malignancy. Urology. 2006;67(1):162–5.
8. Elert A, Olbert P, Hegele A, Barth P, Hofmann R, Heidenreich A. Accuracy of frozen section examination of testicular tumors of uncertain origin. Eur Urol. 2002;41(3):290–3.
9. Leroy X, Rigot J-M, Aubert S, Ballereau C, Gosselin B. Value of frozen section examination for the management of nonpalpable incidental testicular tumors. Eur Urol. 2003;44(4):458–60.
10. Tokuc R, Sakr W, Pontes JE, Haas GP. Accuracy of frozen section examination of testicular tumors. Urology. 1992;40(6):512–6.
11. Mosharafa AA, Foster RS, Bihrle R, Koch MO, Ulbright TM, Einhorn LH, Donohue JP. Does retroperitoneal lymph node dissection have a curative role for patients with sex cord–stromal testicular tumors? Cancer. 2003;98(4):753–7.
12. Di Tonno F, Tavolini IM, Belmonte P, Bertoldin R, Cossaro E, Curti P, D'Incà G, Fandella A, Guaitoli P, Guazzieri S, Mazzariol C, North-Eastern Uro-Oncological Group Italy. Lessons from 52 patients with Leydig cell tumor of the testis: the GUONE (North-Eastern Uro-Oncological Group, Italy) experience. Urol Int. 2009;82(2):152–7.
13. Peschel R, Gettman MT, Steiner H, Neururer R, Bartsch G. Management of adult Leydig-cell testicular tumors: assessing the role of laparoscopic retroperitoneal lymph node dissection. J Endourol. 2003;17(9):777–80.
14. Bertram KA, Bratloff B, Hodges GF, Davidson H. Treatment of malignant Leydig cell tumor. Cancer. 1991;68(10):2324–9.

15. Conkey DS, Howard GCW, Grigor KM, McLaren DB, Kerr GR. Testicular sex cord-stromal tumours: the Edinburgh experience 1988–2002, and a review of the literature. Clin Oncol R Coll Radiol G B. 2005;17(5):322–7.
16. Farkas LM, Székely JG, Pusztai C, Baki M. High frequency of metastatic Leydig cell testicular tumours. Oncology. 2000;59(2):118–21.
17. Davis S, Di Martino NA, Schneider G. Malignant interstitial cell carcinoma of the testis: report of two cases with steroid synthetic profiles, response to therapy, and review of the literature. Cancer. 1981;47(2):425–31.
18. Bokemeyer C, Harstrick A, Gonnermann O, Schober C, Kuczyk M, Poliwoda H, Schmoll H. Metastatic Leydig-cell tumors of the testis – report of 4 cases and review of the literature. Int J Oncol. 1993;2(2):241–4.
19. Basciani S, Brama M, Mariani S, De Luca G, Arizzi M, Vesci L, Pisano C, Dolci S, Spera G, Gnessi L. Imatinib mesylate inhibits Leydig cell tumor growth: evidence for in vitro and in vivo activity. Cancer Res. 2005;65(5):1897–903.
20. Froehner M, Beuthien-Baumann B, Dittert D-D, Schuler U, Wirth MP. Lack of efficacy of imatinib in a patient with metastatic Leydig cell tumor. Cancer Chemother Pharmacol. 2006;58(5):716–8.
21. Ulbright TM, Young RH. Tumors of the testis and adjacent structures, Armed Forces Institute of Pathology (US); American Registry of Pathology. Silver Springs, MD: American Registry of Pathology; 2013.
22. Ulbright TM, Srigley JR, Hatzianastassiou DK, Young RH. Leydig cell tumors of the testis with unusual features: adipose differentiation, calcification with ossification, and spindle-shaped tumor cells. Am J Surg Pathol. 2002;26(11):1424–33.
23. McCluggage WG, Shanks JH, Arthur K, Banerjee SS. Cellular proliferation and nuclear ploidy assessments augment established prognostic factors in predicting malignancy in testicular Leydig cell tumors. Histopathology. 1998;33(4):361–8.
24. Wilson DM, Pitts WC, Hintz RL, Rosenfeld RG. Testicular tumors with Peutz-Jeghers syndrome. Cancer. 1986;57(11):2238–40.
25. Ulbright TM, Amin MB, Young RH. Intratubular large cell hyalinizing Sertoli cell neoplasia of the testis: a report of 8 cases of a distinctive lesion of the Peutz-Jeghers syndrome. Am J Surg Pathol. 2007;31(6):827–35.
26. Gourgari E, Saloustros E, Stratakis CA. Large-cell calcifying Sertoli cell tumors of the testes in pediatrics. Curr Opin Pediatr. 2012;24(4):518–22.
27. Rutgers JL, Scully RE. The androgen insensitivity syndrome (testicular feminization): a clinicopathologic study of 43 cases. Int J Gynecol Pathol. 1991;10(2):126–44.
28. Washecka R, Dresner MI, Honda SAA. Testicular tumors in Carney's complex. J Urol. 2002;167(3):1299–302.
29. Eble JN, World Health Organization, and International Agency for Research on Cancer, editors. Pathology and genetics of tumours of the urinary system and male genital organs. Lyon: Oxford: IARC Press ; Oxford University Press; 2004. distributor.
30. Young RH, Koelliker DD, Scully RE. Sertoli cell tumors of the testis, not otherwise specified: a clinicopathologic analysis of 60 cases. Am J Surg Pathol. 1998;22(6):709–21.
31. Henley JD, Young RH, Ulbright TM. Malignant Sertoli cell tumors of the testis: a study of 13 examples of a neoplasm frequently misinterpreted as seminoma. Am J Surg Pathol. 2002;26(5):541–50.
32. Kratzer SS, Ulbright TM, Talerman A, Srigley JR, Roth LM, Wahle GR, Moussa M, Stephens JK, Millos A, Young RH. Large cell calcifying Sertoli cell tumor of the testis: contrasting features of six malignant and six benign tumors and a review of the literature. Am J Surg Pathol. 1997;21(11):1271–80.
33. Bufo P, Pennella A, Serio G, Mastropasqua MG, Cenacchi G, Rogatsch H, Mikuz G. Malignant large cell calcifying Sertoli cell tumor of the testis (LCCSCTT). Report of a case in an elderly man and review of the literature. Pathologica. 1999;91(2):107–14.
34. Gierke CL, King BF, Bostwick DG, Choyke PL, Hattery RR. Large-cell calcifying Sertoli cell tumor of the testis: appearance at sonography. Am J Roentgenol. 1994;163(2): 373–5.

35. Shin SL, Outwater EK. Benign large cell calcifying Sertoli cell tumor of the testis in a prepubescent patient. Am J Roentgenol. 2007;189(2):W65–6.
36. Drevelengas A, Kalaitzoglou I, Destouni E, Skordalaki A, Dimitriadis A. Bilateral Sertoli cell tumor of the testis: MRI and sonographic appearance. Eur Radiol. 1999;9(9):1934.
37. Silberstein JL, Bazzi WM, Vertosick E, Carver BS, Bosl GJ, Feldman DR, Bajorin DF, Motzer RJ, Al-Ahmadie H, Reuter VE, Sheinfeld J. Clinical outcomes of local and metastatic testicular sex cord-stromal tumors. J Urol. 2014;192(2):415–9.
38. Nicolai N, Necchi A, Raggi D, Biasoni D, Catanzaro M, Piva L, Stagni S, Maffezzini M, Torelli T, Faré E, Giannatempo P, Pizzocaro G, Colecchia M, Salvioni R. Clinical outcome in testicular sex cord stromal tumors: testis sparing vs radical orchiectomy and management of advanced disease. Urology. 2015;85(2):402–6.
39. Compérat E, Tissier F, Vieillefond A. Late metastasis after a testicular Sertoli cell tumour. Ann Pathol. 2004;24(1):45–6.
40. Grem JL, Robins HI, Wilson KS, Gilchrist K, Trump DL. Metastatic Leydig cell tumor of the testis. Report of three cases and review of the literature. Cancer. 1986;58(9):2116–9.
41. Acar C, Gurocak S, Sozen S. Current treatment of testicular sex cord-stromal tumors: critical review. Urology. 2009;73(6):1165–71.
42. Zuckerberg LR, Young RH, Scully RE. Sclerosing Sertoli cell tumor of the testis. A report of 10 cases. Am J Surg Pathol. 1991;15(9):829–34.
43. Kao CS, Kum JB, Idrees MT, Ulbright TM. Sclerosing Sertoli cell tumor of the testis: a study of 20 cases. Am J Surg Pathol. 2014;38(4):510–7.
44. Jacobsen G.K. Malignant Sertoli cell tumors of the testis. J Urol Pathol. 1993;1:233–5.
45. Proppe KH, Dickersin GR. Large-cell calcifying Sertoli cell tumor of the testis: light microscopic and ultrastructural study. Hum Pathol. 1982;13(12):1109–14.
46. De Raeve H, Schoonooghe P, Wibowo R, Van Marck E, Goossens A. Malignant large cell calcifying Sertoli cell tumor of the testis. Pathol Res Pract. 2003;199(2):113–7.
47. Nielsen K, Jacobsen GK. Malignant Sertoli cell tumor of the testis. An immunohistochemical study and a review of the literature. APMIS. 1988;98(8):755–60.
48. Compérat E, Tissier F, Boye K, De Pinieux G, Vieillefond A. Non-Leydig sex-cord tumors of the testis. The place of immunohistochemistry in diagnosis and prognosis. A study of 20 cases. Virchows Arch. 2004;444(6):567–71.
49. Rutgers JL, Scully RE. Pathology of the testis in intersex syndromes. Semin Diagn Pathol. 1987;4(4):275–91.
50. Brown B, Ram A, Clayton P, Humphrey G. Conservative management of bilateral Sertoli cell tumors of the testicle in association with Carney complex: a case report. J Pediatr Surg. 2007;42:E13–5.
51. Venara M, Ray R, Beergada I, Mendilaharzu, Campo S, Chemes H. Sertoli cell proliferations of the infantile testis: an intratubular form of Sertoli cell tumor? Am J Surg Pathol. 2001;25:1237–44.
52. Kara C, Kutlu AO, Tosun MS, Apaydin S, Senel F. Sertoli cell tumor causing prepubertal gynecomastia in a boy with the Peutz-Jeghers syndrome: the outcome of 1-year treatment with the aromatase inhibitor testolactone. Horm Res. 2005;63:252–6.
53. Lawrence WD, Young RH, Scully RE. Juvenile granulosa cell tumor of the infantile testis. A report of 14 cases. Am J Surg Pathol. 1985;9(2):87–94.
54. Fagin R, Berbescu E, Landis S, Strumpf K, Patil U. Juvenile granulosa cell tumor of the testis. Urology. 2003;62(2):351.
55. Schubert TE, Stoehr R, Hartmann A, Schöne S, Löbelenz M, Mikuz G. Adult type granulosa cell tumor of the testis with a heterologous sarcomatous component: case report and review of the literature. Diagn Pathol. 2014;9(1):107.
56. Cornejo KM, Young RH. Adult granulosa cell tumors of the testis: a report of 32 cases. Am J Surg Pathol. 2014;38(9):1242–50.
57. Suppiah A, Musa MM, Morgan DR, North AD. Adult granulosa cell tumour of the testis and bony metastasis. A report of the first case of granulosa cell tumour of the testicle metastasising to bone. Urol Int. 2005;75(1):91–3.

58. Zugor V, Labanaris AP, Witt J, Seidler A, Weingärtner K, Schott GE. Congenital juvenile granulosa cell tumor of the testis in newborns. Anticancer Res. 2010;30(5):1731–4.
59. Bulotta AL, Molinaro F, Angotti R, Ferrara F, Maggio GD, Bindi E, Messina M. Juvenile granulosa cell tumor of the testis: prenatal diagnosis and prescrotal approach. Ital J Pediatr. 2012;38(1):67.
60. Mitra A, Palit V, Paes R, Ferro M. Sonographic features of an adult granulosa cell tumor of the testis. Radiol Case Rep. 2008;3:1–3.
61. Ko K, Itoh N, Sakai S, Sato M. Adult-type testicular granulosa cell tumor: a case report and radiological findings of a rare testicular tumor. BJUI. 2013; DOI: 10.1002/BJUIw-2012-073-web.
62. Thomas JC, Ross JH, Kay R. Stromal testis tumors in children: a report from the prepubertal testis tumor registry. J Urol. 2001;166(6):2338–40.
63. Nieto N, Torres-Valdivieso MJ, Aguado P, Mateos ME, López-Pérez J, Melero C, Vivanco JL, Gómez A. Juvenile granulosa cell tumor of the testis: case report and review of literature. Tumori. 2002;88(1):72–4.
64. Shukla AR, Huff DS, Canning DA, Filmer RB, Snyder HM, Carpintieri D, Carr MC. Juvenile granulosa cell tumor of the testis: contemporary clinical management and pathological diagnosis. J Urol. 2004;171(5):1900–2.
65. Cosentino M, Algaba F, Saldaña L, Bujons A, Caffaratti J, Garat JM, Villavicencio H. Juvenile granulosa cell tumor of the testis: a bilateral and synchronous case. Should testis-sparing surgery be mandatory? Urology. 2014;84(3):694–6.
66. Hanson JA, Ambaye AB. Adult testicular granulosa cell tumor: a review of the literature for clinicopathologic predictors of malignancy. Arch Pathol Lab Med. 2011;135(1):143–6.
67. Jimenez-Quintero LP, Ro JY, Zavala-Pompa A, Amin MB, Tetu B, Ordonez NG, Ayala AG. Granulosa cell tumor of the adult testis: a clinicopathologic study of seven cases and a review of the literature. Hum Pathol. 1993;24(10):1120–6.
68. Due W, Dieckmann KP, Niedobitek G, Bornhoft G, Loy V, Stein H. Testicular sex cord stromal tumor with granulosa cell differentiation: detection of steroid hormone receptors as a possible basis for tumor development and therapeutic management. J Clin Pathol. 1990;43(9):732–7.
69. Matoska J, Ondrus D, Talerman A. Malignant granulosa cell tumor of the testis associated with gynecomastia and long survival. Cancer. 1992;69(7):1769–72.
70. Young RH, Lawrence WD, Scully RE. Juvenile granulosa cell tumor-another neoplasm associated with abnormal chromosomes and ambiguous genitalia. A report of three cases. Am J Surg Pathol. 1985;9(10):737–43.
71. Schenkman NS, Moul JW, Nicely ER, Maggio MI, Ho CK. Synchronous bilateral testis tumor: mixed germ cell and theca cell tumors. Urology. 1993;42(5):593–5.
72. Ueda M, Kanematsu A, Nishiyama H, Yoshimura K, Watanabe K, Yorifuji T, Mikami Y, Kamoto T, Ogawa O. Testicular thecoma in an 11-year-old boy with nevoid basal-cell carcinoma syndrome (Gorlin syndrome). J Pediatr Surg. 2010;45(3):E1–3.
73. Deveci MS, Deveci G, Ongürü O, Kilciler M, Celasun B. Testicular (gonadal stromal) fibroma: case report and review of the literature. Pathol Int. 2002;52(4):326–30.
74. Eble JN, Hull MT, Warfel KA, Donohue JP. Malignant sex cord-stromal tumor of testis. J Urol. 1984;131(3):546–50.
75. Zhang M, Kao C-S, Ulbright TM, Epstein JI. Testicular fibrothecoma: a morphologic and immunohistochemical study of 16 cases. Am J Surg Pathol. 2013;37(8):1208–14.
76. Jones MA, Young RH, Scully RE. Benign fibromatous tumors of the testis and paratesticular region: a report of 9 cases with a proposed classification of fibromatous tumors and tumor-like lesions. Am J Surg Pathol. 1997;21(3):296–305.

Granulosa Cell Tumors of the Testis

17

Winston W. Huh

Introduction

Granulosa cell tumors (GCTs) of the testis are rare testicular neoplasms, and there are less than 200 cases reported in the medical literature (Table 17.1). While sex cord-stromal tumors account for approximately 5 % of testicular tumors, the exact incidence of GCTs is not entirely known [1]. Clinically testicular GCTs are divided into two subgroups, adult-type GCT (AGCT) and juvenile-type GCT (JGCT). In adults Leydig and Sertoli cell tumors are more common than GCT of the testis, while in children JGCTs account for approximately a third of sex cord-stromal tumors of the testis [2, 3]. In AGCTs the tumors typically occur in the early to mid-fifth decade of life, while in JGCTs almost all cases occur in prepubertal males less than 1 year of age [2–6]. A painless scrotal mass is the most common presentation of GCT, while occasional cases have been discovered due to pain resulting from testicular torsion, and metastases to retroperitoneal lymph nodes or other organs at the time of diagnosis can be seen in up to 20 % of adult cases but are rare for JGCT [7, 8]. For JGCT, inguinal and abdominal masses have been reported due to the tumor occurring in an undescended testis [9–11].

Genetics and Clinical Associations

The exact etiology of testicular GCT remains unclear. More biologic and genetic data are available for ovarian GCTs due to their increased frequency over GCTs of the testis, and there have been some studies investigating if ovarian and testicular GCTs share common genetic aberrations. One specific somatic mutation involving

W.W. Huh, MD
Department of Pediatrics, University of Texas MD Anderson Cancer Center,
1515 Holcombe Blvd., Unit 87, Houston, TX 77030, USA
e-mail: whuh@mdanderson.org

L. Pagliaro (ed.), *Rare Genitourinary Tumors*,
DOI 10.1007/978-3-319-30046-7_17

Table 17.1 Summary of largest reported series of granulosa cell tumors of the testis with clinical data in the last 20 years

Study	Number of cases and subtype	Treatment	Comments
Cornejo and Young [4]	32 adult	30 OR, 2 WR/EN	19 patients with follow-up at mean of 51 months. 18 are NED and one patient with alive with lung metastasis
Rane et al. [5]	4 adult/2 juvenile	6 OR and 2 adults received BEP and 1 adult received cisplatin/paclitaxel	4 NED and 1 adult died from embryonal carcinoma
Kao et al. [33]	70 juvenile	62 OR, 6 WR/EN, and 2 biopsy only	24 patients with follow-up at median 61 months and all were NED
Hofmann et al. [3]	16 juvenile		Reported as part of 42-patient cohort of sex cord-stromal tumors. At median follow-up of 3.8 years for the entire cohort, all patients were NED
Cecchetto et al. [2]	4 juvenile	3 OR and 1 WR/EN	Reported as part of 11-patient cohort of sex cord-stromal tumors. At mean follow-up of 59 months for the entire cohort, all patients were NED
Harms and Kock [37]	11 juvenile	8 OR and 1 WR/EN	8 NED at median follow-up 41 months. 3 LTFU
Thomas et al. [6]	9 juvenile	Unknown	All NED at mean follow-up of 25 months

OR orchiectomy, *WR/EN* wedge resection/enucleation, *NED* no evidence of disease, *BEP* bleomycin, etoposide, and cisplatin, *LTFU* lost to follow-up

the transcription factor forkhead box L2 (FOXL2) gene at 402C;G(C134W) has been described to be involved in nearly all ovarian GCTs [12–14]. The presence of the FOXL2 mutation has been demonstrated in both adult and juvenile-type testicular GCTs but at a lower prevalence compared to ovarian GCTs [15, 16]. Kalfa et al. reported aberrant immunohistochemical expression of FOXL2 in three cases of juvenile-type testicular GCT and also noted cytoplasmic expression of SOX9 in two cases instead of the expected nuclear localization [16]. SOX9 is a transcriptional factor that is known to be involved with testis differentiation, but the relationship of the cytoplasmic SOX9 expression is unknown and should be taken with caution given the small sample size [17]. Among the critical functions of the FOXL2 gene is the suppression of transdifferentiation of the ovary to testis [18, 19]. Yet the exact mechanisms involving disruption of normal FOXL2 function leading to formation of either ovarian or testicular GCTs still remain unclear. Boyer et al. also recently demonstrated that dysregulation between the WNT/CTNNB1 and PI3K/AKT pathways may play a synergistic role in the development of testicular GCTs [20]. In a mouse model that expressed CTNNB1 but loss of phosphatase and tensin homolog (PTEN), testicular tumors were generated that histologically appeared similar to GCTs and also expressed FOXL2. Other investigators demonstrated development of similar testicular tumors in murine Sertoli cells through activation of both CTNNB1 and KRAS [21].

Another study noted that in-frame duplications of AKT1 have been found in 60 % of juvenile ovarian GCTs [22]. These tandem duplications resulted in alterations of the pleckstrin-homology domain which resulted in AKT1 activation. Other preclinical studies have examined the role of other genes, such as FOXO1, GATA4, and TGF-beta, for ovarian GCTs, but these studies have not been evaluated for testicular GCT [23–25].

Both adult- and juvenile-type GCTs have not been linked to any familial genetic disorders or syndromes. However, some cases of JGCTs have presented in children with chromosomal abnormalities involving either the Y chromosome, chromosome 4, or X/XY mosaicism presenting with ambiguous genitalia [3, 10, 26–29]. As previously mentioned, JGCT has also been associated with undescended testis. No consistent chromosomal aberrations have been noted for adult-type testicular GCTs. Gynecomastia as a presenting symptom at diagnosis has been reported in several cases of AGCT, but gynecomastia and other hormonal disorders have not been reported in juvenile cases [30–32].

Pathologic Findings

On gross examination adult-type testicular GCTs tend to be well circumscribed and solid, while JGCTs can be more multicystic. One clinicopathologic study of 70 cases of juvenile GCT of the testis noted that 63 % of the tumors were multicystic [33]. Involvement of the seminiferous tubules is often seen for both types of testicular GCTs, while lymphovascular invasion is uncommon. Invasion of the rete testis appears to be more common in AGCTs. Under microscopic examination AGCTs mainly exhibit a diffuse, solid histologic pattern of tumor cells, but spindled (Fig. 17.1), insular, corded, and microfollicular patterns of tumor cells often can be observed in tumors [4]. This variability of histologic patterns is comparable to what has been observed in ovarian GCTs. Juvenile-type GCTs are more likely to exhibit a mixed follicular and solid pattern of tumor cells (Fig. 17.2). The tumor cells tend to be small to medium in size and contain round or oval nuclei with variable amounts of somewhat eosinophilic cytoplasm. Mitotic rate of visualized tumor cells tends to be variable for both adult- and juvenile-type GCTs, but one study of JGCTs did find abundant apoptotic bodies in almost half of the examined tumor samples [33].

Both adult and juvenile testicular GCTs display strong positivity to inhibin, vimentin, calretinin, WT1, steroidogenic factor-1 (SF-1), and FOXL2 on immunohistochemistry. However, inhibin and FOXL2 are not just specific for GCTs. Inhibin has been found to be expressed in fibrothecomas, Leydig cell tumors, and Sertoli cell tumors [2, 34]. FOXL2 expression has also been found on sclerosing stromal tumors, Leydig cell tumors, and Sertoli cell tumors [12]. Interestingly, one study of

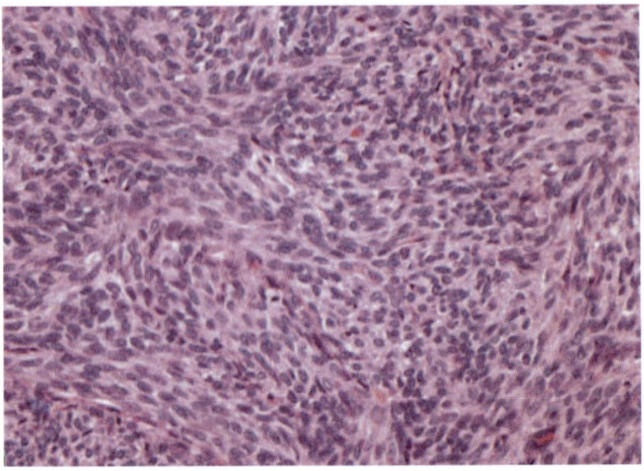

Fig. 17.1 Spindle pattern of tumor cells seen in adult granulosa cell tumor of testis (From Cornejo and Young. Permission obtained from Lippincott Williams and Wilkins)

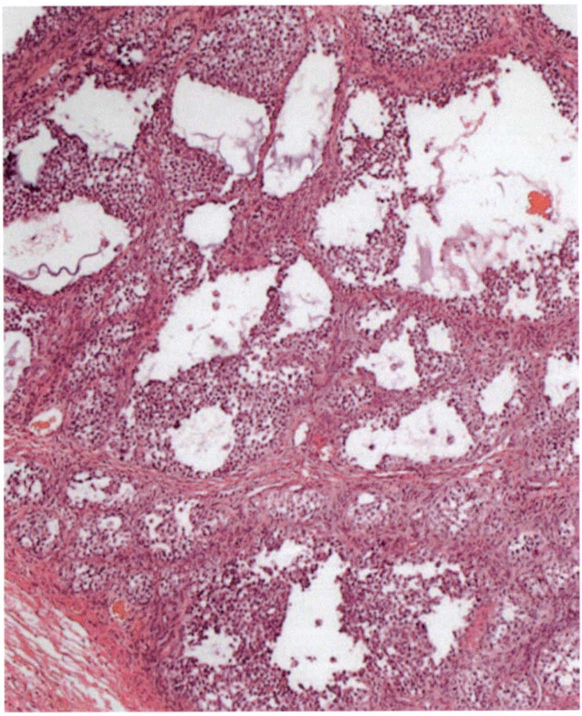

Fig. 17.2 Low power microscopic view of juvenile granulosa cell tumor of testis exhibiting variable-sized follicles (From Kao et al. Permission obtained from Lippincott Williams and Wilkins)

adult testicular GCTs found that tumors displayed FOXL2 immunohistochemical expression, but most of the tumors were negative for the somatic mutation [35]. Alpha-fetoprotein (AFP), SALL4, desmin, and epithelial membrane antigen (EMA) staining tend to be negative [36, 37].

The differential diagnosis for GCTs is quite extensive and includes seminomas, germ cell tumors, teratomas, and other sex cord-stromal tumors, such as Leydig cell tumors, Sertoli cell tumors, and thecomas. The majority of these entities have histologic characteristics that are distinct from GCTs. In children there are several small, round cell malignancies that can mimic JGCTs including paratesticular rhabdomyosarcoma or metastases from neuroblastoma or lymphoma. Primitive neuroectodermal tumors have been found in testicular tumors but usually as a component of a mixed germ cell tumor [38]. However, these malignancies will also have distinct histologic and immunohistochemical characteristics that differentiate them from GCTs, such as myogenin and desmin positivity in rhabdomyosarcomas.

Clinical Management and Prognosis

Complete surgical resection of tumor is considered the mainstay of therapy. Most reported cases have been treated with orchiectomy via a high inguinal approach. Enucleation/testis-sparing surgery has also been reported in a few cases in which there was enough normal-appearing testicular tissue to consider this approach [2, 4, 33]. For JGCTs, however, special attention should be given to the serum AFP level, since yolk sac tumors are in the differential diagnosis. For those patients with suspected retroperitoneal lymph node involvement, then lymph node dissection can be considered. However, there are not enough cases with sufficient long-term data to determine if this approach truly improves survival [39].

Overall the prognosis for cure is excellent for those patients with localized testicular GCT. In the largest series of reported JGCTs, follow-up data and disease status were available for 24 patients, and there were no deaths at a median follow-up interval of 61 months [33]. In adult patients similar results were seen for those with localized disease [4]. For those patients who have exhibited metastatic disease or recurrence, the most common clinical feature has been a primary tumor larger than 5 cm at the time of initial diagnosis [5, 40]. However, there are too few cases to determine significant clinical or pathologic prognostic indicators, such as lymphovascular invasion or high mitotic rate.

In patients with metastatic or unresectable disease, the role and efficacy of conventional cytotoxic chemotherapy is not clear. Ovarian GCTs have been treated with cisplatin-based regimens, such as bleomycin, etoposide, and cisplatin (BEP) or cisplatin, vinblastine, and bleomycin [41–43]. Thus, a regimen, such as BEP, would be considered acceptable for treatment of testicular GCTs. There has been one report of an adult patient with recurrent, metastatic disease with partial response to pazopanib, an anti-angiogenic tyrosine kinase inhibitor, for 5 months, but there are scant data regarding the role of targeted agents for testicular GCTs [44]. Less data are available regarding the utility of chemotherapy in an adjuvant role. Isolated cases have been reported, but the follow-up intervals are relatively short [5, 37].

There are also no definitive data regarding the utility of radiation therapy especially for those patients with retroperitoneal lymph node involvement, although there has been one case report in which radiation therapy was used following orchiectomy and retroperitoneal lymph node dissection in an adult patient with no evidence of disease recurrence after 14 years of follow-up [30].

Conclusion

In summary granulosa cell tumors of the testis are rare neoplasms in both children and adults. While there have been recent data regarding some genetic findings, such as aberrations involving the FOXL2 gene, much is still unknown regarding the pathophysiology of this disease. Surgery remains the primary mode of therapy for GCTs, and the overall prognosis for cure is very good, especially for those with localized disease that is completely resected. New therapies are needed for those patients with distant metastatic disease.

References

1. Dilworth JP, Farrow GM, Oesterling JE. Non-germ cell tumors of testis. Urology. 1991;37:399–417.
2. Cecchetto G, Alaggio R, Bisogno G, et al. Sex cord-stromal tumors of the testis in children. A clinicopathologic report from the Italian TREP project. J Pediatr Surg. 2010;45:1868–73.
3. Hofmann M, Schlegel PG, Hippert F, et al. Testicular sex cord stromal tumors: analysis of patients from the MAKEI study. Pediatr Blood Cancer. 2013;60:1651–5.
4. Cornejo KM, Young RH. Adult granulosa cell tumors of the testis: a report of 32 cases. Am J Surg Pathol. 2014;38:1242–50.
5. Rane SU, Menon S, Desai S, Bakshi G, Joshi A. Granulosa cell tumor of testis: clinicopathological correlation of a rare tumor. Indian J Pathol Microbiol. 2014;57:564–73.
6. Thomas JC, Ross JH, Kay R. Stromal testis tumors in children: a report from the prepubertal testis tumor registry. J Urol. 2001;166:2338–40.
7. Hammerich KH, Hille S, Ayala GE, et al. Malignant advanced granulosa cell tumor of the adult testis: case report and review of the literature. Hum Pathol. 2008;39:701–9.
8. Suppiah A, Musa MM, Morgan DR, North AD. Adult granulosa cell tumour of the testis and bony metastasis. A report of the first case of granulosa cell tumour of the testicle metastasising to bone. Urol Int. 2005;75:91–3.
9. May D, Shamberger R, Newbury R, Teele RL. Juvenile granulosa cell tumor of an intraabdominal testis. Pediatr Radiol. 1992;22:507–8.
10. Yu DC, Pathak B, Vargas SO, et al. Congenital intra-abdominal bilateral juvenile granulosa cell tumors of the testis associated with constitutional loss of material from chromosome 4. Pediatr Dev Pathol. 2011;14:224–7.
11. Partalis N, Tzardi M, Barbagadakis S, Sakellaris G. Juvenile granulosa cell tumor arising from intra-abdominal testis in newborn: case report and review of the literature. Urology. 2012;79:1152–4.
12. Al-Agha OM, Huwait HF, Chow C, et al. FOXL2 is a sensitive and specific marker for sex cord-stromal tumors of the ovary. Am J Surg Pathol. 2011;35:484–94.
13. Jamieson S, Butzow R, Andersson N, et al. The FOXL2 C134W mutation is characteristic of adult granulosa cell tumors of the ovary. Mod Pathol. 2010;23:1477–85.
14. Shah SP, Kobel M, Senz J, et al. Mutation of FOXL2 in granulosa-cell tumors of the ovary. N Engl J Med. 2009;360:2719–29.

15. Lima JF, Jin L, de Araujo AR, et al. FOXL2 mutations in granulosa cell tumors occurring in males. Arch Pathol Lab Med. 2012;136:825–8.
16. Kalfa N, Fellous M, Boizet-Bonhoure B, et al. Aberrant expression of ovary determining gene FOXL2 in the testis and juvenile granulosa cell tumor in children. J Urol. 2008;180:1810–3.
17. Li Y, Zheng M, Lau YF. The sex-determining factors SRY and SOX9 regulate similar target genes and promote testis cord formation during testicular differentiation. Cell Rep. 2014;8:723–33.
18. Uhlenhaut NH, Jakob S, Anlag K, et al. Somatic sex reprogramming of adult ovaries to testes by FOXL2 ablation. Cell. 2009;139:1130–42.
19. Ottolenghi C, Pelosi E, Tran J, et al. Loss of Wnt4 and Foxl2 leads to female-to-male sex reversal extending to germ cells. Hum Mol Genet. 2007;16:2795–804.
20. Boyer A, Paquet M, Lague MN, Hermo L, Boerboom D. Dysregulation of WNT/CTNNB1 and PI3K/AKT signaling in testicular stromal cells causes granulosa cell tumor of the testis. Carcinogenesis. 2009;30:869–78.
21. Richards JS, Fan HY, Liu Z, et al. Either Kras activation or Pten loss similarly enhance the dominant-stable CTNNB1-induced genetic program to promote granulosa cell tumor development in the ovary and testis. Oncogene. 2012;31:1504–20.
22. Bessiere L, Todeschini AL, Auguste A, et al. A hot-spot of in-frame duplications activates the oncoprotein AKT1 in juvenile granulosa cell tumors. EBioMed. 2015;2:421–31.
23. Mansouri-Attia N, Tripurani SK, Gokul N, et al. TGF beta signaling promotes juvenile granulosa cell tumorigenesis by suppressing apoptosis. Mol Endocrinol. 2014;28:1887–98.
24. Liu Z, Ren YA, Pangas SA, et al. FOXO1/3 and PTEN depletion in granulosa cells promotes ovarian granulosa cell tumor development. Mol Endocrinol. 2015;29:1006–24.
25. Anttonen M, Pihlajoki M, Andersson N, et al. FOXL2, GATA4, and SMAD3 co-operatively modulate gene expression, cell viability and apoptosis in ovarian granulosa cell tumor cells. PLoS ONE. 2014;9, e85545.
26. Cortez JC, Kaplan GW. Gonadal stromal tumors, gonadoblastomas, epidermoid cysts, and secondary tumors of the testis in children. Urol Clin N Am. 1993;20:15–26.
27. Raju U, Fine G, Warrier R, Kini R, Weiss L. Congenital testicular juvenile granulosa cell tumor in a neonate with X/XY mosaicism. Am J Surg Pathol. 1986;10:577–83.
28. Tanaka Y, Sasaki Y, Tachibana K, Suwa S, Terashima K, Nakatani Y. Testicular juvenile granulosa cell tumor in an infant with X/XY mosaicism clinically diagnosed as true hermaphroditism. Am J Surg Pathol. 1994;18:316–22.
29. Young RH, Lawrence WD, Scully RE. Juvenile granulosa cell tumor – another neoplasm associated with abnormal chromosomes and ambiguous genitalia. A report of three cases. Am J Surg Pathol. 1985;9:737–43.
30. Matoska J, Ondrus D, Talerman A. Malignant granulosa cell tumor of the testis associated with gynecomastia and long survival. Cancer. 1992;69:1769–72.
31. Mostofi FK, Theiss EA, Ashley DJ. Tumors of specialized gonadal stroma in human male patients. Androblastoma, Sertoli cell tumor, granulosa-theca cell tumor of the testis, and gonadal stromal tumor. Cancer. 1959;12:944–57.
32. Cohen J, Diamond I. Leontiasis ossea, slipped epiphyses, and granulosa cell tumor of testis with renal disease; report of a case with autopsy findings. AMA Arch Pathol. 1953;56:488–500.
33. Kao CS, Cornejo KM, Ulbright TM, Young RH. Juvenile granulosa cell tumors of the testis: a clinicopathologic study of 70 cases with emphasis on its wide morphologic spectrum. Am J Surg Pathol. 2015;39:1159–69.
34. Zhang M, Kao CS, Ulbright TM, Epstein JI. Testicular fibrothecoma: a morphologic and immunohistochemical study of 16 cases. Am J Surg Pathol. 2013;37:1208–14.
35. Hes O, Vanecek T, Petersson F, et al. Mutational analysis (c.402C>G) of the FOXL2 gene and immunohistochemical expression of the FOXL2 protein in testicular adult type granulosa cell tumors and incompletely differentiated sex cord stromal tumors. Appl Immunohistochem Mol Morphol. 2011;19:347–51.

36. Bai S, Wei S, Ziober A, Yao Y, Bing Z. SALL4 and SF-1 are sensitive and specific markers for distinguishing granulosa cell tumors from yolk sac tumors. Int J Surg Pathol. 2013;21:121–5.
37. Harms D, Kock LR. Testicular juvenile granulosa cell and Sertoli cell tumours: a clinicopathological study of 29 cases from the Kiel Paediatric Tumour Registry. Virchows Arch. 1997;430:301–9.
38. Ulbright TM, Hattab EM, Zhang S, et al. Primitive neuroectodermal tumors in patients with testicular germ cell tumors usually resemble pediatric-type central nervous system embryonal neoplasms and lack chromosome 22 rearrangements. Mod Pathol. 2010;23:972–80.
39. Mosharafa AA, Foster RS, Bihrle R, et al. Does retroperitoneal lymph node dissection have a curative role for patients with sex cord-stromal testicular tumors? Cancer. 2003;98:753–7.
40. Hanson JA, Ambaye AB. Adult testicular granulosa cell tumor: a review of the literature for clinicopathologic predictors of malignancy. Arch Pathol Lab Med. 2011;135:143–6.
41. Gershenson DM, Morris M, Burke TW, Levenback C, Matthews CM, Wharton JT. Treatment of poor-prognosis sex cord-stromal tumors of the ovary with the combination of bleomycin, etoposide, and cisplatin. Obstet Gynecol. 1996;87:527–31.
42. Zambetti M, Escobedo A, Pilotti S, De Palo G. cis-platinum/vinblastine/bleomycin combination chemotherapy in advanced or recurrent granulosa cell tumors of the ovary. Gynecol Oncol. 1990;36:317–20.
43. Homesley HD, Bundy BN, Hurteau JA, Roth LM. Bleomycin, etoposide, and cisplatin combination therapy of ovarian granulosa cell tumors and other stromal malignancies: a Gynecologic Oncology Group study. Gynecol Oncol. 1999;72:131–7.
44. Harrison MR, Huang W, Liu G, Gee J. Response to antiangiogenesis therapy in a patient with advanced adult-type testicular granulosa cell tumor. Oncology (Williston Park). 2009;23:792–5.

Paratesticular Tumours

18

Robert A. Huddart and Anna Patrikidou

Introduction

The majority of testicular tumours (90–95 %) are germ cell tumours, arising from the germinal epithelium. More rare forms of testicular tumours arise from the sex cord (gonadal stromal tumours such as Sertoli cell tumours and Leydig cell tumours). Paratesticular tumours are defined as an intra-scrotal mass without testicular origin; this includes tumours originating from the spermatic cord, testicular tunics, epididymis, appendices and vestigial remnants. Such tumours occur in all ages, from the infantile period to adult life. This chapter will focus on malignant paratesticular tumours in adolescents/young adults and adults.

Paratesticular tumours arise from histogenetically diverse tissues, notably from mesenchymal, connective or lymphoid tissues. Primary paratesticular tumours are rare, only accounting for 7–10 % of all intra-scrotal tumours [1]. In adults, the vast majority (over 75 %) of paratesticular tumours arise from the spermatic cord [2, 3]. Although infrequent, they have a high incidence of malignancy (approximately 30 %) [5]. Tumour grade, stage, histological type and lymph node involvement are independently p.

The most frequent benign paratesticular tumours are lipomas, leiomyomas and adenomatoid tumours (the latter usually at the head of the epididymis), followed by epididymal cystoadenoma (von Hippel-Lindau syndrome), well-differentiated

R.A. Huddart, MBBS, PhD
Urological Oncology, Department of Radiotherapy, The Institute of Cancer Research and the Royal Marsden NHS Foundation Trust, Downs Road, Sutton SM2 5PT, UK
e-mail: robert.huddart@icr.ac.uk

A. Patrikidou, MD, PhD (✉)
Academic Uro-Oncology Unit, Department of Radiotherapy, The Institute of Cancer Research and the Royal Marsden NHS Foundation Trust, Downs Road, Sutton SM2 5PT, UK
e-mail: anna.patrikidou@icr.ac.uk

L. Pagliaro (ed.), *Rare Genitourinary Tumors*,
DOI 10.1007/978-3-319-30046-7_18

papillary mesothelioma (not related to asbestos exposure), angiomyxoma, angiomyofibroblastoma, haemangioma and fibroma [5].

Generally, paratesticular tumours present as extra-testicular scrotal masses, frequently painless. However, malignant tumours are generally more likely to be symptomatic, large and rapidly growing. A secondary hydrocoele may be occasionally associated. Differential diagnosis includes inguinal hernia, hydrocoele, spermatocoele, hematocoele, cyst, benign tumours or even chronic infections. Ultrasonography has an excellent sensitivity (95–100 %) for distinguishing extra-testicular from intra-testicular tumours [6, 7] and should be always performed, followed by further imaging as indicated.

It should be highlighted that, owing to the rarity of these tumours, most data come from small single-institution series; hence, the level of evidence is low, especially for consensus management recommendations.

A concise outline of aetiology, presentation and management principles of the main entities of paratesticular tumours is presented in Table 18.1.

Sarcomas

Primary paratesticular mesenchymal malignant tumours occur as various histological subtypes (rhabdomyosarcoma, liposarcoma, leiomyosarcoma, fibrosarcoma, chondrosarcoma, peripheral neuroectodermal tumour/PNET, desmoplastic round cell tumour, etc.). In adults, the most common histotype is liposarcoma (20–45 %), followed by leiomyosarcoma (20–30 %) and rhabdomyosarcoma (16–24 %) [5, 8]. In children, the most common malignant tumour is rhabdomyosarcoma (20 %) [9].

In adults, more than 75 % of these lesions arise from the spermatic cord [3]. Spermatic cord sarcomas, which account for 90–95 % of spermatic cord tumours, frequently arise from the distal spermatic cord and appear as a scrotal mass or hydrocoele.

The cornerstone of management with curative intent is surgery, notably complete resection via radical orchidectomy with high ligation of the spermatic cord [4]. However, the anatomical constraints of the area often render difficult obtaining an adequate, oncologically correct surgery as per sarcoma guidelines. Retroperitoneal lymph node dissection (RPLND) has a role in other types of paratesticular sarcomas such as rhabdomyosarcomas, fibrosarcomas and high-grade sarcomas. Adjuvant radiotherapy has an indication in specific subtypes, such as leiomyosarcoma, and in cases of positive margins or local recurrence and poor prognostic factors. With the exception of rhabdomyosarcoma where adjuvant therapy is indicated, chemotherapy has a role only in the metastatic setting in paratesticular sarcomas. Close follow-up is indicated over the first 3 years when most relapses occur, although relapses may be as late as 15 years [10, 11]. Monitoring should be with regular CT scan, chest X-ray and bone scan if clinically indicated (bone pain).

Table 18.1 Aetiology, presentation and management principles of the main entities of malignant paratesticular tumours

Tumour	Epidemiology	Aetiology	Pathology	Prognosis and relapse	Clinical features	Management	Outcome[a]
Paratesticular rhabdomyosarcoma (PT-RMS)	7 % of all RMS 16–24 % of adult paratesticular tumours	t(2;13) or t(1;13) in the alveolar subtype, chr. 11 LOH Association with LFS, von Recklinghausen's disease	Most common subtype: embryonal (70–90 %) Microscopy: small round cells, "tadpole" or "tennis-racket" cells	Favourable prognosis: PT localisation, stage (early), age (children), histology (embryonal), size (<5 cm), age (<10 yrs), local invasiveness (absence), tumour resectability	Commonly spermatic cord Enlarging painless intra-scrotal mass, occasionally associated hydrocoele Tumour size varies Up to 80 % positive LNs, up to 25 % distant metastasis Metastatic sites: liver, bone marrow, lung, LN	Chemotherapy: cardinal (VAC/VAI), neoadjuvant/adjuvant Inguinal orchidectomy Surgery alone: 50 % relapse at 2 yrs RPLND, RT: unnecessary in LN-negative patients Recurrent/relapsed disease: multimodal management	Children: RFS, 80–85 %; OS, 70–90 % (from 25 = 30 % pre-chemo) Adults: 5-yr OS 30–40 %
Paratesticular liposarcoma (PT-LPS)	20–45 % of PT sarcomas Sixth decade of life	Unknown Occasionally malignant transformation of pre-existing lipoma	Positivity for S100 protein, MDM2, CDK4 and desmin in high-grade tumours	Well-differentiated: better prognosis, but local relapse Dedifferentiated and pleomorphic: aggressive, distant metastases	Large palpable scrotal mass Most commonly spermatic cord	Radical inguinal orchi-funicolectomy No established role for RPLND Adjuvant RT discussed if positive margins Role of chemotherapy/RT in metastatic setting	Recurrence rate 46–57 % 5-yr OS: 20–80 % depending on histological subtype

(continued)

Table 18.1 (continued)

Tumour	Epidemiology	Aetiology	Pathology	Prognosis and relapse	Clinical features	Management	Outcome[a]
Paratesticular leiomyosarcoma (PT-LMS)	20–30 % of PT sarcomas Sixth and seventh decade	Unknown, other than certain radiation-induced cases	Originates from smooth muscle of vas deferens canal wall, blood vessels and cremaster muscle Pseudocapsule Typical LMS smooth muscle differentiation features	Tumour dissemination to regional lymph nodes, haematogenous spread and local extension Up to 50 % relapse with surgery alone Radical excision with negative margins cardinal	Painless extra-testicular intra-scrotal mass Occasionally hydrocoele up to 25 % metastatic disease	Radical inguinal orchi-funicolectomy + adjuvant RT RPLND only in N+ patients	5-yr OS, 71 %; 5-yr locoregional control, 81 %
Malignant mesothelioma of the tunica vaginalis (MMTV)	Arises mostly from the TV <5 % of mesotheliomas Median age 60 yrs (range: 7–87 yrs)	Asbestos exposure	Macroscopy: papillary structure or nodules on smooth sac lining Microscopy: solitary, papillary or biphasic pattern	Metastasis at presentation: 15 % Metastatic sites: LN, lung, liver, pleura, local relapse, cerebral (rare)	Hydrocoele associated with a scrotal mass Bilateral involvement: 4 %	Inguinal orchidectomy: optimal Staging/adjuvant RPLND: controversial RT, chemotherapy: in recurrent/metastatic disease	Local recurrence/metastasis after primary surgery: ~50 % >60 % of recurrences within 2 yrs Most recurring pts develop disseminated disease (84 %) 40 % die of disease
Adenocarcinoma of rete testis (ART)	Extremely rare tumour Arises from the testicular collecting system, located in the hilum Median age 60 yrs (17–91 yrs)	Unknown History of undescended testis, chronic epididymitis, trauma	Macroscopy: 1–7 cm; infiltrative tan to grey-white surface Microscopy: tubular, papillary and cystic patterns	Aggressive nature Metastatic sites: LN, liver, lung	Palpable scrotal mass, sometimes pain or hydrocoele	High inguinal orchidectomy/hemiscrotectomy + RPLND Resistant to RT Chemotherapy: metastatic setting (poor efficacy)	3-yr OS: 49 % 5-yr OS: 13 %

Ovarian-type epithelial tumour (OTET) of the epididymis	Mean age 47 yrs (range: 14–68 yrs)	BRAF or KRAS mutations in borderline malignant tumours (mutually exclusive)	Similar to their ovarian counterparts Borderline serous, mucinous, epithelial-stromal (Brenner)	Mostly borderline malignant profile	Painless scrotal mass, occasionally hydrocoele	Radical inguinal high orchidectomy Adjuvant therapy only in carcinomas	Serous borderline tumours: good prognosis/no recurrence if complete excision Mucinous tumours: locally aggressive, usually no metastasis. Brenner tumours: typically benign
Adenocarcinoma of the epididymis (AE)	Extremely rare	Unknown	Typical adenocarcinoma profile Tubular, tubulocystic or tubulopapillary types	Nodal and metastatic spread	Scrotal mass, may invade testis	Inguinal radical orchidectomy ± RPLND Adjuvant chemoradiotherapy? Metastatic setting: platinum-based chemotherapy	Variable, scanty data

AE adenocarcinoma of the epididymis, *ART* adenocarcinoma of the rete testis, *BRAF* murine sarcoma viral oncogene homologue B, *CDK4* cyclin-dependent kinase 4, *chr.* chromosome, *CR* complete response, *CT* chemotherapy, *Gy* grey, *KRAS* Kirsten rat sarcoma viral oncogene homologue, *LFS* Li-Fraumeni syndrome, *LH* luteinising hormone, *LMS* leiomyosarcoma, *LN* lymph nodes, *LOH* loss of heterozygosity, *LPS* liposarcoma, *LVI* lymphovascular invasion, *MDM2* mouse double minute 2 homologue gene, *MMTV* malignant mesothelioma of tunica vaginalis, *mo* months, *OS* overall survival, *OTET* ovarian-type epithelial tumour, *PFS* progression-free survival, *PS* performance status, *PT* paratesticular, *pts* patients, *RFS* relapse-free survival, *RMS* rhabdomyosarcoma, *RPLND* retroperitoneal lymph node dissection, *RT* radiotherapy, *TMs* tumour markers, *TV* tunica vaginalis, *VAC* vincristine/actinomycin/cyclophosphamide, *VAI* vincristine/actinomycin/ifosfamide, *yrs* years

[a]With optimal management

Paratesticular Liposarcoma

Paratesticular liposarcoma (LPS) typically affects adults and has a long clinical history with large palpable scrotal masses and common recurrences [3, 5, 12, 13]. They most commonly arise from the spermatic cord (76 %), testicular tunics (20 %) and epididymis (1.4 %) [14]. Spermatic cord liposarcoma accounts for 37 % of all spermatic cord tumours and 3–7 % of all LPS [1, 15]. Paratesticular LPS may arise de novo from the paratesticular adipose tissue or by malignant transformation of a benign lipoma [5]. In less than 6 % of cases, there is history of scrotal surgery or trauma [15].

The most frequent age of presentation is the sixth decade, with a range of 16–85 years [16]. They may be frequently mistaken for inguinal hernias or hydrocoeles. Specific markers included S100 protein (positive in up to 90 % of cases), MDM2, CDK4 and desmin in high-grade tumours. Treatment relies on radical inguinal orchi-funicolectomy, whilst radiotherapy and chemotherapy do not have established roles in the management of paratesticular LPS [12, 16, 17]. Although liposarcomas (especially myxoid LPS) are one of the most radiosensitive sarcomas, the results are less clear in paratesticular LPS [16, 18]. Adjuvant radiotherapy should be considered in cases of positive margins or high-grade tumours. There is insufficient evidence to support prophylactic RPLND [11, 19].

As for other LPS localisations, there is a correlation between tumour grading, subtype and clinical behaviour and prognosis. Well-differentiated liposarcomas grow slowly, but have a high rate of recurrence especially if excision is insufficient. Dedifferentiation occurs in a minority of cases, and distant metastases may also occur [20]. The pleomorphic liposarcoma is the rarest subtype and considered to be a high-grade sarcoma, with a high rate of recurrence and metastasis [5]. Five-year survival rates are 80 % for the myxoid and well-differentiated subtypes and 20 % for the round cell and pleomorphic liposarcomas [21].

Paratesticular Leiomyosarcoma

Paratesticular LMS originates from the spermatic cord (cremaster muscle and vas deferens), the scrotum (dartous layer) or the epididymis (smooth muscle surrounding the basement membrane). The first two types drain into the retroperitoneal lymph nodes, whilst epididymal LMS drains into the inguinal, external and internal iliac nodes [22]. Spermatic cord LMS corresponds to 24 % of spermatic cord tumours [1]. Peak incidence is in the sixth and seventh decade [23–25]. It typically presents as unilateral, firm, painless extra-testicular, intra-scrotal or inguinal canal mass, occasionally accompanied by a hydrocoele [26]. Its aetiology is unknown, although there are reports of radiation-induced tumours [27, 28] and even one report of an LMS complicating chronic inflammation of the testis [29].

Histologically, such tumours display classic features of soft tissue LMS, i.e. perpendicularly oriented fascicles of cells with brightly eosinophilic cytoplasm containing longitudinal fibrils and blunt-ended nuclei; although some lesions have numerous pleomorphic nuclei, typical features of smooth muscle differentiation are retained [22]. A pseudocapsule that favours a local infiltrative pattern encloses the tumour.

Up to 25 % present with or develop metastatic disease. Survival rate is estimated at 50–80 % [30]. Most cases are low-grade LMS featuring indolent course and a good prognosis; however, high-grade tumours are aggressive and often develop metastases (most commonly to the lungs) with significant mortality [31]. Unlike other LMS localisations, spermatic cord sarcoma frequently disseminates to regional lymphatics, up to 30 %, although this incidence has never been accurately documented [10, 18, 32]. Radical inguinal orchi-funicolectomy is the recommended treatment, but the reported recurrence rates (approximately 50 %), principally due to anatomical difficulties to obtain sufficient excision margins, indicate the need for adjuvant treatment [30]. Higher risk of local recurrence occurs with large tumour size, inguinal location, narrow or positive margins and prior intralesional surgery [33]. Adjuvant radiation seems to effectively prevent recurrence (60–65 Gy in 30–35 fractions to the inguinal canal and ipsilateral pelvis and scrotum) [10, 18, 19]; the 5-year locoregional control, disease-free and overall survival rates following adjuvant RT are reported to be 81 %, 77 % and 71 %, respectively, declining to 61 %, 58 % and 70 %, respectively, at 8 years [18].

Retroperitoneal lymph node dissection is indicated in cases of positive nodes on imaging [22]. No study has shown a significant survival benefit from the addition of RPLND in node-negative patients.

Paratesticular Rhabdomyosarcoma

Paratesticular rhabdomyosarcoma (RMS) corresponds to 7 % of all RMS [34–37] and up to 25 % of adult paratesticular tumours. The majority of these tumours (80 %) occur in the first two decades of life with a bimodal age distribution (5 years, adolescence), whilst the remaining 20 % are distributed across all other ages. The majority of paratesticular RMS occur in the spermatic cord. All known RMS histological subtypes are described in this localisation: embryonal (most common, 70–90 % of paratesticular RMS), alveolar, pleomorphic (rarest), botryoid, undifferentiated and mixed [35, 36, 38, 39].

It clinically presents as an enlarging, most frequently painless intra-scrotal mass, occasionally compressing or invading the testis or epididymis. Cytogenetically, alveolar RMS is characterised by translocations t(2;13)(q35;q14) or t(1;13)(p36;q14), which result in the creation of PAX-FKHR fusion protein [40, 41]. Rhabdomyosarcomas may also occur as part of the Li-Fraumeni syndrome, von Recklinghausen's disease, type 1 neurofibromatosis and Beckwith-Wiedemann, Costello and Noonan syndromes.

On histopathology, it usually presents macroscopically as an encapsulated grey-white mass with areas of haemorrhage and cystic degeneration. Microscopically, it is characterised by small round cells, typically appearing with a "tadpole" or "tennis-racket" configuration [42].

Rhabdomyosarcomas have a high propensity for lymphatic and haematogenous spread. Most patients (up to 80 %) present with metastasis to the regional lymph nodes and up to 25 % present with distant parenchymal metastases [39, 43]. Metastatic sites include the liver, bone marrow and lung.

Given their rarity, adult rhabdomyosarcoma management guidelines stem from the paediatric experience and the respective guidelines. A diagnosis of paratesticular RMS of any variant typically warrants initial treatment with radical inguinal orchidectomy, which allows for confirmation of diagnosis and removal of primary, followed by systemic chemotherapy [44]. Patients aged >10 years have been shown to have a higher risk of lymph node involvement. Retroperitoneal lymph node dissection in these patients led to an improved 5-year survival from 64 to 86 %, although its role remains controversial [45]. The use of a more intense chemotherapy schedule in such patients seems to be superior, as indicated by the IRS-III trial: the 5-year survival rates were 69 % and 96 % in patients with clinically negative nodes treated with and without RPLND followed by chemotherapy, respectively [46]. Radiation therapy for positive lymph nodes appears to improve the 5-year overall survival in older patients [39, 47]. In case of residual disease post-chemotherapy, surgery is indicated prior to growth completion and surgery or radiotherapy in post-pubertal patients (inverted-Y field, 40 Gy) [42].

RMS prognosis is generally more sombre in adults compared to children [39]. Prognosis varies according to histological subtype, with alveolar and pleomorphic RMS having a poor prognosis, whilst embryonal RMS has a more favourable prognosis [39]. A special variant of embryonal RMS, spindle-cell RMS, accounting for 3 % of all adult RMS, has a favourable prognosis in children (5-year survival rate of 95 %), but substantial data are lacking in adults [48, 49]. For this reason, its management is the same as for all paratesticular RMS [50].

About a third of patients with paratesticular sarcomas die from metastatic disease [51]. Five-year survival for adult RMS is 30–40 % [52, 53].

Desmoplastic Round Cell Tumour

Desmoplastic round cell tumour (DRCT) is a highly aggressive sarcoma subtype. They are rare in the paratesticular region and occur in the young adult, with an age distribution of 17–43 years. Cytogenetically, DRCTs have a unique translocation, t(11;22)(p13;p12), that results in fusion of the exon 9 of the EWSR1 gene to exon 9 of the WT1; the EWSR1-WT1 chimera acts as an oncogenic transcription factor [5]. Long-term survivors in DRCT are rare (median survival, 17 months; 5-year OS, 18 %) [54, 55]. Management should be with radical surgery followed by adjuvant chemotherapy. Although DCRTs are sensitive to chemotherapy and radiotherapy, the response is rarely lasting, and most cases recur within 6 months [56].

Malignant Mesothelioma of the Tunica Vaginalis

Malignant mesothelioma of the tunica vaginalis (MMTV) most commonly arises from the tunica vaginalis, which is part of the peritoneum, although it may also arise from the spermatic cord and the epididymis [5]. Asbestos exposure is an established risk factor for malignant mesothelioma. Other suggested, although not confirmed, aetiological factors include chronic immunosuppression, chromosomal abnormalities, radiation, Simian virus, trauma and previous hernia repair [42].

MMTV is extremely rare, corresponding to <5 % of all mesotheliomas [42]. Peak incidence is at 55–75 years (median age, 60 years; range 7–87 years) [5]. The tumour usually presents as a painless scrotal mass associated with a hydrocoele, frequently recurrent [5]. Macroscopically it presents as a papillary structure or nodules on a smooth sac lining. Microscopically it features a solitary, papillary or biphasic pattern [42].

Management is by radical inguinal orchidectomy. Transscrotal procedures are associated with local recurrence. The role of adjuvant treatment is not fully assessed; adjuvant radiotherapy or RPLND has been recommended by some authors but remains controversial [42, 57]. The role of radiotherapy and chemotherapy (pemetrexed, doxorubicin-based regimens) is limited to recurrent and metastatic disease with short-lasting responses.

MMTV is an aggressive tumour, with 15 % of patients being metastatic at presentation, whilst 50 % present with local recurrence or distant metastasis after primary surgery [5]. Locoregional relapses ought to be managed with salvage surgery, with consideration of adjuvant radiotherapy according to margin status [42]. Metastatic sites include the lung, the liver, the pleura and rarely the brain. Patients relapsing with disseminated disease are managed with palliative chemotherapy. Median time to recurrence is 10 months (range, 2–180 months). Approximately 40 % of patients die from their disease, with a median survival of 24 months [58, 59]. Poorer outcome is seen in patients over 60 years, in non-localised disease and with history of asbestos exposure [58].

Adenocarcinoma of the Rete Testis

Adenocarcinoma of the rete testis (ART) is an extremely rare neoplasm (approximately 65 cases in the literature) arising from the non-spermatogenic epithelium of the testicular excretory ducts [60]. It usually occurs in men over the age of 60 years (range of 17–91 years) [61]. Adenocarcinoma of the rete testis is described primarily in Caucasians. Its aetiology is unknown, although associations with history of undescended testes, chronic epididymitis or trauma have been reported [42]. It presents as a scrotal mass (1–7 cm), located in the hilum or epididymis, occasionally painful or associated with a hydrocoele. Differential diagnosis from other paratesticular tumours is difficult, often leading to delayed, histopathology-based diagnosis. The greatest resemblance is with MMTV, but also germ cell tumours. AFP and βHCG levels may aid in the earlier detection [60], and cytological diagnosis may also aid in early diagnosis and treatment planning. Histopathologically, solid, tubular or papillary patterns with stromal invasion are described, with foci of haemorrhage and necrosis. Slit-like spaces in solid nests of tumour and intra-rete growth are common [62, 63].

Management is primarily surgical, by high inguinal orchidectomy/hemiscrotectomy and RPLND [42, 64]. ART is traditionally resistant to adjuvant therapy, notably to radiotherapy and to a lesser degree to chemotherapy. It is an aggressive neoplasm with poor prognosis; 3-year and 5-year OS is 49 % and 13 %, respectively, with up to 40 % of patients dying within the first year of disease [61], although survival up to 7 years has been reported [65]. Frequent metastatic sites include the lymph nodes, liver and lung. Early diagnosis and radical therapy are crucial to improve outcomes, and organ-confined and smaller lesions (<5 cm) have better prognosis.

Adenocarcinoma of the Epididymis

Epididymal tumours are malignant in 25 %, including sarcomas, germ cell tumours, squamous carcinomas, adenocarcinomas and lymphomas [78–80]. Given its rarity, with approximately 25 cases reported in the literature, limited data exist for this paratesticular tumour [5, 78–81]. Histopathologically, these tumours have the microscopic and immunohistochemical profile of adenocarcinomas (positivity for cytokeratin and epithelial membrane antigen), showing tubular, tubulocystic or tubulopapillary patterns [81]. It presents as a scrotal mass or epididymal thickening that may invade the adjacent testicle, with non-specific clinical characteristics to distinguish it from other paratesticular tumours. Differential diagnosis from metastatic adenocarcinoma might be challenging. Management of these tumours in the literature is surgical, by inguinal radical orchidectomy and RPLND in case of positive nodes, although a staging RPLND has also been recommended [79]. Adjuvant radiotherapy or chemoradiotherapy has also been reported. Choice for chemotherapy regimens could be guided by the adenocarcinoma of other localisations, notably platinum-based regimens for the first-line regimens and gemcitabine-based salvage chemotherapy [81]. Data on survival are scanty, ranging from a few months to 30 years [78, 79, 81].

Ovarian-Type Epithelial Tumours of the Testis

The ovarian-type epithelial (Mullerian) tumours (OTETs) are neoplasms occurring rarely in the paratesticular area, histologically corresponding to the respective ovarian tumours [72]. They may arise from the tunica vaginalis, tunica albuginea, epididymis, rete testis and paratesticular soft tissue. The most frequent subtype is the serous tumour of borderline malignancy, but mucinous, endometrioid, Brenner (transitional cell) and squamous subtypes, as well as serous adenocarcinomas, may also occur. OTETs of the testis originate either from the remnants of Mullerian ducts in paratesticular connective tissue, epididymis and spermatic cord, from Mullerian metaplasia of the mesothelium of the tunica vaginalis or from testicular embryonic mesothelial inclusions.

These tumours usually occur in middle-aged man (mean age, 47 years), with reported age of presentation between 14 and 68 years [73, 74]. No specific aetiological factor has been described, although one case with bilateral cryptorchidism has been reported [75]. They present as painless scrotal mass, occasionally associated with a hydrocoele and frequently situated in the epididymo-testicular groove [76]. Normal AFP, HCG and LDH levels aid in the differential diagnosis from germ cell tumours. They express ovarian epithelial tumour markers such as epithelial membrane antigen (EMA), CA-125 (cancer antigen 125), cytokeratin 7, CD15 (Leu-1), Ber-EP4 and PAX8 (paired box gene 8). Differential diagnosis is mainly with MMTV, but also with adenocarcinoma of the rete testis and of the epididymis [73]. Typical microscopical features are the cystic nature and papillary budding of the serous borderline tumours. Detection of BRAF and KRAS mutations has been reported, indicating a common pathogenesis with the ovarian serous borderline tumours [73, 77]. A rare occurrence of a metastatic deposit to the testis from another site ought to be excluded.

Management is by complete surgical excision by radical inguinal high orchidectomy. Adjuvant therapy is indicated only in carcinomas. The prognosis of the borderline tumours is generally good, with low risk of progression or metastasis; most patients with localised disease show no recurrence in the first 2 years, although late recurrences have also been reported [75, 76]. The mucinous subtypes may be locally aggressive, although usually they do not metastasise. Brenner tumours are of a typically benign nature.

Very Rare Paratesticular Tumours

Reports of other very rare malignant paratesticular tumours occurring in adults include primary paratesticular germ cell tumours [66], extra-testicular sex cord-stromal tumours [67], plasmocytoma [68] and extrarenal Wilms' tumour [69].

Metastatic Paratesticular Disease

The testis and paratesticular tissues represent rare sites of metastatic disease. Reported cases of such primary tumours include prostate, lung and gastrointestinal malignancies and melanoma and even more rarely retinoblastoma, neuroblastoma, bladder, ureter and bile duct malignancies and even carcinoid [70]. Infrequently, a testicular mass could even be the only presenting sign of an occult primary [71]. Disease metastatic to the testicle occurs with greater frequency in children rather than adults and it is usually of lymphopoietic origin [7]. Metastatic disease to the testes should also be considered in patients presenting with bilateral intra-scrotal tumours.

Epidemiology of Malignant Paratesticular Tumours: An Update on Incidence and Mortality Trends in the UK

Incidence and mortality data on malignant paratesticular tumours for the period 2001–2013 are presented below, provided by the National Cancer Intelligence Network, Public Health England (data source: United Kingdom National Cancer Registry Service). Data capture was based on the combination of relevant ICD 10 anatomical localisation codes (C62 comprising C620, C621, C629: malignant neoplasm of testis; C630: epididymis; C631: spermatic cord; CC632: scrotum) and of morphology codes corresponding to carcinoma, sarcoma, mesothelioma, Mullerian mixed tumours and all their subtypes (a total of 88 codes). Incidence data has been estimated based on relevant ICD 10 anatomical site codes and morphology codes, whilst mortality data was selected using the ICD 10 codes of interest only, as there are no morphology codes captured for underlying cause of death. Data pertaining to testicular neoplasms of uncertain or unknown behaviour of testis (ICD 10 code D40.1) were excluded from this analysis.

A total of 524 paratesticular tumours of all ages were identified for the prespecified period. Epididymal and spermatic cord tumours accounted for 5 % and 25 % of tumours, respectively, whilst the remaining tumours were recorded as testicular (45 %) or scrotal localisations (25 %), without further precision. Incidence by year of diagnosis, age-standardised incidence rates and incidence by age group in England in the period 2001–2013 are presented in Fig. 18.1. Case numbers and age-standardised rates for the same period are presented in detail in Table 18.2. The vast majority of tumours (92 %) occurred in Caucasian patients (British or other white background).

A graphic representation of the incidence of malignant paratesticular tumours by morphological subtype is shown in Fig. 18.2, confirming the higher percentage of sarcomas amongst all paratesticular tumours (84 %). Similarly, the incidences of the different sarcoma subtypes are also concordant with the international literature, with LPS being the most common histotype (43 %), followed by LMS (22 %) and RMS (19 %) (Fig. 18.2). A detailed account of all recorded tumours by individual morphological type is given in Table 18.3. In terms of histological grade, over half of recorded cases for which information on grade was available were grade 1 tumours (59 %), with grade 2 and 3 tumours accounting for the remaining 15 % and 23 %, respectively.

Sarcoma subtypes constitute the greatest percentage of paratesticular tumours (Fig. 18.2). Despite these types of tumours generally being much more frequent in children, the paratesticular localisation seems to be more frequent in the older age groups, with peak incidence in the eighth decade of life (Fig. 18.1c).

Cancer-specific mortality for the above cohort was 7.8 % (41 of 524 patients) (Table 18.4). Amongst the tumour types, sarcomas (notably LMS and RMS) had the highest mortality incidence (approximately 60 % of all cancer-related deaths), followed by adenocarcinoma (17 %). However, adenocarcinoma was found to be the

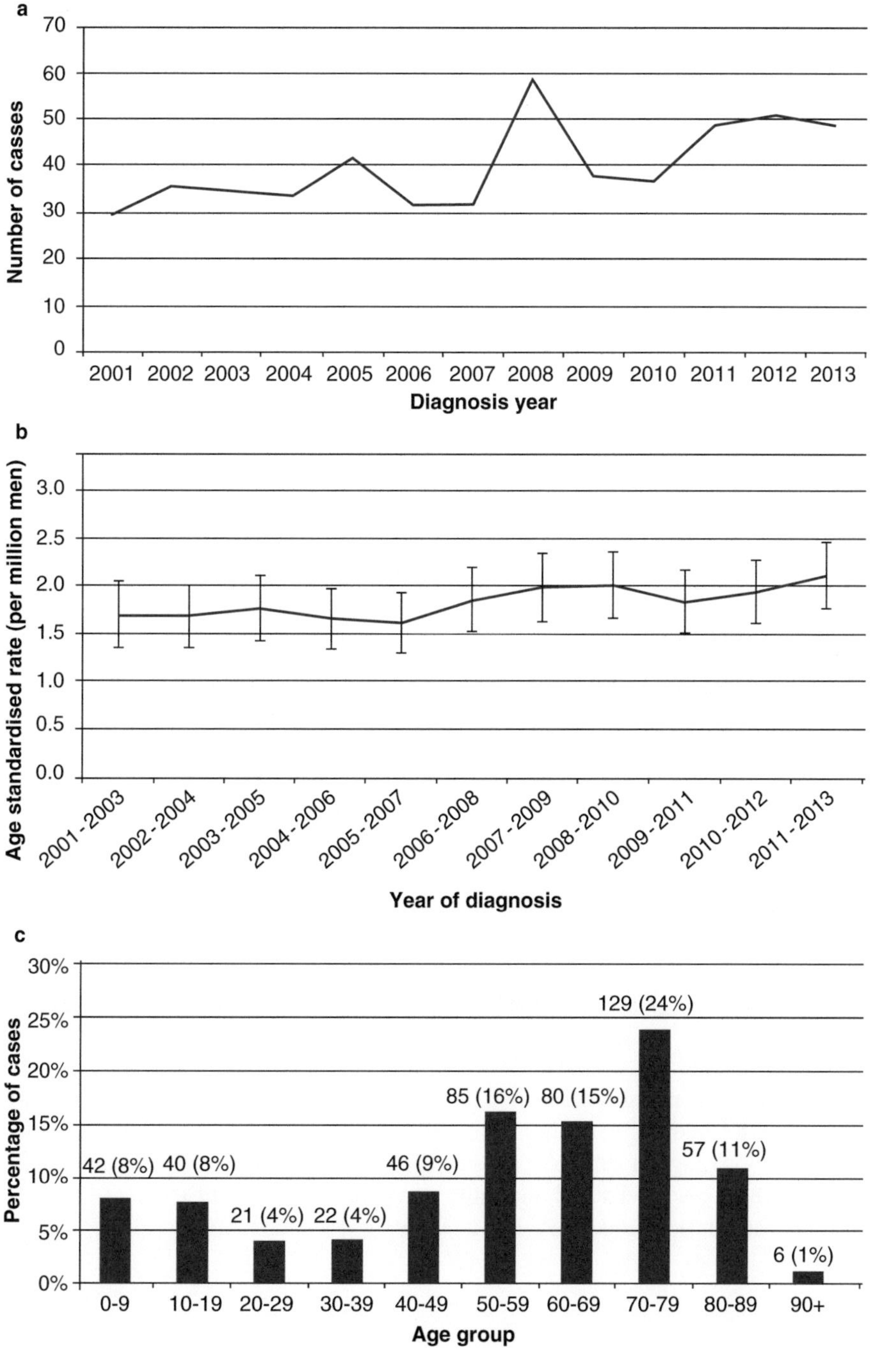

Fig. 18.1 (**a**) Incidence of malignant paratesticular tumours by year of diagnosis in England, 2001–2013. (**b**) Age-standardised incidence rates of malignant paratesticular tumours by year of diagnosis, for rolling three-year periods in England, 2001–2013. (**c**) Incidence of malignant paratesticular tumours by age group in England, 2001–2013. Case numbers are shown (percentages in brackets)

Table 18.2 Age-standardised incidence rates of malignant paratesticular tumours for rolling 3-year periods (per million men) in England, 2001–2013

Year	Cases	ASR	ASR LCI	ASR UCI
2001–2003	101	1.7	1.3	2.0
2002–2004	105	1.7	1.3	2.0
2003–2005	111	1.8	1.4	2.1
2004–2006	108	1.7	1.3	2.0
2005–2007	106	1.6	1.3	1.9
2006–2008	123	1.9	1.5	2.2
2007–2009	129	2.0	1.6	2.3
2008–2010	134	2.0	1.7	2.4
2009–2011	124	1.8	1.5	2.2
2010–2012	137	1.9	1.6	2.3
2011–2013	149	2.1	1.8	2.5

ASR age-standardised rate, *LCI* lower confidence interval, *UCI* upper confidence interval

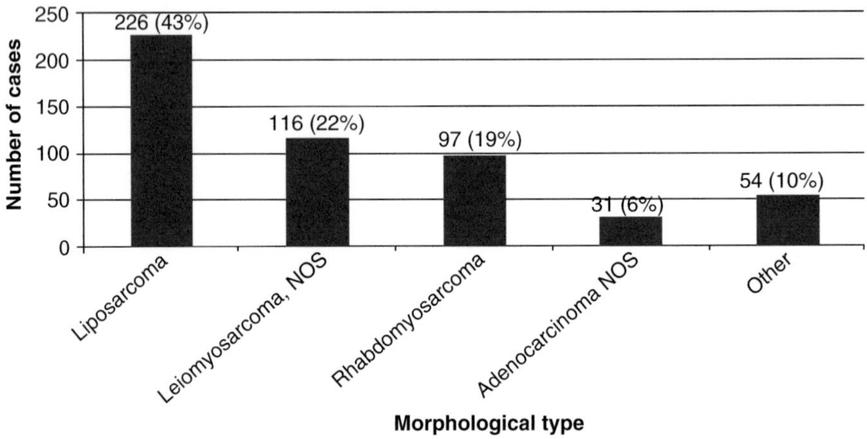

Fig. 18.2 Incidence of malignant paratesticular tumours by morphological type in England, 2001–2013

most aggressive neoplasm, as it featured the highest cancer-specific mortality (22.6 %) as a percentage of individuals with that tumour type (Table 18.4, Fig. 18.4). The rarest histological subtypes, here categorised as Other (and listed individually in Table 18.3), also had a high mortality as a percentage of their incidence (16.7 % [9 of 54 patients]), whereas LPS had a relatively low such mortality (3 %).

Table 18.3 Incidence of malignant paratesticular tumours by morphological type in England, 2001–2013

Morphology code	Morphological type	Cases	Percentage
8890/3	Leiomyosarcoma, NOS	115	21.9
8850/3	Liposarcoma, NOS	98	18.7
8851/3	Liposarcoma, well-differentiated type	78	14.9
8910/3	Embryonal rhabdomyosarcoma/sarcoma botryoides	49	9.4
8858/3	Dedifferentiated liposarcoma	43	8.2
8140/3	Adenocarcinoma, NOS	31	5.9
8900/3	Rhabdomyosarcoma, NOS	24	4.6
8920/3	Alveolar rhabdomyosarcoma	19	3.6
8800/3	Sarcoma NOS	18	3.4
8801/3	Spindle cell sarcoma	10	1.9
8991/3	Embryonal sarcoma	7	1.3
8852/3	Myxoid liposarcoma	5	1.0
8804/3	Epithelioid sarcoma	4	0.8
8810/3	Fibrosarcoma	3	0.6
8830/3	Fibrous histiocytoma	3	0.6
8902/3	Mixed-type rhabdomyosarcoma	3	0.6
8802/3	Giant cell sarcoma	2	0.4
8811/3	Fibromyxosarcoma	2	0.4
8854/3	Pleomorphic liposarcoma	2	0.4
8901/3	Pleomorphic rhabdomyosarcoma	2	0.4
8803/3	Small cell sarcoma	1	0.2
8832/3	Dermatofibrosarcoma, NOS	1	0.2
8891/3	Epithelioid leiomyosarcoma	1	0.2
8950/3	Mullerian mixed tumour	1	0.2
9050/3	Mesothelioma, malignant (C45)	1	0.2
9133/3	Epithelioid hemangioendothelioma	1	0.2
Total	Total	524	100.0

The majority of these deaths (28 patients, 68 %) occurred within 2 years from diagnosis (Fig. 18.3). Cancer-specific survival was 96 %, 94.6 %, 93 % and 92.2 % at 1, 2, 5 and 9 years from diagnosis, respectively. Grade 3 tumours accounted for 50 % of deaths, followed by grade 2 tumours (30 %). When mortality was assessed by age band, the majority of deaths were found to have occurred in the 60–69 years age group (24 %), followed by the 70–79 years (22 %) and 10–19 years (20 %).

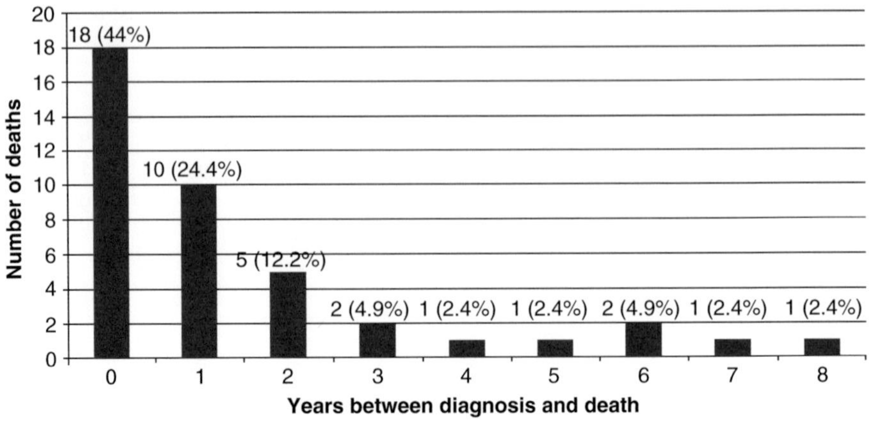

Fig. 18.3 Years between diagnosis and death for men who died from a malignant paratesticular tumour diagnosed between 2001 and 2013, in England

Table 18.4 Cancer-specific mortality of malignant paratesticular tumours (diagnosed 2001–2013), by morphological type, in England

Tumour type	Cases	Percentage of deaths	Percentage of subgroup incidence
Leiomyosarcoma, NOS	9	22	7.7
Rhabdomyosarcoma	9	22	9.3
Adenocarcinoma, NOS	7	17	22.6
Liposarcoma	7	17	3
Other	9	22	16.7
Total	41	100	

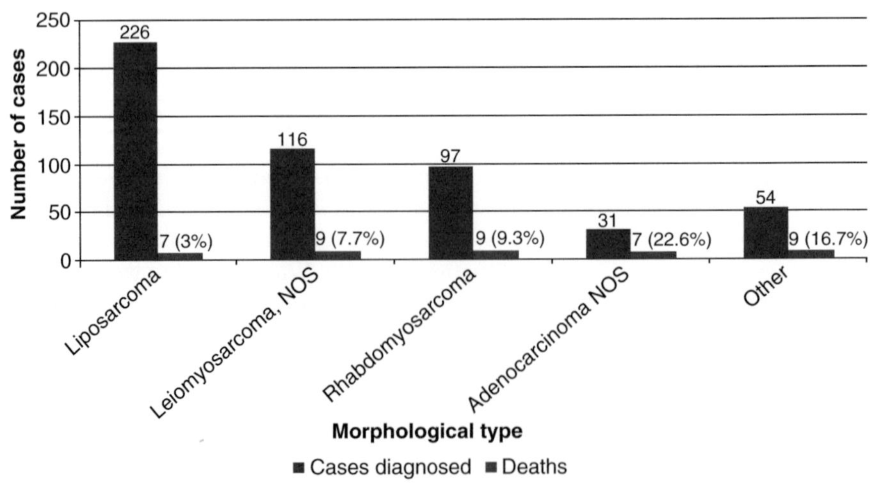

Fig. 18.4 Incidence of paratesticular tumours (diagnosed 2001–2013) and cancer-specific mortality (between 2001 and 2014), by morphological type, in England

References

1. Rodriguez D, Olumi AF. Management of spermatic cord tumours: a rare urological malignancy. Ther Adv Urol. 2012;4(6):325–34.
2. Richie JP. Chapter 78: Neoplasm of testis. In: Walsh PC, Retik AB, Vaughan ED, Wein AJ, editors. Campbell's urology, vol. III. 7th ed. Philadelphia: WB Saunders; 1998. p. 2411–52.
3. Sogani PC, Grabstald H, Whitmore Jr WF. Spermatic cord sarcoma in adults. J Urol. 1978;120:301–5.
4. Merimsky O, Terrier P, Bonvalot S, Le Pechoux C, Delord JP, Le Cesne A. Spermatic cord sarcoma in adults. Acta Oncol. 1999;38:635–8.
5. Khoubehi B, Mishra V, Ali M, Motiwala H, Karim O. Adult paratesticular tumours. BJU Int. 2002;90:707–15.
6. Frates MC, Benson CB, DiSalvo DN, Brown DL, Laing FC, Doubilet PM. Solid extratesticular masses evaluated with sonography: pathologic correlation. Radiology. 1997;204:43–6.
7. Agarwal PK, Palmer JS. Testicular and paratesticular neoplasms in prepubertal males. J Urol. 2006;175:875–81.
8. Rodríguez D, Barrisford GW, Sanchez A, Preston MA, Kreydin EI, Olumi AF. Primary spermatic cord tumors: disease characteristics, prognostic factors, and treatment outcomes. Urol Oncol. 2014;32:52.e19-25.
9. Shapiro E, Strother D. Pediatric genitourinary rhabdomyosarcoma. J Urol. 1992;148:1761.
10. Ballo MT, Zagars GK, Pisters PWT, Feig BW, Patel SR, von Estenbach AC. Spermatic cord sarcoma: outcome, pattern of failure and management. J Urol. 2001;166:1306–10.
11. Coleman J, Brennan MF, Alektiar K, Russo P. Adult spermatic cord sarcomas: management and results. Ann Surg Oncol. 2003;10:669–75.
12. Garcia-Morua A, Lozano Salinas JF, ValdeÅLs SepuÅLlveda F, et al. Liposarcoma of the spermatic cord: our experience and review of the literature. Actas Urol Esp. 2009;33:811–5.
13. Montgomery E, Fisher C. Paratesticular liposarcoma: a clinicopathologic study. Am J Surg Pathol. 2003;27:40–7.
14. Gabriele R, Ferrara G, Tarallo MR, Giordano A, De Gori A, Izzo L, Conte M. Recurrence of paratesticular liposarcoma: a case report and review of the literature. World J Surg Oncol. 2014;12:276–9.
15. Schwartz SL, Swierzewski SJ, Sondak VK, et al. Liposarcoma of the spermatic cord: report of 6 cases and review of the literature. J Urol. 1995;153(1):154–7.
16. Fitzgerald S, MacLennan GT. Paratesticular liposarcoma. J Urol. 2009;181:331–2.
17. Vorstman B, Block NL, Politano VA. The management of spermatic cord liposarcomas. J Urol. 1984;131:66–9.
18. Fagundes MA, Zietman AL, Althausen AF, Coen JJ, Shipley WU. The management of spermatic cord sarcoma. Cancer. 1996;77:1873–6.
19. Catton CN, Cummings BJ, Fornasier V, O'Sullivan B, Quirt I, Warr D. Adult paratesticular sarcomas: a review of 21 cases. J Urol. 1991;146:342–5.
20. Henricks WH, Chu YC, Goldblum JR, Weiss SW. Dedifferentiated liposarcoma: a clinicopathological analysis of 155 cases with a proposal for an expanded definition of dedifferentiation. Am J Surg Pathol. 1997;21:271–81.
21. Alyousef H, Osman EW, Gomha MA. Paratesticular liposarcoma: a case report and review of the literature. Case Rep Urol. 2013: Article ID 806289, 3 pages.
22. Galosi AB, Scarpelli M, Mazzucchelli R, Lopez-Beltran A, Giustini L, Cheng L, Montironi R. Adult primary paratesticular mesenchymal tumors with emphasis on a case presentation and discussion of spermatic cord leiomyosarcoma. Diagn Pathol. 2014;9:90–5.
23. Rao CR, Srinivasulu M, Naresh KN, Doval DC, Hazarika D. Adult paratesticular sarcomas: a report of eight cases. J Surg Oncol. 1994;56:89–93.
24. Weinshank LB, Kellner D, Nash I. Paratesticular leiomyosarcoma: case report and review. Conn Med. 2011;75:399–403.
25. Yuen VT, Kirby SD, Woo YC. Leiomyosarcoma of the epididymis: 2 cases and review of the literature. Can Urol Assoc J. 2011;5:E121–4.

26. Enoch S, Wharton SM, Murray DS. Management of leiomyosarcomas of the spermatic cord: the role of reconstructive surgery. Worl J Surg Oncol. 2005;3:23–9.
27. Lynch Jr DF, Herr HW. Radiation-induced sarcoma following radiotherapy for testicular tumor. J Urol. 1981;126(6):845–6.
28. Stein ME, Leviov M, Drumea K, Goralnik L, Miselevich I, Kuten A. Radiation-induced sarcoma following curative radiotherapy for testicular seminoma: case report and brief review of the literature. Tumori. 1997;83(3):721–3.
29. Ali Y, Kehinde EO, Makar R, Al-Awadi KA, Anim JT. Leiomyosarcoma complicating chronic inflammation of the testis. Med Princ Pract. 2002;11(3):157–60.
30. Blitzer PH, Dosoretz DE, Proppe KH, Shipley WU. Treatment of malignant tumors of the spermatic cord: a study of 10 cases and a review of the literature. J Urol. 1981;126:611–4.
31. Fisher C, Goldblum JR, Epstein JI, Montgomery E. Leiomyosarcoma of the paratesticular region: a clinicopathologic study. Am J Surg Pathol. 2001;25:1143–9.
32. Banowsky LH, Shultz GN. Sarcoma of the spermatic cord and tunics: review of the literature, case report and discussion of the role of retroperitoneal lymph node dissection. J Urol. 1970;103:628–31.
33. Folpe AL, Weiss SW. Paratesticular soft tissue neoplasms. Semin Diagn Pathol. 2000;17:307–18.
34. Raney Jr RB, Hays DM. Paratesticular rhabdomyosarcoma in childhood. Cancer. 1978;42:729–36.
35. Stewart LH, Lioe TF, Johnston SR. Thirty-year review of intrascrotal rhabdomyosarcoma. Br J Urol. 1991;68:418–20.
36. Stewart RJ, Martelli H, Oberlin O, Rey A, Bouvet N, Spicer RD, et al. Treatment of children with nonmetastatic paratesticular rhabdomyosarcoma: results of the malignant mesenchymal tumors studies (MMT 84 and MMT 89) of the International Society of Pediatric Oncology. J Clin Oncol. 2003;21:793–8.
37. De Vries JD. Paratesticular rhabdomyosarcoma. World J Urol. 1995;13:219–25.
38. Dagher R, Helman L. Rhabdomyosarcoma: an overview. Oncologist. 1999;4:34–44.
39. Ferrari A, Bisogno G, Casanova M, Meazza C, Piva L, Cecchetto G, et al. Paratesticular rhabdomyosarcoma: report from the Italian and German Cooperative Group. J Clin Oncol. 2002;20:449–55.
40. Barr FG, Galili N, Holick J, Biegel JA, Rovera G, Emmanuel GS. Rearrangement of the PAX3 paired box gene in the paediatric solid tumour alveolar rhabdomyosarcoma. Nat Genet. 1993;3:113–7.
41. Davis RJ, D'Cruz CM, Lovell MA, Biegel JA, Barr FG. Fusion of PAX7 to FKHR by the variant t(1; 13)(p36;q14) translocation in alveolar rhabdomyosarcoma. Cancer Res. 1994;54:2869–72.
42. Huddart R, Hazell S, Horwich A. Rare tumors of the testis and paratesticular tissues. In: Raghavan D, Blanke CD, Johnson DH, Moots PL, Reaman GH, Rose PG, Sekeres MA editors. Textbook of uncommon cancer. John Wiley and Sons Inc., Hoboken, NJ, USA. 2012.
43. Akbar SA, Sayyed TA, Jafri SZ, Hasteh F, Neill JS. Multimodality imaging of paratesticular neoplasms and their rare mimics. Radiographics. 2003;23:1461–76.
44. Hamilton CR, Pinkerton R, Horwich A. The management of paratesticular rhabdomyosarcoma. Clin Radiol. 1989;40:314–7.
45. Hermans BP, Foster RS, Bihrle R, et al. Is retroperitoneal lymph node dissection necessary for adult paratesticular rhabdomyosarcoma? J Urol. 1998;160:2074–7.
46. Crist W, Gehan EA, Ragab AH, et al. The Third Intergroup Rhabdomyosarcoma Study. J Clin Oncol. 1995;13:610–30.
47. Dang ND, Dang PT, Samuelian J, et al. Lymph node management in patients with paratesticular rhabdomyosarcoma: a population-based analysis. Cancer. 2013;119:3228–33.
48. Newton Jr WA, Gehan EA, Webber BL, et al. Classification of rhabdomyosarcomas and related sarcomas. Pathologic aspects and proposal for a new classification-an Intergroup Rhabdomyosarcoma Study. Cancer. 1995;76:1073–85.
49. Leuschner I, Newton Jr WA, Schmidt D, et al. Spindle cell variants of embryonal rhabdomyosarcoma in the paratesticular region. A report of the Intergroup Rhabdomyosarcoma Study. Am J Surg Pathol. 1993;17:221–30.

50. Carroll SJ, Nodit L. Spindle cell rhabdomyosarcoma: a brief diagnostic review and differential diagnosis. Arch Pathol Lab Med. 2013;137:1155e–8.
51. Dotan ZA, Tal R, Golijanin D, et al. Adult genitourinary sarcoma: the 25-year Memorial Sloan-Kettering experience. J Urol. 2006;176:2033–8.
52. Little DJ, Ballo MT, Zagars GK, Pisters PWT, Patel SR, El-Naggar AK, Garden AS, Benjamin AS. Adult rhabdomyosarcoma. Outcome following multimodality treatment. Cancer. 2002;95(2):377–88.
53. Sultan I, Qaddoumi I, Yaser S, et al. Comparing adult and pediatric rhabdomyosarcoma in the surveillance, epidemiology and end results program, 1973 to 2005: an analysis of 2,600 patients. J Clin Oncol. 2009;27:3391–7.
54. Schwarz RE, Gerald WL, Kushner BH, Coit DG, Brennan MF, La Quaglia MP. Desmoplastic small round cell tumors: prognostic indicators and results of surgical management. Ann Surg Oncol. 1998;5(5):416–22.
55. Hassan I, Shyyan R, Donohue JH, Edmonson JH, Gunderson LL, Moir CR. Intraabdominal desmoplastic small round cell tumors: a diagnostic and therapeutic challenge. Cancer. 2005;104(6):1264–70.
56. Livaditi E, Mavridis G, Soutis M, Papandreou E, Moschovi M, Papadakis V. Diffuse intraabdominal desmoplastic small round cell tumor: a ten-year experience. Eur J Pediatr Surg. 2006;16(6):423–7.
57. Smith III JJ, Malone MJ, Geffin J, Silverman ML, Libertino JA. A retroperitoneal lymph node dissection in malignant mesothelioma of tunica vaginalis testis. J Urol. 1990;144:1242–3.
58. Plas E, Riedl CR, Pfluger H. Malignant mesothelioma of the tunica vaginalis testis. Review of literature and assessment of prognostic parameters. Cancer. 1998;83:2437–46.
59. Jones MA, Young RH, Scully RE. Malignant mesothelioma of the tunica vaginalis. A clinicopathologic analysis of 11 cases with review of the literature. Am J Surg Pathol. 1995;19:815–25.
60. Tian Y, Yao W, Yang L, Wang J, Wazir R, Wang K. Primary adenocarcinoma of the rete testis: a case report and review of the literature. Oncol Lett. 2014;7:455–7.
61. Sánchez-Chapado M, Angulo JC, Haas GP. Adenocarcinoma of the rete testis. Urology. 1995;46:468–75.
62. Haas GP, Ohorodnik JM, Farah RN. Cystadenocarcinoma of the rete testis. J Urol. 1987;137(6):1232–3.
63. Crisp-Lindgren N, Travers H, Wells MM. Papillary adenocarcinoma of rete testis: autopsy findings, histochemistry, immunohistochemistry, ultrastructure and clinical correlations. Am J Surg Pathol. 1988;12(6):492–501.
64. Perimenis P, Speakman M. Primary adenocarcinoma of the rete testis. Int Urol Nephrol. 2004;35(3):373–4.
65. Glazier DB, Vates TS, Cummings KB, Antoun S. Adenocarcinoma of rete testis. World J Urol. 1996;14(6):397–400.
66. Dichmann O, Engel U, Jensen DB, et al. Juxtatesticular seminoma. Br J Urol. 1990;66: 324–5.
67. Hartwick RW, Srigley JR, Burns B, et al. A clinicopathologic review of 112 paratesticular tumours [Abstract]. Laboratory Invest. 1987. 56:30A.
68. Ferry JA, Young RH, Scully RE. Testicular and epididymal plasmacytoma: a report of 7 cases, including 3 that were the initial manifestation of plasma cell lymphoma. Am J Surg Pathol. 1997;21:590–8.
69. Ulbright TM, Srigley JR, Reuter VE, Wojno K, Roth LM, Young RH. Sex cord-stromal tumors of the testis with entrapped germ cells: a lesion unclassified mixed germ cell sex cord-stromal tumors. Am J Surg Pathol. 2000;24:535–42.
70. Choudhary ND, Kadri SM, Tasleem SA, Reshi A, Besina S, Choudhary QA. Testicular and paratesticular neoplasms in old patients. JK Science. 2003;5(2):58–62.
71. Haupt HM, Mann RB, et al. Metastatic carcinoma involving the testis. Cancer. 1984;54:709.
72. Guarch R, Rivas A, Puras A, Pesce C. Papillary serous carcinoma of ovarian type of the testis with borderline differentiation. Histopathology. 2005;46(5):588–90.

73. Burger T, Schildhaus HU, Inniger R, Hansen J, Mayer P, Schweyer S, Radzun HJ, Strobel P, Bremmer F. Ovarian-type epithelial tumours of the testis: immunohistochemical and molecular analysis of two serous borderline tumours of the testis. Diagn Pathol. 2015;10:118–23.
74. Young RH, Scully RE. Testicular and paratesticular tumors and tumour-like lesions of ovarian common epithelial and mullerian types. A report of four cases and review of literature. Am J Clin Pathol. 1990;198:146–52.
75. Di Franco CA, Porru D, Viglio A, Paulli M, Rovereto B. Primary paratesticular mucinous "ovarian-type" adenocarcinoma: a rare case of scrotal tumor in a patient with history of bilateral cryptorchidism. World J Nephrol Urol. 2015;4(4):260–3.
76. Jones MA, Young RH, Srigley JR, Scully RE. Paratesticular serous papillary carcinoma. Am J Surg Pathol. 1995;19:1359–65.
77. Singer G, Oldt 3rd R, Cohen Y, Wang BG, Sidransky D, Kurman RJ, et al. Mutations in BRAF and KRAS characterize the development of low-grade ovarian serous carcinoma. J Natl Cancer Inst. 2003;95(6):484–6.
78. Ganem JP, Jhaveri FM, Marroum MC. Primary adenocarcinoma of the epididymis: case report and review of the literature. Urology. 1998;52(5):904–8.
79. Chauhan RD, Gingrich JR, Eltorky M, Steiner MS. The natural progression of adenocarcinoma of the epididymis. J Urol. 2001;166:608–10.
80. Alleman WG, Gorman B, King BF, Larson DR, Chrville JC, Nehra A. Benign and malignant epididymal masses evaluated with scrotal sonography. Clinical and pathologic review of 85 patients. J Ultrasound Med. 2008;27:1195–202.
81. Jones MA, Yong RH. Adenocarcinoma of the epididymis: a report of four cases and review of the literature. Am J Surg Pathol. 1997;21(12):1474–80.

Squamous Cell Carcinoma of the Penis and Scrotum

19

Lance Pagliaro

Introduction

Penile and scrotal cancers are rare in developed countries. In the United States, the estimated number of new cases of penile cancer for 2015 was 1,820 [1]. Scrotal cancer is even less common, with an incidence rate of about one case per million men per year [2]. New cases of male genital cancers are estimated to number approximately 26,000 per year worldwide, and by far the most common histologic classification is squamous cell carcinoma (SCC) [3]. The incidence increases with age and is highest between 50 and 70 years.

SCC of the Penis

Epidemiology

Penile cancer occurs almost exclusively in men who did not undergo circumcision at birth [3]. The disease is especially rare among religious groups that practice childhood circumcision [4]. Among Israeli Jews, for example, the incidence rate is 0.1 per 100,000 per year [5]. The highest reported incidence is from Brazil, where the rate is 2.9–6.8 per 100,000 per year and affects predominantly low-income, Caucasian, uncircumcised men [6]. In the United States, Hispanics and African Americans appear to be at higher risk than non-Hispanic Caucasians. Lower rates of childhood circumcision among Hispanic men may explain the higher reported incidence of penile cancer compared to non-Hispanic men [3].

The overall incidence rate for penile cancer in the United States, where it accounts for just under 1 % of new cancers in men, was 0.58 per 100,000 per year in

L. Pagliaro, MD
Division of Medical Oncology, Department of Oncology,
Mayo Clinic, Rochester, MN 55905, USA
e-mail: pagliaro.lance@mayo.edu

L. Pagliaro (ed.), *Rare Genitourinary Tumors*,
DOI 10.1007/978-3-319-30046-7_19

the period 1993–2002 and 0.81 cases per 100,000 per year in the period 1998–2003. The most likely explanation for the apparent rise in incidence is higher exposure to human papillomavirus (HPV) brought about by changes in sexual behavior [3]. A similar trend was seen in the United Kingdom (UK). In Europe there is considerable geographic variation, with incidence of penile cancer that is highest in Spain and lowest in Italy.

Aside from HPV exposure and lack of childhood circumcision, other risk factors for penile cancer include phimosis, lichen sclerosis, tobacco use, poor personal hygiene, penile trauma, sexual history, marital status, and a history of treatment with ultraviolet A photochemotherapy (PUVA) [7]. Phimosis is seen in 35–90 % of men diagnosed with penile cancer. Phimosis prevents adequate penile hygiene, leading to accumulation of smegma in the preputial sac. Circumcision allows better penile hygiene and may also lower the risk of HPV infection. These are potential mechanisms for the protective effect of circumcision, but it is unclear whether circumcision is beneficial when adequate penile hygiene is being practiced [3]. Treatment of psoriasis with PUVA was associated with a higher risk of genital tumors [8]. In a study of men receiving methoxsalen and PUVA for psoriasis, the incidence of penile and scrotal cancer was 1.6 %. The incidence of penile neoplasms among the subgroup who had received high levels of exposure to PUVA was 7.1 times greater than those who had received lower levels, showing that the effect was dose dependent.

The cancer risk associated with lack of circumcision, phimosis, and inadequate genital hygiene suggests that chronic inflammation is important for the pathogenesis of penile cancer. Penile cancer has also been reported in patients with longstanding lichen sclerosis, a chronic inflammatory skin disease that affects the anogenital area.

Pathology

There are several histologic variants of penile SCC. These included basaloid, warty, and verrucous subtypes, which are collectively referred to as "unusual" SCC variants, and the remainder are the majority of cases, which are termed "usual" type, or keratinizing SCC [7]. Within a tumor, there may be more than one histologic pattern (Fig. 19.1).

Role of HPV

Human papillomavirus is the principal etiologic agent in a number of sexually transmitted diseases including genital condylomata, cervical dysplasia, and SCC of the cervix. Of the many serotypes of HPV, types 16, 18, 31, 33, 35, and 39 are most associated with malignant disease. Evidence of HPV infection has been found in SCC of the penis, including both the usual-type SCC and unusual histologic variants. Approximately 31–66 % of all penile SCC tumors are HPV related, with type 16 virus being the most prevalent [9, 10]. The basaloid and warty subtypes are associated with HPV in 80–100 % of cases, whereas usual-type SCC is less commonly associated and the verrucous subtype is least associated [11, 12].

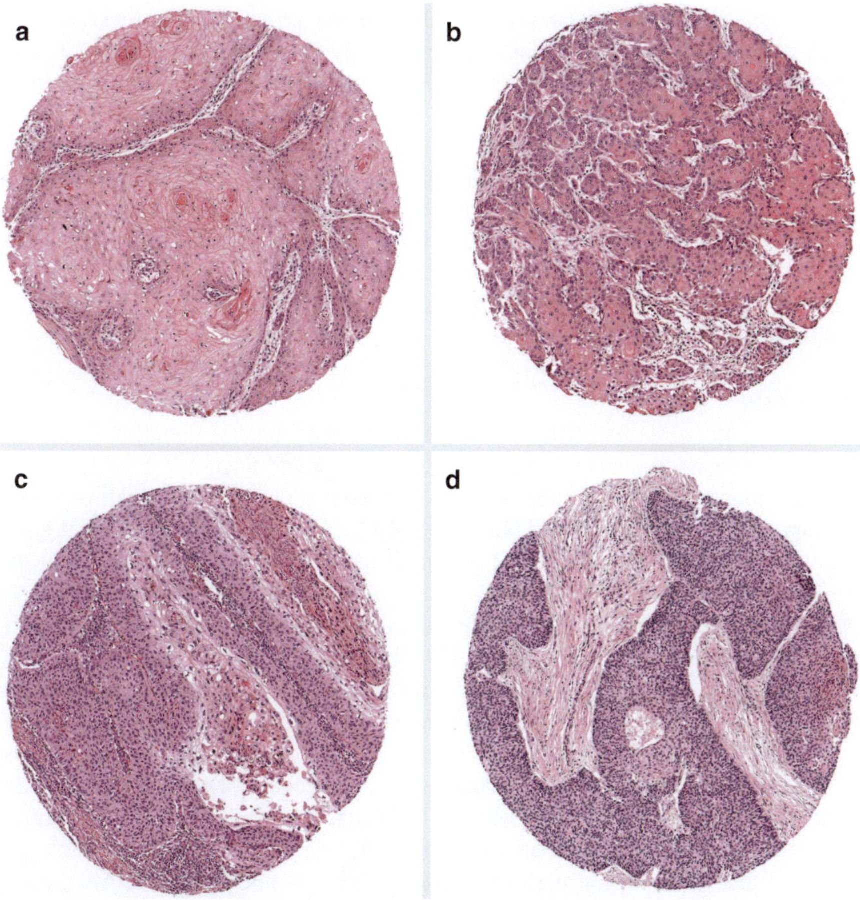

Fig. 19.1 Tissue microarray spots of penile tumors with and without basaloid/warty features. (**a**) Grade 1, usual-type squamous cell carcinoma. (**b**) Grade 3, usual-type squamous cell carcinoma. (**c**) Warty-basaloid carcinoma. (**d**) Basaloid carcinoma (Reproduced with permission from Chaux et al. [12])

The viral genes *E6* and *E7* are expressed in HPV-transformed cells and are known to interact with the *RB1* and *TP53* tumor suppressor pathways [11]. These pathways are therefore implicated in penile cancer. Mutations of *TP53* are found in a subset of penile SCC and were associated with higher incidence of lymph node metastasis and lower overall survival [13, 14]. It is likely that somatic mutations in the *RB1* and *TP53* pathway genes are more common in HPV-unrelated tumors where those pathways are not already inactivated by viral proteins [15]. Thus, there are possibly distinct molecular mechanisms underlying HPV-related and HPV-unrelated penile cancer. A similar dichotomy has been proposed in HPV-related and HPV-unrelated oropharyngeal SCC [16].

HPV-related penile cancers appear to have better prognosis than those that are unrelated. For example, one population-based study found that the detection of HPV DNA in penectomy specimens was associated with 96 % disease-specific survival versus 82 % for HPV-negative tumors [9]. Clinical determination of HPV-"positive" or HPV-"negative" penile SCC, however, is not straightforward [12]. In situ hybridization assays for HPV DNA are limited by poor sensitivity. Immunohistochemical detection of p16 as a marker of HPV infection has been utilized, with positive staining for p16 protein also associated with improved survival [17].

Evaluation and Staging

Diagnosis

The primary tumor is often symptomatic with either a nonhealing flat/ulcerative lesion or exophytic mass located in the glans, foreskin, or coronal sulcus [7]. It is often clinically obvious but may be hidden under a nonretractable foreskin. Small or occult primary tumors can present with bulky inguinal lymphadenopathy as the chief complaint. Physical examination should include careful inspection and palpation of the penis and inguinal regions [18]. Enlarged inguinal lymph nodes indicate the likely presence of metastatic disease, although reactive lymph nodes are also common in this location. Computed tomography (CT) or magnetic resonance imaging (MRI) may be necessary in obese patients in whom inguinal palpation is unreliable. Suspicious lymph nodes should be biopsied to confirm metastatic involvement.

A personal history of genital HPV infection, (e.g., genital condylomata) or phimosis, should increase diagnostic suspicion for penile cancer. Less common patterns of presentation include tumors located on the shaft of the penis or at the penoscrotal junction. While most men presenting with penile SCC are uncircumcised, it should be noted that circumcision performed after puberty is not protective. Also, occasional cases have occurred despite neonatal circumcision. Care should be taken not to confuse SCC of the urethra (a variant of urothelial carcinoma) with penile SCC. This may be challenging for tumors located at or near the urethral meatus.

Staging and Prognostic Factors

Depending on the pattern of presentation, biopsy for establishing tissue diagnosis may consist of shave biopsy, needle biopsy, or excisional biopsy of a penile lesion, circumcision, or fine-needle aspirate of inguinal lymph node. Prognostic predictors include perineural and lymphatic invasion, grade (G2–3), and stage (T2–4) [18–20]. Basaloid, sarcomatoid, and poorly differentiated types are also high risk. Verrucous, papillary, and warty types are low risk for metastasis, although they can be locally destructive [7]. The more common usual-type SCCs are associated with an intermediate risk, with presence of inguinal lymph node metastases having adverse prognosis. Invasive lymph node staging is recommended for patients with clinically negative inguinal lymph nodes and high-risk pathology [21, 22]. For those with enlarged inguinal lymph nodes, the number, size, and mobility should be noted, and CT or MRI should be done to assess the pelvic lymph nodes [23]. Patients with evidence of regional lymph node metastasis should also have chest x-ray or CT.

Treatment

Localized Disease

Treatment of the primary tumor is aimed at radical removal of the tumor and, when possible, organ preservation. Factors affecting the choice of treatment include tumor size, proximal or distal location, risk factors such as stage and grade, confinement to the foreskin, and patient preference. Topical chemotherapy such as imiquimod or 5-fluorouracil (5-FU) is first-line treatment in cases of carcinoma in situ (CIS) [24]. Other options are laser ablation or total or partial glans resurfacing [25, 26]. For Ta/T1a lesions, circumcision may be sufficient, or glansectomy with intraoperative assessment of surgical margins. Penis-sparing techniques allow better quality of life than with partial penectomy [27]. While there are no controlled trials to compare different treatment methods, local recurrence rates are generally higher with organ-sparing compared with partial penectomy (5–12 % vs 5 %) but with good salvage results and minimal impact on survival. Larger (T3–T4) or more proximal tumors may require total penectomy with perineal urethrostomy [18].

Radiotherapy is another penis-sparing option for tumors that are less than 4 cm and T2 or less [28, 29]. Circumcision must be performed prior to radiotherapy as a prophylactic measure, regardless of tumor involvement, for prevention of phimosis. Treatment consists of either brachytherapy or external beam radiotherapy with a brachytherapy boost. Potential complications include glans necrosis, meatal stenosis, and urethral stenosis.

Metastatic Disease: Regional Lymph Nodes

Some patients with regional lymph node metastases are curable, and radical inguinal lymphadenectomy (ILND) is the mainstay of treatment [18]. Multimodal treatment is often indicated, and controversy exists over the optimal treatment strategy for pelvic lymph node involvement. Lymphatic spread occurs first to uni- or bilateral superficial and deep inguinal lymph nodes. Pelvic lymph nodes are the second regional group to be involved, and metastasis to pelvic lymph nodes does not appear to occur without ipsilateral inguinal node involvement (Fig. 19.2). Patients with pelvic lymph node metastases are rarely cured with surgery alone, so the role of pelvic lymph node dissection remains controversial. Some authors recommend neoadjuvant chemotherapy followed by unilateral or bilateral pelvic lymph node dissections in patients with stable or responding disease [30, 31]. Spread to lymph nodes above the aortic bifurcation is classified as distant metastasis; those patients are not considered curable with current treatment methods [20].

Non-palpable Inguinal Nodes (cN0)

The choice in management of patients with clinically negative groins is between surgery (staging ILND) or surveillance and intervention at the point of recurrence (therapeutic ILND). There is currently no role for adjuvant radiotherapy to lymph nodes or chemotherapy in patients with clinically nonmetastatic (cN0) penile cancer. The risk of nodal recurrence for this group is about 25 % and varies according to low-, intermediate-, and high-risk features in the primary [18]. In comparative series for higher-risk tumors, invasive staging with early ILND gives survival

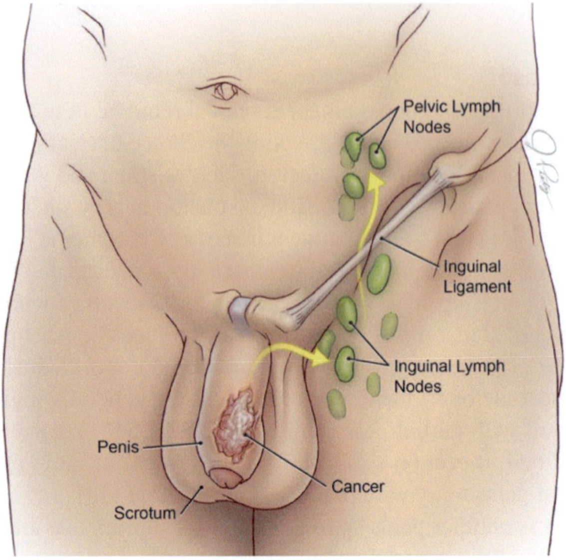

Fig. 19.2 The pattern of lymphatic metastasis in penile cancer

>90 %, whereas surveillance and therapeutic ILND for clinical recurrence carries survival <40 % [21]. Accordingly, only patients with clinically negative inguinal nodes and low-risk primary tumors should be offered surveillance.

Palpable Inguinal Nodes (cN1/cN2)

Ultrasound-guided fine-needle aspirate biopsy is recommended when there is reasonable doubt as to whether enlarged inguinal nodes are reactive or malignant. Biopsy is generally not required when there is obvious metastatic disease such as a bulky, fixed, or ulcerated inguinal mass. Radical ILND can be curative in a subset of patients with nodal metastases. Postoperatively, patients with finding of one involved inguinal lymph node without extranodal extension (pN1) can be observed. Patients with two or more nodes involved (pN2), bilateral, or with extranodal extension (pN3), however, are at higher risk of recurrence and death (Fig. 19.3) [20, 32]. Several multimodal treatment strategies have been studied in this N2/N3 patient set, whether they are identified on the basis of pathologic staging (post-ILND) or by clinical criteria (e.g., two or more nodes involved, or enlarged pelvic lymph nodes on CT or MRI) [30, 33–36]. Patients with inguinal recurrence after a therapeutic ILND have a poor prognosis, with reported 5-year overall survival of 16 % [37].

Multimodal Therapy for Advanced Nodal Disease (N2 or N3)

The standard of care for patients with pN2-N3 disease found on ILND is ipsilateral PLND, which may be performed at the same time or as a second procedure [18, 31]. Unfortunately, the finding of positive pelvic lymph node involvement carries a poor prognosis for survival [32]. Potentially effective strategies to improve the survival

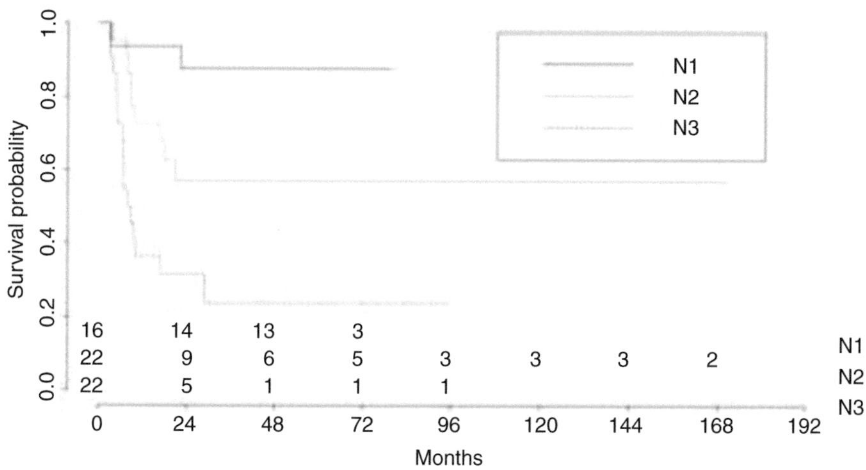

Fig. 19.3 Survival curves of patient subgroups by 7th AJCC N staging system (staged with upfront surgery) (Reproduced with permission from Zhu et al. [32])

for such patients include (1) adjuvant chemotherapy following upfront PLND, (2) neoadjuvant chemotherapy before PLND based on the high-risk ILND pathology results, or (3) neoadjuvant chemotherapy prior to ILND or PLND based on clinical staging [30, 38, 39]. The lack of randomized controlled trials in penile cancer has led to some variation in published guidelines and treatment practice.

Evidence to support neoadjuvant chemotherapy with paclitaxel, ifosfamide, and cisplatin (TIP) consists of a phase 2 clinical trial in patients with clinical N2-3 M0 metastatic penile cancer [30]. Importantly, this prospective trial included some patients who were not necessarily candidates for upfront surgery, for example, those with an initially nonmobile (unresectable) groin mass or enlarged pelvic lymph nodes on CT or MRI. Objective response with clinically meaningful downstaging was observed in 50 % of patients, and 73 % of patients in the study were able to complete 4 courses of TIP and undergo post-chemotherapy surgery (bilateral ILND and uni- or bilateral PLND, usually in the same procedure). Ten percent (3/30) of patients enrolled had a pathologic complete response. Long-term disease-free survival was observed in 37 % of these high-risk patients. In a univariable analysis, objective response to neoadjuvant TIP was significantly associated with overall and progression-free survival.

Both the European Association of Urology and National Comprehensive Cancer Network (NCCN) endorse neoadjuvant TIP for initially unresectable or very advanced regional nodal disease [18, 31]. There is also general acceptance of upfront ILND and surveillance in the postoperative period for cN1/pN1 disease. There are differences, however, in the approach to regional lymph node metastases that are resectable but also high risk. In the United States, patients who are clinical N2-3 and technically resectable often receive neoadjuvant TIP prior to any surgery, as was done in the phase 2 clinical trial, and likewise for those found to be pN2-3 on the basis of ILND and before a prophylactic PLND [38]. The European Association of Urology guidelines, on the other hand, advocate upfront surgery (ILND ± PLND) for all patients with initially resectable disease and adjuvant 5-FU and cisplatin for those found on pathology to have pelvic nodal involvement [39].

Advantages of neoadjuvant chemotherapy compared to adjuvant include the opportunity to observe the tumor response during treatment. Response to neoadjuvant TIP can be assessed with CT or MRI after two cycles (6 weeks) and a different strategy chosen if there is no response. Also tolerance of chemotherapy is better prior to surgery. One disadvantage of neoadjuvant chemotherapy is that potentially curative surgery is delayed. It is therefore best reserved for those patients who are unlikely to be cured with surgery alone, such as those with enlarged pelvic lymph nodes. Also, patient selection can be refined by first performing ILND and identifying those with extranodal extension (pN3) or bilateral inguinal nodes involved (pN2), as they have a high risk of pelvic nodal involvement and should receive neoadjuvant TIP prior to PLND.

By comparison, the individual response to adjuvant chemotherapy is impossible to assess because in that setting, there is no measurable disease. Patients may already be cured and survive despite the chemotherapy. Only a randomized controlled trial can prove a clinical benefit for adjuvant chemotherapy. Moreover, adjuvant chemotherapy is often not possible in the postoperative period if the recovery time is prolonged or there are other complications. Retrospective data with adjuvant 5-FU and cisplatin [39] must be interpreted with caution for these reasons and also because of the inherent patient selection bias.

Chemoradiotherapy to the pelvis has been suggested as an alternative to PLND in patients with metastatic penile cancer. There is a lack of positive evidence for this approach in penile cancer specifically [40]. By way of extrapolation, however, successful use of radiotherapy instead of PLND for women with metastatic SCC of the vulva [41] has generated interest in this approach for penile cancer. At the present time, chemoradiotherapy to the pelvis remains a valuable option for men with metastatic penile cancer who are not operable, refuse surgery, or do not respond to neoadjuvant TIP [42, 43].

Metastatic Disease: Distant and/or Visceral

Advanced metastatic penile cancer is rapidly lethal. It is an aggressive disease typically with rapid progression, involvement of lungs, liver, bone, skin, muscles, and other unusual sites. It is often associated with hypercalcemia. In the non-curative setting, goals of treatment are palliation of symptoms and improved survival duration.

Chemotherapy

Chemotherapy-naïve patients with distant metastases may respond initially to cisplatin-based chemotherapy. There have been no randomized controlled trials for treatment of metastatic penile cancer and hence no single standard chemotherapy regimen. As previously discussed, TIP was studied prospectively in a phase 2, single-center trial for patients with regional lymph node metastases

(N2-3 M0), and while none had clinical evidence of distant metastasis at the time of study entry, all of them had measurable disease in lymph nodes [30]. The objective response rate by RECIST (CR + PR) was 50 % (15/30) with median overall survival of 17 months.

The 5-FU and cisplatin combination was studied retrospectively in a small series of patients from several institutions, with a reported overall response rate of 32 % (8/25) and median overall survival of 8 months [44]. These were patients with either regional lymph node or distant metastases. Published guidelines endorse either TIP or 5-FU and cisplatin as first-line chemotherapy for patients with metastatic penile cancer [31]. Small phase 2 trials with other platinum-based regimens have demonstrated a comparatively higher risk of toxicity compared to TIP or 5-FU/cisplatin, without improved efficacy [34, 45–49]. Whenever possible, patients should be encouraged to participate in clinical trials.

There is no standard second-line chemotherapy for metastatic penile cancer [31]. In a small phase 2 study, paclitaxel single-agent therapy (175 mg/m^2 every 3 weeks) as second line after 5-FU and cisplatin had a response rate of 20 % (5/25); all were partial responses and the median overall survival was 23 weeks [50]. A retrospective study of treatment in the second line from MD Anderson Cancer Center found a median overall survival of 5.7 months (range, 1.4–30 months) from the time of first-treatment failure [51]. The study group consisted of 19 patients who had initially received neoadjuvant TIP for regional lymph node metastasis (N2-N3 M0) and had progressed, recurred, or never completed the treatment. A variety of secondary treatments had been attempted, including surgery, chemoradiotherapy, other cisplatin-based chemotherapy, and investigational therapies. Two patients had received supportive care only. In a comparison of those who received some form of platinum-based systemic therapy (after TIP) versus those who had received other treatment or supportive care, there was no discernible difference in median overall survival of less than 6 months.

Targeted Therapy

Several case reports and two case series have reported on the antitumor activity of EGFR-targeted therapies in metastatic penile SCC [52–57]. While none of these studies is conclusive, they do collectively point to a meaningful clinical benefit for a subset of patients. Studies of EGFR expression by immunohistochemistry show high levels of expression in the majority of penile SCC tumors [58].

Cetuximab

Case reports of cetuximab alone or in combination are summarized in Table 19.1 [52, 53]. In a series reported from MD Anderson, 20 patients had been treated with cetuximab alone, cetuximab plus cisplatin, or cetuximab plus TIP (Table 19.2) [54]. Of the 17 patients who had received cetuximab with or without cisplatin, there were four partial responses (24 %). Most patients in that series had received at least one prior cisplatin-based regimen. Patients with only lymph node metastases had significantly better overall survival than patients with visceral or bone metastases (median 49.9 weeks and 24.7 weeks, respectively).

Table 19.1 Case reports of cetuximab treatment for penile cancer

Author (year)	Drug(s)	Prior systemic chemotherapy	Site(s) of metastasis	Best response	Time to progression	Overall survival (months)
Rescigno et al. (2012)	Cetuximab and docetaxel	Yes	Inguinal lymph nodes	PR	NR	NR
Brown et al. (2014)	Cetuximab	Yes	Inguinal and pelvic lymph nodes	PR	Censored at 12 weeks[a]	>42
Brown et al. (2014)	Cetuximab	Yes	Inguinal, pelvic, and mediastinal lymph nodes	Progression	4 weeks	8

PR partial response, *NR* not reported
[a]The patient received radiotherapy to inguinal and pelvic lymph nodes

Table 19.2 MD Anderson series of 20 patients treated with cetuximab alone or with chemotherapy

Treatment	No. patients	Prior systemic chemotherapy	Response (PR/CR)	Response rate (%)	Median TTP (range), weeks
Cetuximab	5	5	1/0	20	8.1 (6.7–40.1)
Cetuximab + cisplatin	12	11	3/0	25	13.6 (1.6–27)
Cetuximab + TIP	3	2	2/0	67	12.3 (10.4–27.3)

PR partial response, *CR* complete response, *TTP* time to progression, *TIP* paclitaxel, ifosfamide, and cisplatin

Panitumumab

Published reports of panitumumab alone or in combination are summarized in Table 19.3 [53, 55, 56]. A series was reported from the Istituto Nazionale dei Tumori in Milan, in which 11 previously treated patients with metastatic penile cancer received panitumumab 6 mg/kg every 2 weeks [56]. There were one partial and two complete responses, for an overall response rate of 27 %. Responses were seen in skin and lymph node metastases. The median overall survival was 9.5 months; the subgroup of patients with visceral metastases had shorter survival, as had been observed with cetuximab in the MD Anderson study.

Future Directions

Looking ahead, further research into the role of HPV in penile cancer is likely to reveal distinct molecular pathways for the pathogenesis of HPV-related and HPV-unrelated penile cancer. The HPV-related tumors appear to have a slightly better prognosis overall, but so far the association with HPV is not predictive of response to treatment. HPV-related penile and scrotal tumors may be more

Table 19.3 Reports of panitumumab plus or minus chemotherapy

Author (year)	Drug(s)	Type of report	Prior systemic chemotherapy	Site(s) of metastasis	Response	Time to progression	Overall survival
Necchi et al. (2011)	Panitumumab	Case report	Yes (TPF)	Skin and base of penis	Yes (PR)	NR	NR
Brown et al. (2014)	Panitumumab and cisplatin	Case report	Yes (TIP, TPF)	Lymph nodes and base of penis	Yes (PR)	Censored at 15 weeks[a]	NR
Necchi et al. (2015)	Panitumumab	Pilot study $N=11$	10/11	Lymph nodes ($N=8$), skin ($N=4$), viscera ($N=6$)	3/11 (2 CR, 1 PR)	Median 1.9 months	Median 9.5 months

TPF docetaxel, cisplatin, and 5-FU, *TIP* paclitaxel, ifosfamide, and cisplatin, *PR* partial response, *CR* complete response

[a]The patient underwent consolidative surgical resection of all visible disease; he recurred 2 months later

immunogenic than their HPV-negative counterparts. New oncology drugs that target the programmed cell death-1 (PD-1) protein will presumably be studied in penile cancer. PD-1 is a co-inhibitory receptor found on B cells, T cells, and NK cells. Interaction of PD-1 with its ligand (programmed cell death-1 ligand [PD-L1]) results in inhibition of T-cell proliferation and cytokine production. Immunohistochemistry has revealed that a subpopulation of tumor cells express PD-L1 in penile cancer, and it was seen in both HPV-related and HPV-unrelated penile SCC tumors [59]. Other solid tumors that express PD-L1 have been successfully treated with anti-PD-1 monoclonal antibodies [60]. Indeed, an expansion cohort of patients with oropharyngeal SCC was treated in the KEYNOTE-012 study with pembrolizumab, irrespective of their tumor PD-L1 expression level or HPV status [61]. The investigators reported preliminary results at a meeting presentation in 2015; they had observed an overall response rate of 24.8 % and stable disease in 25 %, adding to an approximately 50 % disease control rate. Moreover, the response rates for HPV-positive and HPV-negative oropharyngeal carcinoma were similar (20.6 % and 26.3 %, respectively). This finding in an HPV-related cancer is analogous to penile cancer, and the results of PD-L1 immunohistochemistry in penile SCC suggest that future trials of anti-PD-1 or anti-PD-L1 immune checkpoint inhibitors should include men with both HPV-related and HPV-unrelated penile cancer.

Future efforts to control penile cancer should include measures aimed at cancer prevention. Neonatal circumcision is protective but is unlikely to be widely accepted as a public health measure because of cultural attitudes. Multivalent vaccines for HPV are also protective, both for the vaccinated individual and for his or her sexual contacts [62]. Unfortunately, cultural attitudes have in some cases opposed the widespread vaccination of boys and girls against HPV infection, despite multiple health benefits that include prevention of cancer.

There have been no randomized controlled trials of treatment for penile cancer. An international, multicenter, randomized trial is in development and hopefully will answer basic questions about the optimal management of locally advanced SCC of the penis. The **In**ternational **P**enile **A**dvanced **C**ancer **T**rial (InPACT; NCT02305653) is a 400-patient trial to be conducted in the United Kingdom, the United States, and Canada [63]. The trial has two independent randomizations, addressing key questions in the clinical pathway: first, the role of neoadjuvant therapy before standard surgery, by randomizing to chemotherapy, chemoradiotherapy, or no neoadjuvant therapy, and second, the role of prophylactic PLND following the standard surgery with therapeutic ILND. The primary outcome measure is overall survival.

SCC of the Scrotum

Scrotal SCC is less common than penile cancer; however, SCC is the most prevalent histologic pattern found in scrotal tumors. Scrotal SCC was historically linked to occupational exposure to carcinogens. In 1775, Sir Percivall Pott was first to describe an apparent cause and effect between soot lodged in the scrotal skin of chimney sweeps and their risk of scrotal cancer [2]. The carcinogen was later identified as 3,4-benzpyrene [64]. Other occupational groups at risk for this disease include paraffin and tar workers, creosote workers, shale oil workers, pitch workers, machine tool setters and operators, and lathe workers.

Etiology

The incidence of scrotal cancer has remained stable over time despite improved occupational health measures and avoidance of carcinogens [65]. Although not proven, some have speculated that the reason for the sustained incidence over time has been the emergence of newer causes such as HPV exposure and PUVA treatment for psoriasis [2, 66]. The Photochemotherapy Follow-up Study [8] was a prospective study of 892 men who had undergone prolonged ultraviolet radiation for psoriasis, of whom 5 developed scrotal SCC. Patients who had received high levels of exposure to PUVA had 286 times the general population risk of invasive genital SCC (scrotal or penile).

Detection of HPV in scrotal tumors has been reported in only a few cases, and its actual significance has not been fully characterized. As was reported for penile cancer, HPV-related scrotal cancers are more likely to display a basaloid or warty histologic pattern and p16 positivity [67, 68]. The frequency of HPV detection in two small case series of scrotal SCC was 24–42 %.

Other suspected contributing factors include chronic mechanical irritation, poor hygiene, smoking, ionizing radiation, exposure to carcinogenic metals (arsenic, nickel, chromium), and chronic scrotal lymphedema [2].

Pathology

Scrotal SCC occurs more commonly in the left scrotum and in lower/anterior areas [2, 69]. The most common presentation is as an erythematous nodule or plaque and may be accompanied by pruritus. Presentation as an abscess or ulcerative lesion is uncommon [70]. Multiple scrotal SCCs in the same patient have been reported. Scrotal SCC in situ has been rarely reported. The differential diagnosis includes extramammary Paget's disease, verrucous carcinoma, and Bowenoid papulosis.

Epidemiology

The incidence of scrotal cancer is about 1 case per million men per year. Median age at diagnosis of SCC of the scrotum is 52–57 years [67, 71]. The incidence in Caucasian men exceeds that of men who are African American, Asian, and other ethnicities. There have been, however, several reports of scrotal SCC from Japan, Africa, and the Indian subcontinent [66, 72, 73]. Immunosuppressed men appear to be at increased risk, including transplant patients and those with acquired or inherited immunodeficiency [2].

Evaluation and Staging

There are notable differences in the staging of penile and scrotal cancers. The American Joint Committee on Cancer (AJCC) TNM classification for scrotal cancer designates any nodal metastasis as N1, N2 or N3 based on size, and there is no site-specific classification as there is for penile cancer. The T classification is based on both size and invasiveness: T1 $\leq$ 2 cm, T2 >2 cm and <5 cm, T3 $\geq$5 cm, and T4 describing invasion into any of the deeper extradermal structures. The Lowe staging is another system for scrotal cancer; developed in 1983, it is still in use (Table 19.4) [74].

Depth of invasion can be assessed with ultrasound or MRI of the scrotum. Clinical staging of lymph nodes includes a physical examination of inguinal lymph nodes, ultrasound-guided biopsy of suspicious or enlarged lymph nodes, and CT scan or MRI for evaluation of both the pelvic lymph nodes and inguinal nodes. In selected cases, PET/CT may be helpful based on extrapolation from published results in penile cancer [2, 75].

Table 19.4 Lowe system for staging scrotal cancer

A1	Disease localized to scrotum
A2	Locally extensive disease involving adjacent structures (penis, perineum, testis or cord, and pubic bone) by continuity but without evident metastasis
B	Superficial lymph node metastasis, resectable
C	Pelvic lymph node metastasis or any unresectable metastasis
D	Distant metastasis beyond regional nodes

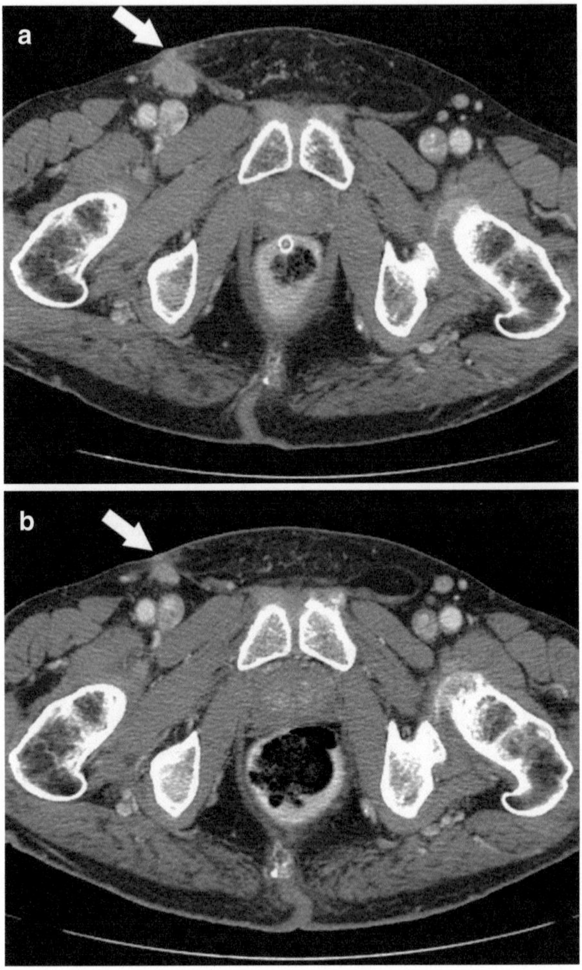

Fig. 19.4 Right inguinal metastasis (*arrows*) from squamous cell carcinoma of the scrotum. The metastasis had recurred after a primary inguinal resection. (**a**) Appearance on computed tomography scan after two courses of paclitaxel, ifosfamide, and cisplatin chemotherapy (TIP) without response. (**b**) Appearance on computed tomography scan after two courses of cetuximab plus TIP (Reproduced with permission from Carthon et al. [54])

Treatment

For the primary tumor, wide local excision is the mainstay of treatment. Primary closure is often possible owing to the redundancy and laxity of scrotal skin [76]. Hemiscrotectomy may be necessary for larger tumors. There does not appear to be a benefit from postoperative radiotherapy, although the experience with it in scrotal SCC is very limited [68]. One study estimated the 5-year overall survival for scrotal SCC was 77 % [71].

For treatment of locally advanced and metastatic scrotal SCC, there are too few studies to develop an algorithm specific to the disease. Treatment essentially follows the algorithm for penile cancer. For example, systemic chemotherapy is appropriate for inoperable scrotal SCC. Platinum-based chemotherapy regimens such as TIP for 5-FU/cisplatin are reasonable options, although neither has been evaluated systematically in patients with scrotal cancer. Carthon et al. reported a series of 24 men with invasive genital SCC who received EGFR-targeted therapies [54]. One of these patients had SCC of the scrotum with primary tumor excised and metastasis in the right groin. He had first received two courses of TIP with no response. Cetuximab was added, and after two courses of TIP + cetuximab, followed by cetuximab monotherapy, there had been a clinically meaningful response allowing surgical resection of residual tumor from the groin (Fig. 19.4). This patient was reported to be disease-free on surveillance at 38 months after receiving EFGR-targeted therapy.

Conclusion

Squamous cell carcinoma of the penis and scrotum are rare malignancies with a distinctive pathogenesis. Preventive strategies are now possible, such as HPV vaccination, genital shielding during prolonged ultraviolet radiation exposure, and neonatal circumcision. Treatment has become more standardized with the first publication of NCCN guidelines for penile cancer in 2012. Improved understanding of molecular heterogeneity in genital SCCs has led to refinements in the interpretation of pathology and identification of potential therapeutic targets. Without the benefit of randomized controlled trials, the evolution of new treatment strategies has been slow, but it has occurred nevertheless, and we may see the first randomized clinical trial for penile cancer opening in the near future.

References

1. Siegel RL, Miller KD, Jemal A. Cancer statistics, 2015. CA Cancer J Clin. 2015;65(1):5–29.
2. Vyas R, et al. Squamous cell carcinoma of the scrotum: a look beyond the chimneystacks. World J Clin Cases. 2014;2(11):654–60.
3. Christodoulidou M, et al. Epidemiology of penile cancer. Curr Probl Cancer. 2015; 39(3):126–36.
4. Dillner J, et al. Etiology of squamous cell carcinoma of the penis. Scand J Urol Nephrol. Supplementum. 2000;205:189–93.
5. Licklider S. Jewish penile carcinoma. J Urol. 1961;86:98.
6. Favorito LA, et al. Epidemiologic study on penile cancer in Brazil. Int Braz J Urol: Off J Braz Soc Urol. 2008;34(5):587–91. discussion 591–3.
7. Chaux A, Cubilla AL. Advances in the pathology of penile carcinomas. Hum Pathol. 2012; 43(6):771–89.
8. Stern RS. Genital tumors among men with psoriasis exposed to psoralens and ultraviolet A radiation (PUVA) and ultraviolet B radiation. The photochemotherapy follow-up study. N Engl J Med. 1990;322(16):1093–7.
9. Djajadiningrat RS, et al. Human papillomavirus prevalence in invasive penile cancer and association with clinical outcome. J Urol. 2015;193(2):526–31.
10. de Sousa ID, et al. Prevalence of human papillomavirus in penile malignant tumors: viral genotyping and clinical aspects. BMC Urol. 2015;15:13.
11. Chaux A, Cubilla AL. The role of human papillomavirus infection in the pathogenesis of penile squamous cell carcinomas. Semin Diagn Pathol. 2012;29(2):67–71.

12. Chaux A, et al. Combining routine morphology, p16(INK4a) immunohistochemistry, and in situ hybridization for the detection of human papillomavirus infection in penile carcinomas: a tissue microarray study using classifier performance analyses. Urol Oncol. 2014;32(2):171–7.
13. Rocha RM, et al. A clinical, pathologic, and molecular study of p53 and murine double minute 2 in penile carcinogenesis and its relation to prognosis. Hum Pathol. 2012;43(4):481–8.
14. Lopes A, et al. p53 as a new prognostic factor for lymph node metastasis in penile carcinoma: analysis of 82 patients treated with amputation and bilateral lymphadenectomy. J Urol. 2002;168(1):81–6.
15. Mannweiler S, et al. Two major pathways of penile carcinogenesis: HPV-induced penile cancers overexpress p16ink4a, HPV-negative cancers associated with dermatoses express p53, but lack p16ink4a overexpression. J Am Acad Dermatol. 2013;69(1):73–81.
16. Dillon MT, Harrington KJ. Human papillomavirus-negative pharyngeal cancer. J Clin Oncol: Off J Am Soc Clin Oncol. 2015;33(29):3251–61.
17. Gunia S, et al. p16(INK4a) is a marker of good prognosis for primary invasive penile squamous cell carcinoma: a multi-institutional study. J Urol. 2012;187(3):899–907.
18. Hakenberg OW, et al. EAU guidelines on penile cancer: 2014 update. Eur Urol. 2015;67(1):142–50.
19. Cubilla AL. The role of pathologic prognostic factors in squamous cell carcinoma of the penis. World J Urol. 2009;27(2):169–77.
20. Edge S, Byrd D, Compton C. Penis. In: AJCC Cancer Staging Manual. 7th ed. New York: Springer; 2010.
21. Leijte JA, et al. Recurrence patterns of squamous cell carcinoma of the penis: recommendations for follow-up based on a two-centre analysis of 700 patients. Eur Urol. 2008;54(1):161–8.
22. Alkatout I, et al. Squamous cell carcinoma of the penis: predicting nodal metastases by histologic grade, pattern of invasion and clinical examination. Urol Oncol. 2011;29(6):774–81.
23. Lont AP, et al. A comparison of physical examination and imaging in determining the extent of primary penile carcinoma. BJU Int. 2003;91(6):493–5.
24. Alnajjar HM, et al. Treatment of carcinoma in situ of the glans penis with topical chemotherapy agents. Eur Urol. 2012;62(5):923–8.
25. Meijer RP, et al. Long-term follow-up after laser therapy for penile carcinoma. Urology. 2007;69(4):759–62.
26. Shabbir M, et al. Glans resurfacing for the treatment of carcinoma in situ of the penis: surgical technique and outcomes. Eur Urol. 2011;59(1):142–7.
27. Li J, et al. Organ-sparing surgery for penile cancer: complications and outcomes. Urology. 2011;78(5):1121–4.
28. de Crevoisier R, et al. Long-term results of brachytherapy for carcinoma of the penis confined to the glans (N- or NX). Int J Radiat Oncol Biol Phys. 2009;74(4):1150–6.
29. Crook J, Jezioranski J, Cygler JE. Penile brachytherapy: technical aspects and postimplant issues. Brachytherapy. 2010;9(2):151–8.
30. Pagliaro LC, et al. Neoadjuvant paclitaxel, ifosfamide, and cisplatin chemotherapy for metastatic penile cancer: a phase II study. J Clin Oncol: Off J Am Soc Clin Oncol. 2010;28(24):3851–7.
31. National Comprehensive Cancer Network. NCCN Clinical Practice Guidelines in Oncology, Penile cancer, version 1.2016; http: NCCN.org, accessed March 22, 2016.
32. Zhu Y, et al. New N staging system of penile cancer provides a better reflection of prognosis. J Urol. 2011;186(2):518–23.
33. Bermejo C, et al. Neoadjuvant chemotherapy followed by aggressive surgical consolidation for metastatic penile squamous cell carcinoma. J Urol. 2007;177(4):1335–8.
34. Djajadiningrat RS, et al. Neoadjuvant taxane-based combination chemotherapy in patients with advanced penile cancer. Clin Genitourin Cancer. 2015;13(1):44–9.
35. Pizzocaro G, Piva L. Adjuvant and neoadjuvant vincristine, bleomycin, and methotrexate for inguinal metastases from squamous cell carcinoma of the penis. Acta Oncol. 1988;27(6b):823–4.

36. Leijte JA, et al. Neoadjuvant chemotherapy in advanced penile carcinoma. Eur Urol. 2007;52(2):488–94.
37. Graafland NM, et al. Inguinal recurrence following therapeutic lymphadenectomy for node positive penile carcinoma: outcome and implications for management. J Urol. 2011; 185(3):888–93.
38. Dickstein RJ, et al. Prognostic factors influencing survival from regionally advanced squamous cell carcinoma of the penis after preoperative chemotherapy. BJU Int. 2016;117(1): 118–25.
39. Sharma P, et al. Adjuvant chemotherapy is associated with improved overall survival in pelvic node-positive penile cancer after lymph node dissection: a multi-institutional study. Urol Oncol. 2015;33(11)):496 e17–23.
40. Burt LM, Shrieve DC, Tward JD. Stage presentation, care patterns, and treatment outcomes for squamous cell carcinoma of the penis. Int J Radiat Oncol Biol Phys. 2014;88(1):94–100.
41. Kunos C, et al. Radiation therapy compared with pelvic node resection for node-positive vulvar cancer: a randomized controlled trial. Obstet Gynecol. 2009;114(3):537–46.
42. Pagliaro LC, Crook J. Multimodality therapy in penile cancer: when and which treatments? World J Urol. 2009;27(2):221–5.
43. Pond GR, et al. Concurrent chemoradiotherapy for men with locally advanced penile squamous cell carcinoma. Clin Genitourin Cancer. 2014;12(6):440–6.
44. Di Lorenzo G, et al. Cisplatin and 5-fluorouracil in inoperable, stage IV squamous cell carcinoma of the penis. BJU Int. 2012;110(11 Pt B):E661–6.
45. Haas GP, et al. Cisplatin, methotrexate and bleomycin for the treatment of carcinoma of the penis: a Southwest Oncology Group study. J Urol. 1999;161(6):1823–5.
46. Theodore C, et al. A phase II multicentre study of irinotecan (CPT 11) in combination with cisplatin (CDDP) in metastatic or locally advanced penile carcinoma (EORTC PROTOCOL 30992). Ann Oncol: Off J Eur Soc Med Oncol/ESMO. 2008;19(7):1304–7.
47. Nicholson S, et al. Phase II trial of docetaxel, cisplatin and 5FU chemotherapy in locally advanced and metastatic penis cancer (CRUK/09/001). Br J Cancer. 2013;109(10):2554–9.
48. Zhang S, Zhu Y, Ye D. Phase II study of docetaxel, cisplatin, and fluorouracil in patients with distantly metastatic penile cancer as first-line chemotherapy. Oncotarget. 2015;6(31):32212–9.
49. Houédé N, et al. Intermediate analysis of a phase II trial assessing gemcitabine and cisplatin in locoregional or metastatic penile squamous cell carcinoma. BJU Int. 2016;117:444–9.
50. Di Lorenzo G, et al. Paclitaxel in pretreated metastatic penile cancer: final results of a phase 2 study. Eur Urol. 2011;60(6):1280–4.
51. Wang J, Pettaway CA, Pagliaro LC. Treatment for metastatic penile cancer after first-line chemotherapy failure: analysis of response and survival outcomes. Urology. 2015;85(5):1104–10.
52. Rescigno P, et al. Combination of docetaxel and cetuximab for penile cancer: a case report and literature review. Anti-Cancer Drugs. 2012;23(5):573–7.
53. Brown A, et al. Epidermal growth factor receptor-targeted therapy in squamous cell carcinoma of the penis: a report of 3 cases. Urology. 2014;83(1):159–65.
54. Carthon BC, et al. Epidermal growth factor receptor-targeted therapy in locally advanced or metastatic squamous cell carcinoma of the penis. BJU Int. 2014;113(6):871–7.
55. Necchi A, et al. Proof of activity of anti-epidermal growth factor receptor-targeted therapy for relapsed squamous cell carcinoma of the penis. J Clin Oncol: Off J Am Soc Clin Oncol. 2011;29(22):e650–2.
56. Necchi, A, et al. Panitumumab Treatment for Advanced Penile Squamous Cell Carcinoma When Surgery and Chemotherapy Have Failed. Clin Genitourin Cancer. 2015; online ahead of print.
57. Men HT, et al. A case of penile squamous cell carcinoma treated with a combination of anti-epidermal growth factor receptor antibody and chemotherapy. Anti-Cancer Drugs. 2014;25(1):123–5.
58. Chaux A, et al. The epidermal growth factor receptor is frequently overexpressed in penile squamous cell carcinomas: a tissue microarray and digital image analysis study of 112 cases. Hum Pathol. 2013;44(12):2690–5.

59. Wang J, et al. Programmed death ligand-1 (PD-L1) expression in penile squamous cell carcinoma (meeting abstract). J Clin Oncol. 2015;33(suppl 7):abstr 393.
60. Sharma P, Allison JP. The future of immune checkpoint therapy. Science. 2015;348(6230): 56–61.
61. Starr P. Encouraging results for pembrolizumab in head and neck cancer. Am Health Drug Benefits. 2015;8(Spec Issue):16.
62. Flaherty A, et al. Implications for human papillomavirus in penile cancer. Urol Oncol. 2014;32(1):53 e1–8.
63. Barber J. The development of a clinical trial protocol to test the timing and effectiveness of adjuvant and neoadjuvant therapy in locally advanced penile cancer. Curr Probl Cancer. 2015;39(3):173–85.
64. Boffetta P, Jourenkova N, Gustavsson P. Cancer risk from occupational and environmental exposure to polycyclic aromatic hydrocarbons. Cancer Causes Control: CCC. 1997;8(3): 444–72.
65. Roush GC, Schymura MJ, Flannery JT. Secular and age distribution of scrotal cancer in Connecticut and a review of United States literature. Cancer. 1984;54(3):596–601.
66. Taniguchi S, et al. Squamous cell carcinoma of the scrotum. Dermatology. 1996;193(3): 253–4.
67. Matoso A, et al. Squamous neoplasia of the scrotum: a series of 29 cases. Am J Surg Pathol. 2014;38(7):973–81.
68. Andrews PE, Farrow GM, Oesterling JE. Squamous cell carcinoma of the scrotum: long-term followup of 14 patients. J Urol. 1991;146(5):1299–304.
69. McDonald MW. Carcinoma of scrotum. Urology. 1982;19(3):269–74.
70. Huen KH, et al. Scrotal abscess as initial presentation of squamous cell carcinoma. Case Rep Urol. 2013;2013:807346.
71. Verhoeven RH, et al. Scrotal cancer: incidence, survival and second primary tumours in the Netherlands since 1989. Br J Cancer. 2010;103(9):1462–6.
72. Oluwasanmi JO, Williams AO, Alli AF. Superficial cancer in Nigeria. Br J Cancer. 1969;23(4):714–28.
73. Criton S, Aravindan KP. Bowenoid papulosis turning to squamous cell carcinoma. Indian J Dermatol Venereol Leprol. 1998;64(1):37–9.
74. Lowe FC. Squamous cell carcinoma of the scrotum. J Urol. 1983;130(3):423–7.
75. Rosevear HM, et al. Utility of (1)(8)F-FDG PET/CT in identifying penile squamous cell carcinoma metastatic lymph nodes. Urol Oncol. 2012;30(5):723–6.
76. Azike JE. A review of the history, epidemiology and treatment of squamous cell carcinoma of the scrotum. Rare Tumors. 2009;1(1):e17.

Basal Cell Carcinoma of the Male External Genitalia

20

Priyadharsini Nagarajan and Victor G. Prieto

Introduction

Basal cell carcinomas (BCCs) are the most common malignant (cutaneous) neoplasms worldwide, with an incidence of approximately 2.8 million in the United States [1]. The lifetime risk of developing a BCC is about 30 % in Caucasians, and most of the tumors develop in patients older than 50 years of age [2]. Individuals with Fitzpatrick type I and II complexions have the highest risk of developing BCC [3]. Though exposure to the ultraviolet component of sunlight is the most common cause, about 0.27 % cases of BCC occur in the non-sun-exposed genital skin [4, 5].

Etiopathogenesis

Intermittent, intense exposure to ultraviolet light at younger age is the most common cause of BCC. However, in sun-shielded regions, other factors including poor hygiene, smoking, exposure to ionizing radiation, combination of oral methoxsalen (psoralen) and ultraviolet A radiation (PUVA therapy), arsenic, polycyclic aromatic hydrocarbons and other chemicals including coal tar-derived compounds, chronic irritation (e.g., long-term use of diapers), and even immune deficiency have been implicated to be causative and/or permissive for development of BCC [5–7]. Some BCCs have developed at scars or sites of prior trauma caused by burns, vaccination, varicella, venous stasis ulcer, tattoo, and other conditions such as pilonidal sinuses [8–10], suggesting that chronic inflammation and the resultant tissue regeneration/remodeling may be contributing factors. In addition to Gorlin (basal cell nevus) syndrome, there are other genodermatoses that also increase the risk of developing

P. Nagarajan, MD, PhD • V.G. Prieto, MD, PhD (✉)
Department of Pathology, University of Texas MD Anderson Cancer Center,
1515 Holcombe Blvd., Unit 0085, Houston, TX 77030, USA
e-mail: pnagarajan@mdanderson.org; vprieto@mdanderson.org

L. Pagliaro (ed.), *Rare Genitourinary Tumors*,
DOI 10.1007/978-3-319-30046-7_20

BCC including xeroderma pigmentosum, Rombo syndrome, Bazex-Dupré-Christol syndrome, Dowling-Meara-type epidermolysis bullosa simplex, or multiple hereditary infundibulocystic BCC [5, 11–18].

Most BCCs likely originate from the hair follicle bulge stem cells or from the interfollicular epidermal progenitor cells [19, 20]. Activation of the sonic hedgehog-signaling pathway is the most common genetic event in the development of BCCs, and about up to 90 % of sporadic BCCs exhibit this abnormality. Loss-of-function mutations of the PTCH1 (most common), activating mutations of SMO, and overexpression of GLI1 or GLI2 likely contribute to basal cell carcinogenesis. Mutations of the p53 gene have also been identified in approximately 50 % of the cases [21]. Polymorphisms of glutathione S-transferase and the cytochrome p450 enzyme CYP2D6 have also been associated with increased risk of developing BCC [22]. Human papillomavirus (HPV) DNA has been detected in BCCs although a causative role of HPV has not been demonstrated in BCC [23, 24].

Clinical Features

The diagnosis of genital BCC is almost never made on the grounds of clinical examination alone, even when there is a history of a defined cancer susceptibility syndrome. The lesions are typically slow growing and painless and may ulcerate after a long period of time because patients usually do not present early in the course of the disease. The diagnosis may be delayed further since the differential diagnoses of a long-standing lesion at these anatomic sites typically do not include BCC. Therefore, there should be a low threshold for biopsy of such lesions. Itching is the most common presenting symptom, followed by local discomfort, pain, mass, ulcer, bleeding, or rarely even genital swelling.

Clinically, BCCs of the genitalia, when presenting as single or discrete lesions, often evoke the possibility of a syphilitic chancre, lichen simplex chronicus, squamous cell carcinoma, or melanoma. When the lesions are more numerous or diffuse, the initial clinical diagnoses include candidiasis and inflammatory dermatoses such as psoriasis, contact dermatitis, lichen sclerosus, and Paget disease. Several clinical variants have been described: nodular/ulcerative, superficial/multifocal, diffuse/infiltrating/morpheaform, pigmented, polypoid, and fibroepithelioma of Pinkus. Of these the former two constitute the most common types seen in the genitalia (see also Pathology features; Figs. 20.1, 20.2, and 20.3).

Pathologic Features

Grossly, the lesions can be vegetating, ulcerated, infiltrative, nodular, pigmented, or pedunculated. Histologic features are similar to BCCs found elsewhere [25]. Of the several histologic variants, superficial and nodulocystic patterns are most prevalent in the genitalia (Figs. 20.1, 20.2, and 20.3) [26]. As with most BCCs, the tumor is composed of nests of small basaloid cells displaying high nuclear-to-cytoplasmic

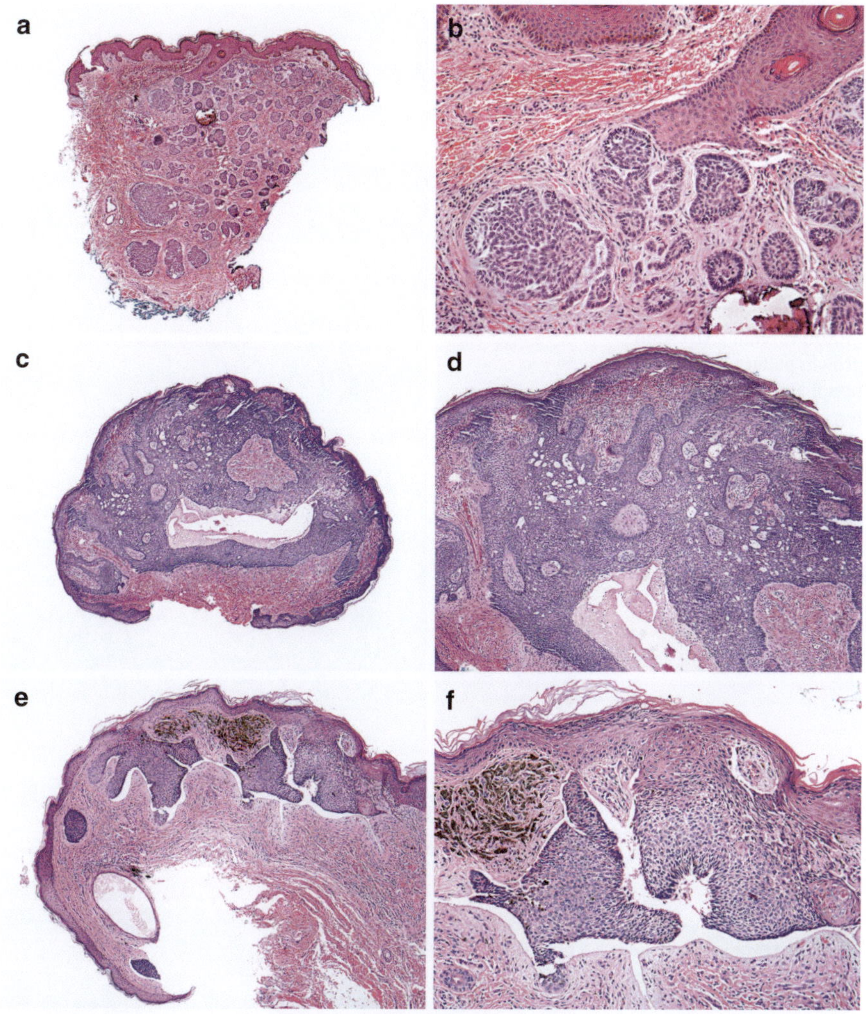

Fig. 20.1 Penile basal cell carcinoma. Hematoxylin- and eosin-stained sections show the most common types of BCCs at this site. (**a**, **b**) Nodular type with focal micronodular pattern, (**b**) focal epidermal connection can be seen, (**c**, **d**) nodulocystic variant, (**e**, **f**) superficial variant with pigmentation of the tumor cells. Peripheral palisading and retraction artifact are seen mostly in superficial and nodular variants. Magnifications: (**a**, **c**, **e**) 20×, (**b**) 200×, (**d**, **f**) 100×

ratio, with monomorphic ovoid hyperchromatic nuclei and scant cytoplasm. Epidermal connection can often be identified. Mitotic figures and apoptotic cells are frequently seen within the same nest. Although peripheral palisading of the tumor cells is a typical characteristic, it may be inconspicuous in infiltrative lesions and those with smaller nests. The stroma surrounding the tumor cells is loose and mucin-rich, with an abundance of hyaluronic acid, leading to retraction artifacts due to mucin shrinkage during tissue processing. The presence of perineural infiltration

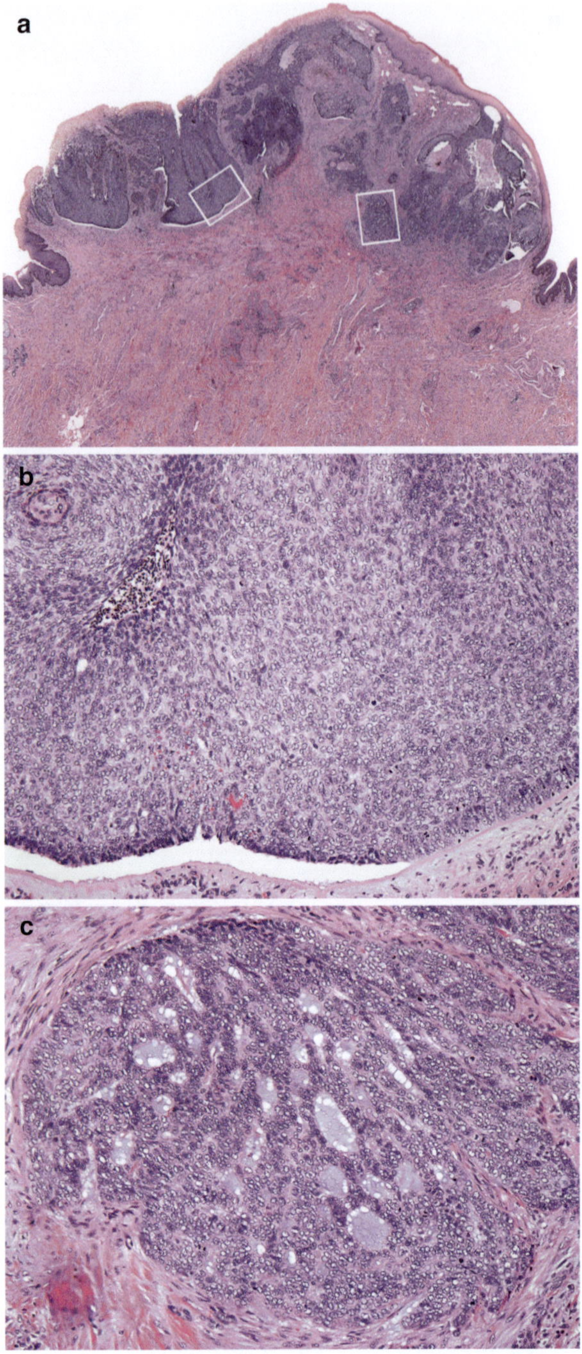

Fig. 20.2 Scrotal basal cell carcinoma. Hematoxylin- and eosin-stained sections show (**a**) a nodular basal cell carcinoma overlying the smooth muscle fibers of dartos muscle (bottom half, magnification: 20×). The areas marked by the white rectangles are seen at higher magnifications (400×) revealing (**b**) solid growth pattern with peripheral palisading and retraction artifact and (**c**) adenoid growth pattern within the same tumor

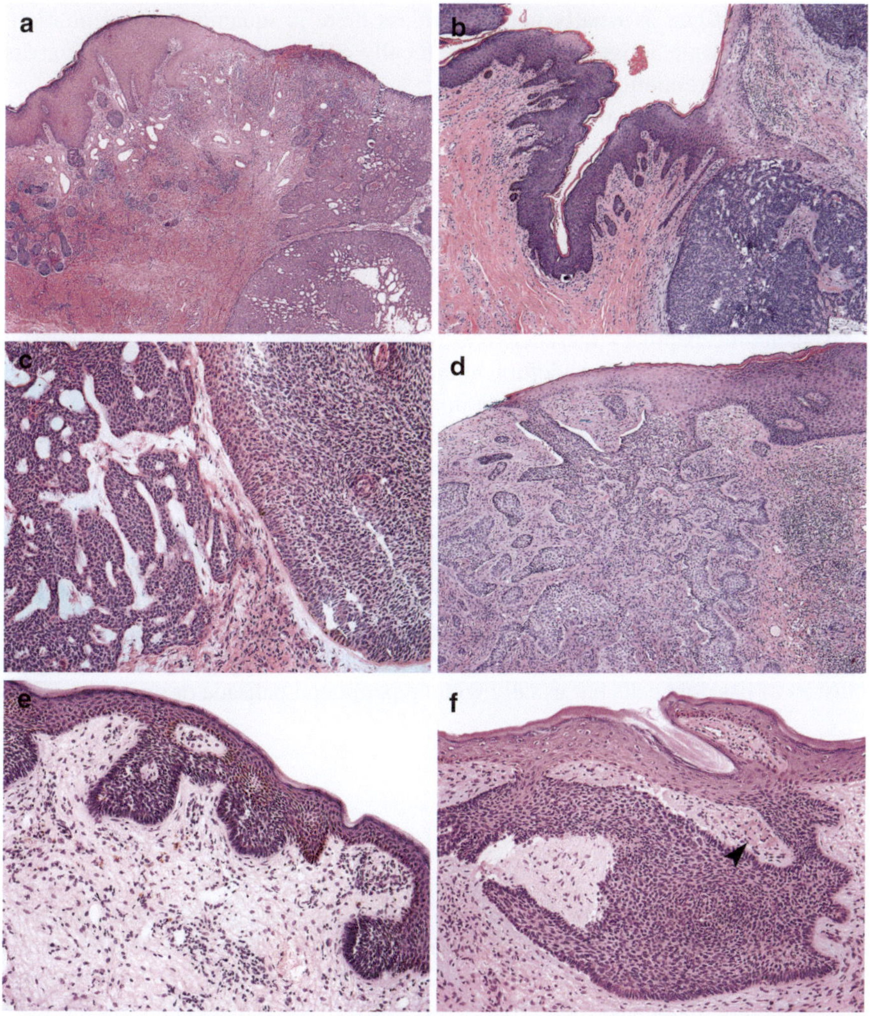

Fig. 20.3 Scrotal basal cell carcinomas. Hematoxylin- and eosin-stained sections show various patterns of BCC (**a**) nodular and focal infiltrative patterns with focal epidermal ulceration, (**b**) nodular pattern without ulceration, (**c**) adenoid and solid patterns with mucinous peritumoral stroma, (**d**) nodular pattern with focal retraction artifact and peripheral palisading, (**e**) superficial pattern with focal pigmentation, and (**f**) superficial with focal deposition of keratin-derived amyloid within the peritumoral stroma. Magnifications: (**a**) 20×, (**b**) 40×, (**c**) 400×, (**d**, **e**) 40×, (**e**, **f**) 100×

and lymphovascular space involvement may be associated with an aggressive behavior. Also, dartos muscle involvement has been seen more frequently in metastatic BCC [27].

The tumor cells are diffusely positive for keratin (e.g., with a pancytokeratin cocktail), high-molecular-weight cytokeratin, cytokeratin 5/6, p53, p63, p40, epithelial cell adhesion molecule, and B-cell CLL/lymphoma 2. Epithelial membrane antigen is usually negative unless there is squamous differentiation. Carcinoembryonic antigen is expressed focally only in the rare cases with areas of eccrine differentiation [28].

Histologic differential diagnoses include other basaloid neoplasms such as trichoblastoma, trichoepithelioma, desmoplastic trichoepithelioma, basaloid squamous cell carcinoma, and cutaneous neuroendocrine (Merkel cell) carcinoma [29]. In general, all these lesions typically lack the peripheral palisade, clefting along the tumor-stroma interface, and myxoid stroma characteristic of BCC. Trichoblastoma is a neoplasm of basaloid cells showing primitive follicular differentiation. Trichoepithelioma is another lesion showing more advanced follicular differentiation, including papillary mesenchymal bodies and fibrotic stroma. Desmoplastic trichoepithelioma shows, in addition to the features of a standard trichoepithelioma, thin infiltrating strands of epithelium in a markedly fibrotic stroma resembling an infiltrative BCC. It is very important to distinguish between BCC and basaloid squamous cell carcinoma and Merkel cell carcinoma, since the latter two entities have more aggressive behavior than BCC. Although BCC may occasionally have neuroendocrine immunohistochemical features [30], Merkel cell carcinoma shows not only expression of synaptophysin and chromogranin but also commonly of CK20, with a perinuclear dot-like pattern, a finding not characteristic of BCC. Basaloid squamous cell carcinoma is another aggressive lesion, typically involving the cutaneous-mucosal interface (as in the mouth, anus, and urethra) with variably sized clusters of basaloid cells but usually without peripheral palisade or myxoid stroma.

Specific Genital Locations

Penis

BCCs are uncommon tumors of the penis and comprise 0.5–5 % of all malignant neoplasms at this site [31]. While majority of the cases are seen in elderly white males, the age at diagnosis ranges from 22 to 87 years [26, 32], and they are rarely seen in darkly pigmented men [26, 33, 34]. Most of the tumors occur on the shaft [35, 36], and less likely on the glans, prepuce, base of the penis, or the urethral meatus [33, 36–38]. Most of tumors are usually superficially invasive, involving the dartos or sometimes Buck fascia. Rarely, large tumors may invade deep into the underlying structures including tunica albuginea involving corpus cavernosum, even up to the urethra [39]. Average duration of tumor before presentation/diagnosis is quite variable, ranging from 3 months to 50 years. Findings associated with some of these cases include local trauma, phimosis, dermatitis, usage of truss for inguinal hernia, remote surgery, chronic balanoposthitis, syphilis, and exposure to sunlight, pesticides, and wood products [26].

Most patients complain of slow-growing lesions with late ulceration and rarely bleeding or discharge. Clinically the lesions are erythematous and/or pigmented, irregularly shaped, fairly well-demarcated, thin plaques to large ulcerated nodules. The lesions are typically single ranging in size from 0.7 to 5 cm and only rarely multifocal BCC [40]. Elevated, rolled, pearly tumor borders and telangiectasia may be conspicuous. The tumors are usually freely mobile, since most are superficially invasive. Induration should raise the concern for deeper invasion. Metastases from the penile BCCs are rare, and the site of metastases is usually inguinal or other regional lymph nodes [41, 42].

Scrotum

BCCs constitute 5–18 % of all scrotal neoplasms [27, 43] and usually develop in elderly Caucasian males (age range: 42–82 years). Scrotal BCCs have also been described in the Asian population [27, 44, 45]. While majority of the cases have a long duration of at least a few years (1–51 years), some patients may seek clinical advice within 3–6 months of noticing the lesion [46–48]. Though obvious contributing factors are not present in most of the cases, some patients report chronic exposure to arsenic, cleaning chemicals used in laundry, coal dust, organic solvents, and ultraviolet rays or local radiation therapy [46–50].

Most patients present with a history of long-standing pruritic, plaque-like lesions that then develop focal erosions and ulcerations. In such cases, the patients are treated usually for a long period of time for dermatitis before a biopsy is performed. Patients may also present with single, painless, ulcerated nodules. The lesions are typically 0.5–5.5 cm in size [47, 51]. A rare case of giant, ulcerated BCC (40 × 20 cm) involving the entire genital and lower abdominal area has been reported with deep invasion and extensive involvement of external iliac and femoral vessels [52]. Clinically, the lesions range in appearance from erythematous plaques with scattered erosions to papulo-nodular lesions to frank ulcers. There may be pigmentation and lichenification of the lesions. Uncommon variants including linear and polypoid BCCs have also been reported at this anatomic location [44, 53]. Local recurrence is extremely rare after complete excision of the lesion with adequate margins.

BCCs arising from the scrotum may develop metastasis at a rate higher than that seen in other sites (10.7–13 % vs 0.0028–0.5 %) [54–56]. Most of the metastases occur as recurrence of the disease a few months after wide local resection, frequently to the inguinal lymph nodes but also to lung [27, 48, 55, 57–62], with or without simultaneous local recurrence [62]. Larger size of the primary tumor and infiltrative growth patterns are associated with metastases [27].

Management

A thorough physical examination and imaging studies including CT scan, PET-CT, and MRI can be helpful in determining the extent of the disease and in examining for the presence of metastases [39]. Most cases of BCCs arising in the genital areas are small and have a low risk for local or distant recurrence. However, complete removal of the tumor, while preserving normal function and optimal cosmesis, can be a challenge.

Surgical resection has long been the standard of care for treatment of genital BCC [63, 64]. Wide local excision to include up to 2 cm margin for scrotal BCCs and to the depth of tunica albuginea, where possible, usually has resulted in excellent local control of disease [27]. With penile lesions, a margin of at least 2–5 mm is recommended. Mohs micrographic surgery or surgical excision with frozen section examination is a reliable mode of resection and is associated with lower recurrence rates for both primary and secondary lesions [27, 39, 65]. Inguinofemoral lymph node sampling may also be considered for deep and/or large tumors, but regional node dissection is usually not recommended unless there is documented metastasis [63]. Curettage and electrodessication is rarely used as a primary modality of treatment at this site.

Radiation therapy is typically not recommended in the genital area due to poor cosmetic outcome [66], although rarely adjuvant or palliative radiation therapy may be used in patients who refuse surgical excision or in those that are poor surgical candidates. History of basal cell nevus syndrome and xeroderma pigmentosum are absolute contraindications for radiation. Age less than 60 years is a relative contraindication due to the increased risk of developing secondary tumors [27, 47].

Cryotherapy using liquid nitrogen and laser therapy as well as topical therapy using immunomodulators such as topical imiquimod, 5-fluorouracil, and photodynamic therapy are usually not recommended in the treatment of genital BCCs [67, 68]. In the past, immunotherapy with Bacillus Calmette-Guerin administered by scarification has also been used for treatment of multifocal scrotal BCC [48, 69]. Some cases of metastatic BCC have been shown to respond to combination chemotherapy using cisplatin, bleomycin, doxorubicin, cyclophosphamide, and 5-fluorouracil [48, 57]. Inhibition of sonic hedgehog signaling by utilizing SMO antagonists, such as vismodegib, has been approved by the FDA only for recurrent and/or metastatic BCCs that cannot be treated with surgery or radiation [70].

References

1. Rogers HW, Weinstock MA, Harris AR, et al. Incidence estimate of nonmelanoma skin cancer in the United States, 2006. Arch Dermatol. 2010;146(3):283–7.
2. Miller DL, Weinstock MA. Nonmelanoma skin cancer in the United States: incidence. J Am Acad Dermatol. 1994;30(5 Pt 1):774–8.
3. Khalesi M, Whiteman DC, Tran B, Kimlin MG, Olsen CM, Neale RE. A meta-analysis of pigmentary characteristics, sun sensitivity, freckling and melanocytic nevi and risk of basal cell carcinoma of the skin. Cancer Epidemiol. 2013;37(5):534–43.
4. Gibson GE, Ahmed I. Perianal and genital basal cell carcinoma: a clinicopathologic review of 51 cases. J Am Acad Dermatol. 2001;45(1):68–71.
5. Rubin AI, Chen EH, Ratner D. Basal-cell carcinoma. N Engl J Med. 2005;353(21):2262–9.
6. Dourmishev LA, Rusinova D, Botev I. Clinical variants, stages, and management of basal cell carcinoma. Indian Dermatol Online J. 2013;4(1):12–7.
7. Nijsten TE, Stern RS. The increased risk of skin cancer is persistent after discontinuation of psoralen+ultraviolet A: a cohort study. J Invest Dermatol. 2003;121(2):252–8.
8. Noodleman FR, Pollack SV. Trauma as a possible etiologic factor in basal cell carcinoma. J Dermatol Surg Oncol. 1986;12(8):841–6.

9. Alarcon-Del Agua I, Bernardos-Garcia C, Bustos-Jimenez M, Serrano-Borrero I, Casado-Maestre MD, Docobo-Durantez F. Malignant degeneration in pilonidal disease. Cir Cirujanos. 2011;79(4):346–50.
10. Kasper M, Jaks V, Are A, et al. Wounding enhances epidermal tumorigenesis by recruiting hair follicle keratinocytes. Proc Natl Acad Sci U S A. 2011;108(10):4099–104.
11. Bree AF, Shah MR, Group BC. Consensus statement from the first international colloquium on basal cell nevus syndrome (BCNS). Am J Med Genet A. 2011;155A(9):2091–7.
12. Michaelsson G, Olsson E, Westermark P. The Rombo syndrome: a familial disorder with vermiculate atrophoderma, milia, hypotrichosis, trichoepitheliomas, basal cell carcinomas and peripheral vasodilation with cyanosis. Acta Derm Venereol. 1981;61(6):497–503.
13. Glaessl A, Hohenlautner U, Landthaler M, Vogt T. Sporadic bazex-dupre-christol-like syndrome: early onset basal cell carcinoma, hypohidrosis, hypotrichosis, and prominent milia. Dermatol Surg Off Publ Am Soc Dermatol Surg. 2000;26(2):152–4.
14. Fine JD, Johnson LB, Weiner M, Li KP, Suchindran C. Epidermolysis bullosa and the risk of life-threatening cancers: the National EB Registry experience, 1986–2006. J Am Acad Dermatol. 2009;60(2):203–11.
15. Castori M, Morrone A, Kanitakis J, Grammatico P. Genetic skin diseases predisposing to basal cell carcinoma. Eur J Dermatol EJD. 2012;22(3):299–309.
16. Parren LJ, Frank J. Hereditary tumour syndromes featuring basal cell carcinomas. Br J Dermatol. 2011;165(1):30–4.
17. Requena L, Farina MC, Robledo M, et al. Multiple hereditary infundibulocystic basal cell carcinomas: a genodermatosis different from nevoid basal cell carcinoma syndrome. Arch Dermatol. 1999;135(10):1227–35.
18. Halkud R, Shenoy AM, Naik SM, Chavan P, Sidappa KT, Biswas S. Xeroderma pigmentosum: clinicopathological review of the multiple oculocutaneous malignancies and complications. Indian J Surg Oncol. 2014;5(2):120–4.
19. Youssef KK, Van Keymeulen A, Lapouge G, et al. Identification of the cell lineage at the origin of basal cell carcinoma. Nat Cell Biol. 2010;12(3):299–305.
20. Thieu K, Ruiz ME, Owens DM. Cells of origin and tumor-initiating cells for nonmelanoma skin cancers. Cancer Lett. 2013;338(1):82–8.
21. Ziegler A, Leffell DJ, Kunala S, et al. Mutation hotspots due to sunlight in the p53 gene of nonmelanoma skin cancers. Proc Natl Acad Sci U S A. 1993;90(9):4216–20.
22. Lear JT, Smith AG, Strange RC, Fryer AA. Detoxifying enzyme genotypes and susceptibility to cutaneous malignancy. Br J Dermatol. 2000;142(1):8–15.
23. Wieland U, Ritzkowsky A, Stoltidis M, et al. Communication: papillomavirus DNA in basal cell carcinomas of immunocompetent patients: an accidental association?TITLE. J Invest Dermatol. 2000;115(1):124–8.
24. Meyer T. Molecular pathogenesis of basal cell carcinoma. Cancer Treat Res. 2009;146:193–204.
25. Tumors of the surface epithelium. In: Calonje E, Brenn T, Lazar A, McKee PH, editors. McKee's pathology of the skin. Elsevier Saunder, Philadelphia, USA. 2012; p. 1076–149.
26. Nguyen H, Saadat P, Bennett RG. Penile basal cell carcinoma: two cases treated with Mohs micrographic surgery and remarks on pathogenesis. Dermatol Surgery Off Publ Am Soc Dermatol Surg. 2006;32(1):135–44.
27. Dai B, Kong YY, Ye DW, Xu XW, Yao XD, Zhang SL. Basal cell carcinoma of the scrotum: clinicopathologic analysis of 10 cases. Dermatol Surg Off Publ Am Soc Dermatol Surg. 2012;38(5):783–90.
28. Chang YT, Liu HN, Wong CK. Penile basal cell carcinoma with eccrine differentiation. Clin Exp Dermatol. 1995;20(6):487–9.
29. Carr RA, Sanders DSA. Basaloid skin tumours: mimics of basal cell carcinoma. Curr Diagn Pathol. 2007;13(4):273–300.
30. Foschini MP, Eusebi V. Divergent differentiation in endocrine and nonendocrine tumors of the skin. Semin Diagn Pathol. 2000;17(2):162–8.
31. Brady KL, Mercurio MG, Brown MD. Malignant tumors of the penis. Dermatol Surg Off Publ Am Soc Dermatol Surg. 2013;39(4):527–47.

32. Fegen JP, Beebe D, Persky L. Basal cell carcinoma of the penis. J Urol. 1970;104(6):864–6.
33. Greenbaum SS, Krull EA, Simmons EB. Basal cell carcinoma at the base of the penis in a black patient. J Am Acad Dermatol. 1989;20(2 Pt 2):317–9.
34. Alvarez-Arguelles H, Castro Diaz DM, Casteneda Suardiaz J, et al. Basal cell carcinoma of the penis. Actas Urol Esp. 1987;11:93–6.
35. Hartman DL. Basal cell epithelioma of the penis. Arch Dermatol. 1966;94(3):326–7.
36. Jeck H. Unusual tumours of the penis. Trans Am Assoc Genitourin Surg. 1931;24:315–21.
37. Fox JM. Basal cell epithelioma of the glans penis. Arch Dermatol. 1966;94(6):807–9.
38. Kalensky J. Carcinoma of the penis. Cesk Dermatol. 1960;35:115–7.
39. Suyama T, Teramoto Y, Yamamoto A, Kuroda I, Yoshikawa S, Kiyohara Y. Case of giant basal cell carcinoma around the base of the penis in an elderly patient. J Dermatol. 2014;41(5):439–42.
40. Peison B, Benisch B, Nicora B. Multicentric basal cell carcinoma of penile skin. Urology. 1985;25(3):322–3.
41. Doolittle KH, Klotz D, Bennett JE, Heisel EB, Winter CC. The management of extensive lesions of the male genitalia. Am Pract Dig Treat. 1962;13:655–8.
42. Jones VS, Chandra S, Smile SR, Narasimhan R. A unique case of metastatic penile basal cell carcinoma. Indian J Pathol Microbiol. 2000;43(4):465–6.
43. Wright JL, Morgan TM, Lin DW. Primary scrotal cancer: disease characteristics and increasing incidence. Urology. 2008;72(5):1139–43.
44. Iga N, Sakurai K, Fujii H, Kore-eda S. Linear basal cell carcinoma at the external genitalia. J Dermatol. 2014;41(3):275–6.
45. Jianwei W, Libo M, Jianwei W, Liqun Z, Lihua G. Basal cell carcinoma of the scrotum with a lesion of 51 years' duration. Int J Dermatol. 2012;51(6):752–4.
46. Staley TE, Nieh PT, Ciesielski TE, Cieplinski W. Metastatic basal cell carcinoma of the scrotum. J Urol. 1983;130(4):792–4.
47. Vandeweyer E, Deraemaecker R. Basal cell carcinoma of the scrotum. J Urol. 2000;163(3):914.
48. Cieplinski W. Combination chemotherapy for the treatment of metastatic basal cell carcinoma of the scrotum. A case report. Clin Oncol. 1984;10(3):267–72.
49. Koc E, Arca E, Dincer D, Acikcoz G, Turan Y, Demiriz M. A case of scrotal superficial basal cell carcinoma caused by chronic arsenic exposure. G Ital Dermatol Venereol Organo Ufficiale Soc Ital Dermatol Sifilografia. 2014;149(1):157–9.
50. Izikson L, Vanderpool J, Brodsky G, Mihm Jr MC, Zembowicz A. Combined basal cell carcinoma and langerhans cell histiocytosis of the scrotum in a patient with occupational exposure to coal tar and dust. Int J Dermatol. 2004;43(9):678–80.
51. Handa Y, Kato Y, Ishikawa H, Tomita Y. Giant superficial basal cell carcinoma of the scrotum. Eur J Dermatol EJD. 2005;15(3):186–8.
52. Kikuchi M, Yano K, Kubo T, Hosokawa K, Yamaguchi Y, Itami S. Giant basal cell carcinoma affecting the lower abdominal, genital and bilateral inguinal regions. Br J Plast Surg. 2002;55(5):445–8.
53. Ouchi T, Sugiura M. Polypoid basal cell carcinoma on the scrotum. J Dermatol. 2008; 35(12):804–5.
54. Esquivias Gomez JI, Gonzalez-Lopez A, Velasco E, Pozo T, del Villar A. Basal cell carcinoma of the scrotum. Australas J Dermatol. 1999;40(3):141–3.
55. Nahass GT, Blauvelt A, Leonardi CL, Penneys NS. Basal cell carcinoma of the scrotum. Report of three cases and review of the literature. J Am Acad Dermatol. 1992;26(4):574–8.
56. Mohan SV, Chang AL. Advanced Basal Cell Carcinoma: epidemiology and therapeutic innovations. Curr Dermatol Rep. 2014;3:40–5.
57. Costanza ME, Dayal Y, Binder S, Nathanson L. Metastatic basal cell carcinoma: review, report of a case, and chemotherapy. Cancer. 1974;34(1):230–5.
58. Curry MC, Montgomery H, Winkelmann RK. Giant basal cell carcinoma. Arch Dermatol. 1977;113(3):316–9.
59. Kinoshita R, Yamamoto O, Yasuda H, Tokura Y. Basal cell carcinoma of the scrotum with lymph node metastasis: report of a case and review of the literature. Int J Dermatol. 2005;44(1):54–6.

60. Ribuffo D, Alfano C, Ferrazzoli PS, Scuderi N. Basal cell carcinoma of the penis and scrotum with cutaneous metastases. Scand J Plast Reconstr Surg Hand Surg/Nord Plastikkirurgisk Foren Nord Klubb Handkirurgi. 2002;36(3):180–2.
61. Schleicher SM, Milstein HJ, Ilowite R. Basal cell carcinoma of the scrotum. Cutis. 1997;59(3):116.
62. Hughes JM. Metastatic basal cell carcinoma. A report of two cases and a review of literature. Clin Radiol. 1973;24(3):392–3.
63. Clark CM, Furniss M, Mackay-Wiggan JM. Basal cell carcinoma: an evidence-based treatment update. Am J Clin Dermatol. 2014;15(3):197–216.
64. Smeets NW, Krekels GA, Ostertag JU, et al. Surgical excision vs mohs' micrographic surgery for basal-cell carcinoma of the face: randomised controlled trial. Lancet. 2004; 364(9447):1766–72.
65. Wells MJ, Taylor RS. Mohs micrographic surgery for penoscrotal malignancy. Urol Clin N Am. 2010;37(3):403–9.
66. Veness M, Richards S. Role of modern radiotherapy in treating skin cancer. Australas J Dermatol. 2003;44(3):159–66. quiz 167-158.
67. Gruber W, Frischauf AM, Aberger F. An old friend with new skills: imiquimod as novel inhibitor of hedgehog signaling in basal cell carcinoma. Oncoscience. 2014;1(9):567–73.
68. Berking C, Hauschild A, Kolbl O, Mast G, Gutzmer R. Basal cell carcinoma-treatments for the commonest skin cancer. Deutsches Arzteblatt Int. 2014;111(22):389–95.
69. Hortobagyi GN, Richman SP, Dandridge K, Gutterman JU, Blumenschein GR, Hersh EM. Immunotherapy with BCG administered by scarification: standardization of reactions and management of side effects. Cancer. 1978;42(5):2293–303.
70. Basset-Seguin N, Sharpe HJ, de Sauvage FJ. Efficacy of hedgehog pathway inhibitors in basal cell carcinoma. Mol Cancer Ther. 2015;14(3):633–41.

Extramammary Paget's Disease

21

Fardod O'Kelly, Dara Lundon, and Paul K. Hegarty

Epidemiology

Extramammary Paget's disease (EMPD) is a rare intraepithelial malignancy that has only been a few hundred times in the literature with level 4 evidence. The precise incidence is unknown. However, little is known regarding optimal treatment and prognostic factors. Due to poor understanding of the condition, it can remain undiagnosed for a number of years prior to treatment, and with individual patient numbers remaining small across centers, it becomes difficult to build up a true understanding of the disease process.

Crocker first described this epithelial adenocarcinoma with a predilection for apocrine glands in 1889, affecting the scrotum and penis [1]. The disease commonly affects patients in the sixth to eighth decades with a female predominance of 3:1 [2]. The most common sites affected are the vulval, perianal, axillae, and inguinoscrotal regions [3]. Clinically, EMPD frequently presents as a pink eczematoid area with white islands of hyperkeratosis that is accompanied by pruritus. Although this condition is most commonly reported in postmenopausal Caucasian females, there is also a growing body of evidence that the condition may be more common in Asian men, in which the disease acts less aggressively [4, 5].

Disease Associations

This disease occurs most commonly in the anogenital region and was originally described as occurring anywhere along the "milk line"; however, it can arise in any area of the skin or mucosa. Although the disease arises most frequently on the vulva

F. O'Kelly, MD • D. Lundon, PhD • P.K. Hegarty, MD (✉)
Department of Andrology, Urological and Reconstructive Surgery,
Mater Misericordiae University Hospital, Eccles. St. 7, Dublin 7, Republic of Ireland
e-mail: paul.hegarty@materprivate.ie

L. Pagliaro (ed.), *Rare Genitourinary Tumors*,
DOI 10.1007/978-3-319-30046-7_21

of postmenopausal women, it comprises 2 % or less of primary vulval neoplasms, and extramammary Paget's disease arising in other sites is even rarer. There are reports of the disease arising in other apocrine gland-rich areas, such as the axilla and ear, with a reported case from 1955 on the eyelid being associated with a Moll's gland carcinoma [6, 7]. Extramammary Paget's disease of the external male and female genitalia may be associated with neoplasms arising from the bladder and urethra and kidney and in the prostate in males [4]. Extramammary Paget's disease of the perianal skin is often associated with colorectal neoplasia. Occasional cases have involved the skin of the extremities and abdomen. Cases have occurred in the squamous epithelial lining of an ovarian teratoma and in the lining of an epidermal cyst [8, 9]. The differential for this disease includes:

- Basal cell carcinoma
- Bowen's disease (squamous cell carcinoma in situ)
- Melanoma in situ
- Cutaneous candidiasis
- Contact dermatitis
- Seborrheic dermatitis
- Lichen simplex chronicus
- Plaque psoriasis
- Tinea cruris
- Intertrigo
- Langerhans cell histiocytosis

Cytogenetics and Pathogenesis

EMPD usually arises as a primary cutaneous adenocarcinoma. The epidermis becomes infiltrated with neoplastic cells demonstrating glandular differentiation (see section "Histopathological features"). Tumor cells may originate from apocrine gland ducts or from keratinocytic stem cells. Approximately 25 % of the cases of EMPD are associated with an underlying in situ or invasive neoplasm. In all patients, the neoplasm most likely to be associated with EMPD is an adnexal apocrine carcinoma. This associated neoplasm may represent infiltration of the deeper adnexal tissues by epidermal Paget cells [10, 11].

c-erbB-2 expression can be found in EMPD, but the staining patterns are not as intense as those found in Paget's disease of the nipple. There is, however, discordance among authors as to whether this oncogene, which is overexpressed in 15–20 % invasive breast cancers, actually plays any role in EMPD. However, there is recent evidence to demonstrate that it may in fact confer a worse prognosis with EMPD [12]. Studies have also demonstrated a role for the ras p21 oncogene in mammary and extramammary Paget's disease. Strong expression was found in mammary Paget's disease (which was all associated with invasive carcinoma) and those cases of EMPD demonstrating invasion, and therefore it has been suggested that p21 staining positivity may be able to be used as a prognostic marker [13].

p-FAK and p-ERK1/2 overexpression have also been shown to play a role in the tumorigenesis and malignant transduction of EMPD [14]. Flow cytometry has also shown 50–64 % cases of EMPD to be diploid. Aneuploidy in this condition has been found to be associated with aggressive biological behavior (recurrence, stromal and lymphatic invasion, and metastasis) [15].

The proposal of EMPD arising as an intraepidermal adenocarcinoma from glandular was based on the high expression of carcinoembryonic antigen (CEA) in this condition. It was then illustrated that antibodies to GCDFP-15 were found to react with both Paget cells and apocrine gland cells, but not with cells of eccrine glands [16, 17]. Further evidence for EMPD arising as an apocrine carcinoma stems from immunohistochemistry in which they usually stain positive for the androgen receptor (AR), but negative for both the estrogen (ER) and progesterone receptor (PR) [18]. Another study suggested that EMPD may be a proliferation of adnexal stem cells residing in the infundibulosebaceous unit of hair follicles and adnexal structures, since they both express the cytokeratins typical for follicular differentiation [19].

Two other proposed mechanisms of pathogenesis exist: It has been suggested that EMPD arises from the malignant transformation in situ of a basal stem cell that expresses apocrine gland differentiation based on the theory that the squamous epithelium and pilar apparatus, including apocrine and eccrine sweat glands, are derived from the pluripotent embryonal cell. This is supported by the strong expression of CK7, CEA, and CAM in both Paget's disease and areas of full-thickness atypia in Bowen's disease [20, 21]. The second mechanism suggests the migration of mammary ectopic cells (Toker cells) from the nipple. These cells have been regarded, on a morphological, histological, and ultrastructural point of view, to be EMPD precursors and have been found in association with mammary-like glands of the vulva [22–24].

Gross Appearance and Clinical Variants

The most common symptoms are pruritus, burning pain, and occasionally a painful erosion. A visible lesion, typically an erythematous plaque, is present in almost all patients (Fig. 21.1). The average lesion's dimension is of about 5 cm, and the lesion is in the most of cases unilateral with no side prediction. Major labia are the most often involved site, followed by minor labia, clitoris, perineum, and the perineal area [25]. The usual clinical eczematous appearance of EMPD and other signs, such as localized depigmentation in the genital area, can however often lead to misdiagnosis [26].

If a mass is palpable, invasive disease or underlying adenocarcinoma must be clinically suspected. There is an association with underlying adnexal carcinoma in up to 30 % cases [27]. Clinical variants include:

- General/classical
- Apocrine carcinoma
- Depigmented
- Fibroepithelioma

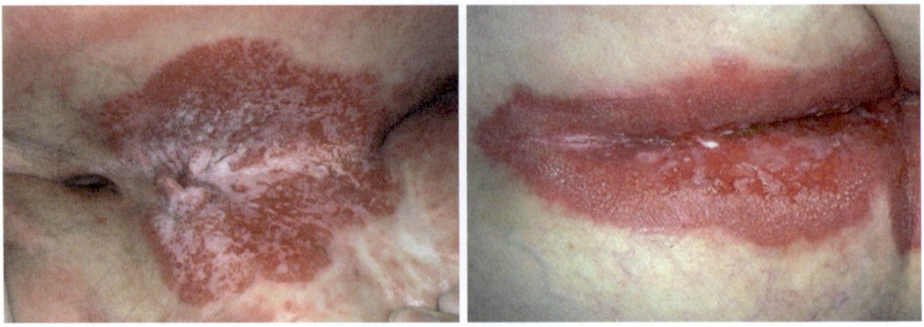

Fig. 21.1 Clinical manifestation of EMPD with classical erythematous plaque formation

Histopathological Features

Mammary Paget's disease was first described by James Paget, in 1874. He stated that the malignancy originated in large lactiferous ducts from where it extended into the overlying epidermis and considered that the changes in the skin preceded and induced malignant change in the underlying breast tissue [28]. The histological findings in EMPD are almost identical. Paget cells are large cells with abundant basophilic or amphophilic, finely granular cytoplasm, which tend to stand out in contrast to the surrounding epithelial cells. On close inspection the nucleus is usually large, centrally situated, and sometimes contains a prominent nucleolus. Pronounced nuclear atypia and pleomorphism are also present. Signet ring cells might be present in small numbers, and mitotic figures are frequent. The Paget cells might be dispersed singly or form clusters, glandular structures, or solid nests. There may be infiltration into upper strata of the epidermis, but most cells are concentrated in the lower portion, often being observed in the pilosebaceous apparatus. A dense inflammatory infiltrate is often seen associated with the epidermal malignancy. In >90 % of cases of extramammary Paget's disease, the tumor cells contain cytoplasmic mucin, staining positively with mucicarmine and periodic acid-Schiff reagent (Fig. 21.2a–c).

Cytological examination of skin scrapings from lesions of Paget's disease reveals single malignant cells with vacuolated cytoplasm and eccentric nuclei, three-dimensional cell aggregates, and acinar groups consistent with glandular differentiation. However, the material obtained is variably cellular and often shows a background of keratinous debris, which may lead to confusion with inflammatory skin conditions or squamous neoplasia [29–31]. There are a number of diagnostic criteria, which aid in the diagnosis of EMPD:

- *Intraepithelial population of large atypical cells (Paget cells) distinct from surrounding normal epithelial cells*: Formation of large nuclei, with prominent nucleoli, and abundant pale cytoplasm. These may be scattered individually and in clusters or may form small acini. They lack features of squamous differentiation, with no visible intercellular bridges and no transition to surrounding squamous cells.

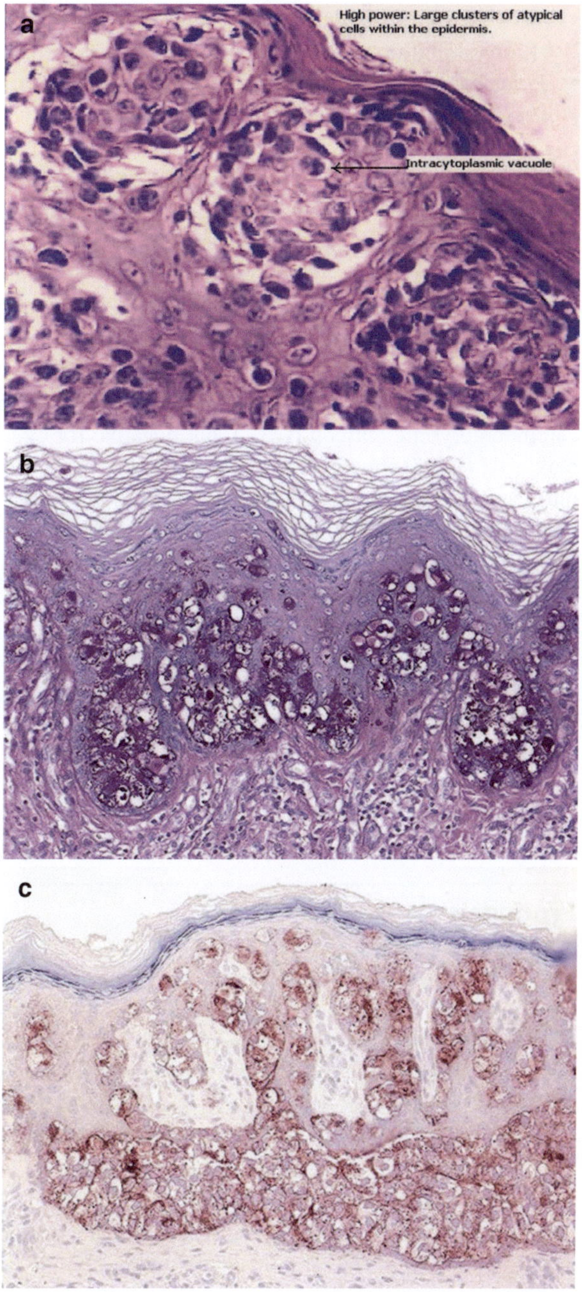

Fig. 21.2 (**a**) High-powered microscopic view of EMPD demonstrating clusters of intraepidermal atypical cells and intracytoplasmic vacuolation. (**b**) Microscopic view of EMPD. Positive staining with periodic acid-Schiff (PAS). (**c**) Microscopic view of EMPD. Positive staining with carcinoembryonic antigen (CEA)

- *Most cases are mucin positive*: They may form signet rings and underlying chronic inflammation common.
- *Epidermal hyperplasia and hyperkeratosis and parakeratosis frequently occur*: Present in half of cases (>90 % of anal cases).

Although traditionally considered a single disease process, EMPD represents several distinct entities and has been subclassified into two distinct types, specifically primary (of cutaneous origin) or secondary (of non-cutaneous origin) [32]. Each classification has three subtypes. The primary is divided into intraepithelial cutaneous Paget's disease of the usual type, intraepithelial cutaneous Paget's disease with invasion, and intraepithelial cutaneous Paget's disease as a manifestation of underlying adenocarcinoma of skin appendage or vulval glands. The cells are immunoreactive for cytokeratin 7(CK7), gross cystic disease fluid protein 15 (GCDFP-15), and carcinoembryonic antigen (CEA), but negative for cytokeratin 20 (CK20) and uroplakin III (UPK). Invasion is uncommon, but can occur. The secondary is divided into Paget's disease of anorectal origin that demonstrates CK20 and CEA immunoreactivity but is usually nonreactive for CK7 and consistently non-immunoreactive for GCDFP-15 and UPK; Paget's disease of urothelial origin, which is immunoreactive for CK7 and UPK, may express CK20 but non-immunoreactive for GCDFP-15 and CEA and Paget's disease of other origin [33, 34].

Another method used to identify invasive Paget cells is a combination of immunohistochemical staining for MUC1 and MUC5AC. Reduced expression of MUC5AC demonstrates increasing malignant potential and consequently a higher tendency of Paget cells to invasion. A more noteworthy difference is met in the Ki67, and cyclin D1 expression levels are also significantly higher in invasive lesions than in situ lesions [35, 36].

Prognosis

The prognosis of EMPD is generally favorable, especially with disease confined to the epidermis. There is an overall disease-specific mortality rate of 26 %, and those patients with an underlying cutaneous adnexal carcinoma have an odds ratio of 2.6 of risk of death, with progression dependent on the underlying malignancy [37]. Progression is usually slow and may last 10–15 years without evidence of invasive cancer or metastatic spread. It has been shown that in patients without dermal invasion, only a small percentage develops a local recurrence. Reciprocally, lymph node metastases were found in patients with reticular dermis or subcutaneous tissue invasion. Furthermore, those with positive lymph nodes had a very poor outcome, with a 5-year survival of 0 % in those with inguinal lymph node metastases [38–40].

The mean time to disease recurrence following treatment is 2.5 years. When EMPD reappears after 6 months from initial treatment, it is called recurrent; however, if the relapse happens within 6 months, it is termed persistent [41]. Recurrence of EMPD occurs in up to 40 % cases as a result of the disease's multifocality and its behaviors to encroach over clinically visible borders. Clear surgical margins,

Table 21.1 Proposed staging system for extramammary Paget's disease (EMPD)

Stage	Description
I	Disease in dermis without visceral/adnexal carcinoma
IIA	EMPD associated with adnexal carcinoma
IIB	EMPD associated with visceral carcinoma
III	EMPD with involved regional lymph nodes
IV	EMPD with distant metastases

tumor cell DNA ploidy, ER receptor status, and p53 immunohistochemical expression are independent of disease recurrence [42]. Factors which positively correlate with disease recurrence include epidermal acanthosis, chronic inflammation, and parakeratosis [43].

Formal staging systems for EMPD do not exist, and currently two have been described. The first dates to 1977 and was originally described for scrotal carcinoma. The second and more modern applied specifically to perianal disease (Table 21.1) [44, 45].

Treatment

Surgery remains the treatment of choice for EMPD. There have been reports of spontaneous regression; however, these are very rare [46]. Due to the multifocality of the disease, much like penile, bladder, and prostate, as well as the ability to extend out beyond clinical visibility, wide lateral margin control remains an issue. There have been reports of positive margin rates as high as 40 % with 2 cm visible margins and up to 74 % in the presence of palpable erythematous patches [47]. There have been two surgical modifications in an attempt to reduce this unacceptably high positive margin rate. The use of intraoperative frozen section (IOFS) has been shown to reduce the positive margin rate in one study to 13 % with no evidence of recurrence after follow-up of up to 2 years [48]. One issue with IOFS is its ability to lead to false-negative results with multifocal disease. This has been reduced further with the use of wire localization; however, a further surgical modification has been adopted for this disease in the form of Mohs micrographic surgery (MMS). This technique has been shown to assist in the microscopic evaluation of the entire lateral margin and has been shown to be equivalent to IOFS after 2 years median follow-up, with positive margin rates of up to 27 % [49, 50]. This type of dermatological surgery however is highly specialized, with limited availability and extremely time-consuming, and costly. It has also been generally withdrawn as a viable option in the treatment of penile cancer. The use of fluorescein has also been described to improve margin delineation with a sensitivity of 99.8 % and specificity of 98 % [51]. As inguinal lymphadenectomy is associated with significant morbidity in older patients, sentinel lymph node biopsy might be an appropriate procedure in those cases with dermal invasion. However, the survival benefit of early lymphadenectomy currently needs further evaluation [52].

There are a number of nonsurgical modalities which exist, such as radiation therapy, chemotherapy, carbon dioxide (CO_2) laser ablation, and photodynamic therapy

(5-aminolevulinic acid), that have been used as both primary and adjuvant treatment. However, there is no consensus as to which of these provide an optimal treatment modality, and no controlled trials exist. It would appear that radiation therapy provides reasonable results and is certainly an option for those deemed to be nonoperative candidates. However, there are also reports that radiation therapy may increase the aggressiveness of the disease [53–56]. Other proposed treatment options include chemotherapeutic regimes such as antineoplastic drugs (5-fluorouracil, mitomycin C, cisplatin, etoposide), immunomodulators (imiquimod), hormonal therapy (LHRH analogues), and trastuzumab for those lesions, which are erbB-2 positive. More studies are required to determine the efficacy of these agents. Antineoplastic agents have been proposed for use in the adjuvant setting, especially in those with invasive adenocarcinoma or lymph node positivity [57].

The largest series to date of 495 patients demonstrates that the incidence rates of EMPD in the USA have been increasing with an annual percent change of +3.2 % since 1978, while a relative incidence of EMPD in blacks was nearly four times lower and in Asians/Pacific islanders four times higher relative to whites. Overall survival among 495 patients was 60.2 % at 120 months post diagnosis and treatment. On multivariate analysis, significant factors negatively impacting survival were primary site in the perianal region compared to penoscrotal and truncal lesions, age older than 75 years, and the presence of distant versus localized disease [58]. The second largest series from Asia demonstrated that clinical lymphadenopathy was strongly correlated with pathological LN metastasis; however, the rate of occult LN metastasis detected by sentinel lymph node biopsy (SLNB) was 15 %. Survival was not affected by SLN status even when an advanced primary tumor was present in patients with positive SLN. The data indicated that SLNB should be considered for invasive EMPD even if clinical lymphadenopathy is not appreciated [59]. Following radical excision and regional lymph node dissection, it was demonstrated on univariate analysis that patients with one of the following poor prognostic factors, depth of invasion of lower dermis or deeper, the presence of lymphovascular invasion, and regional lymph node metastasis at diagnosis, had significantly shorter cancer-specific survival time. Multivariate analysis found that depth of invasion was the only independent prognostic factor [60].

References

1. Crocker HR. Paget's disease affecting the scrotum and penis. Trans Pathol Soc. 1889;40:187–91.
2. Zollo JD, Zeitouni NC. The Roswell Park Cancer Institute experience with extramammary Paget's disease. Br J Dermatol. 2000;142(1):59–65.
3. Chanda JJ. Extramammary Paget's disease: prognosis and relationship to internal malignancy. J Am Acad Dermatol. 1985;13:1009e14.
4. Young DC, Nam HC, Young SP, et al. Lymphovascular and marginal invasion as useful prognostic indicators and the role of c-erbB-2 in patients with male extramammary Paget's disease: a study of 31 patients. J Urol. 2005;174:561–5.
5. Lai YL, Yang WG, Tsang PK, et al. Penoscrotal extramammary Paget's disease: a review of 33 cases in a 20 year experience. Plast Reconstr Surg. 2003;112:1017–23.

6. Fligiel Z, Kaneko M. Extramammary Paget's disease of the external ear canal in association with ceruminous gland carcinoma. Cancer. 1975;36:1072–6.
7. Whorton CM, Patterson JB. Carcinoma of Moll's glands with extramammary Paget's disease of the eyelid. Cancer. 1955;8:1009–15.
8. Theaker JM. Extramammary Paget's disease of the oral mucosa with in situ carcinoma of minor salivary gland ducts. Am J Surg Pathol. 1988;12:890–5.
9. Shimizu S, Kobayashi H, Suchi T, et al. Extramammary Paget's disease arising in mature cystic teratoma of the ovary. Am J Surg Pathol. 1991;15:1002–6.
10. Lai YL, Yang WG, Tsay PK, Swei H, Chuang SS, Wen CJ. Penoscrotal extramammary Paget's disease: a review of 33 cases in a 20-year experience. Plast Reconstr Surg. 2003;112: 1017–23.
11. Parker LP, Parker JR, Bodurka-Bevers D, et al. Paget's disease of the vulva: pathology, pattern of involvement, and prognosis. Gynecol Oncol. 2000;77:183–9.
12. Tanaka R, Sasajima Y, Tsuda H, Namikawa K, Tsutsumida A, Otsuka F, Yamazaki N. Human epidermal growth factor receptor 2 protein overexpression and gene amplification in extramammary Paget disease. Br J Dermatol. 2013;168(6):1259–66.
13. Mori O, Hachisuka H, Nakano S, et al. Expression of ras p21 in mammary and extramammary Paget disease. Arch Pathol Lab Med. 1990;114:858–61.
14. Chen S-Y, Moroi Y, Urabe K, Takeuchi S, Kido M, et al. Concordant overexpression of p-FAK and p-ERK1/2 in extramammary Paget's disease. Arch Dermatol Res. 2008;300(4):195–201.
15. Scheistroen M, Trope C, Kaern J, et al. DNA ploidy and expression of p53 and c-erbB-2 in extramammary Paget's disease of the vulva. Gynecol Oncol. 1997;1:88–92.
16. Nadji M, Morales AR, Girtanner RE, Ziegels-Weissman J, Penneys NS. Paget's disease of the skin. a unifying concept of histogenesis. Cancer. 1982;50:2203–6.
17. Mazoujian G, Pinkus GS, Haagensen DE. Extramammary Paget's disease–evidence for an apocrine origin. An immunoperoxidase study of gross cystic disease fluid protein-15, carcinoembryonic antigen, and keratin proteins. Am J Surg Pathol. 1984;8:43–50.
18. Iijima M, Uhara H, Ide Y, Sakai S, Onuma H, Muto M, Hayashi K, Mitsura F, Kobayashi S, Yoshizawz A, Saida T. Estrogen receptor alpha positive extramammary paget's disease treated with hormonal therapy (case report). Dermatology. 2006;213:144–6.
19. Regauer S. Extramammary paget's disease–a proliferation of adnexal origin? Histopathology. 2006;48:723–9.
20. Quinn AM, Sienko A, Basrawala Z, Campbell SC. Extramammary Paget disease of the scrotum with features of Bowen disease. Arch Pathol Lab Med. 2004;128:84–6.
21. Neilson D, Woodruff JD. Electron microscopy in in situ and invasive vulvar paget's disease. Am J Obstet Gynecol. 1972;113:719–32.
22. Willman JH, Golitz LE, Fitzpatrick JE. Vulvar clear cells of toker: precursors of extramammary paget's disease. Am J Dermatopathol. 2005;27:185–8.
23. Calanog A. Vulvar paget's disease: the need to exclude an invasive lesion. Gynecol Oncol. 1990;38:81–9.
24. Di Tommaso L, Franchi G, Destro A, Broglia F, Minuti F, Rahal D, Roncalli M. Toker cells of the breast. Morphological and immunohistochemical characterization of 40 cases. Hum Pathol. 2008;39(9):1295–300.
25. Shaco-Levy R, Bean SM, Vollmer RT, Jewell E, Jones EL, Valdes CL, Bentley RC, Selim MA, Robboy SJ. Paget disease of the vulva: a study of 56 cases. Eur J Obstet Gynecol Reprod Biol. 2010;149:86–91.
26. Yang C, Lee J, Wong T. Depigmented extramammary paget's disease. Br J Dermatol. 2004;151:1049–53.
27. Louis-Sylvestre C, Haddad B, Paniel BJ. Paget's disease of the vulva: results of different conservative treatments. Eur J Obstet Gynecol Reprod Biol. 2001;99:253–5.
28. Paget J. On disease of the mammary areola preceding cancer of the mammary gland. St Bartholemew Hosp Res Lond. 1874;10:87–9.
29. Jones Jr RE, Austin C, Ackerman AB. Extramammary Paget's disease. A critical reexamination. Am J Dermatopathol. 1979;1:101–32.

30. Sitalkin C, Ackerman AB. Mammary and extramammary Paget's disease. Am J Dermatopathol. 1985;7:335–40.
31. Samarasinghe D, Frost F, Sterrett G, et al. Cytological diagnosis of Paget's disease of the nipple by scrape smears—a report of five cases. Diagn Cytopathol. 1993;3:291–5.
32. Wilkinson EJ, Brown HM. Vulvar paget disease of urothelial origin: a report of three cases and a proposed classification of vulvar paget disease. Hum Pathol. 2002;33:549–54.
33. Lloyd J, Flanagan AM. Mammary and extramammary Paget's disease. Clin Pathol. 2000;53: 742–9.
34. Londero AP, Bertozzi S, Salvadore S, Fruscalzo A, D'Aietti V. A review of extramammary paget's disease: clinical presentation, diagnosis, management and prognosis. J Med Med Sci. 2013;4(4):134–48.
35. Yoshii N, Kitajima S, Yonezawa S, Matsukita S, Setoyama M, Kanzaki T. Expression of mucin core proteins in extramammary Paget's disease. Pathol Int. 2002;52:390–9.
36. Aoyagi S, Akiyama M, Shimizu H. High expression of ki-67 and cyclin d1 in invasive extramammary paget's disease. J Dermatol Sci. 2008;50:177–84.
37. Chanda JJ. Extramammary paget's disease: prognosis and relationship to internal malignancy. J Am Acad Dermatol. 1985;13:1009–14.
38. Tsutsumida A, Yamamoto Y, Minakawa H, Yoshida T, Kokubu I, Sugihara T. Indications for lymph node dissection in the treatment of extramammary Paget's disease. Dermatol Surg. 2003;29:21–4.
39. Lu H, Zhang W, Zhang R, Bai P, Li H. Clinical analysis of extramammary Paget's disease of vulva. Chin J Cancer Res. 2004;16:212–5.
40. Hatta N, Morita R, Yamada M, et al. Sentinel lymph node biopsy in patients with extramammary Paget's disease. Dermatol Surg. 2004;30:1329–34.
41. Tebes S, Cardosi R, Hoffman M. Paget's disease of the vulva. Am J Obstet Gynecol. 2002;187:281–4.
42. Molinie V, Paniel BJ, Lessana-Leibowitch M, Moyal-Barracco M, Pelisse M, Escande JP. Paget disease of the vulva. 36 cases. Ann Dermatol Venereol. 1993;120:522–7.
43. Shaco-Levy R, Sharabi S, Piura B, Sion-Vardy N. Mmp-2, timp- 1, e-cadherin, and beta-catenin expression in endometrial serous carcinoma compared with low-grade endometrial endometrioid carcinoma and proliferative endometrium. Acta Obstet Gynecol Scand. 2008;87:868–74.
44. Shutze WP, Gleysteen JJ. Perianal Paget's disease: classification and a review of management. Report of two cases. Dis Colon Rectum. 1990;33:502–7.
45. Ray B, Whitmore WF. Experience with carcinoma of the scrotum. J Urol. 1977;117(6): 741–5.
46. Archer B, Lonback JB, MacDonald DM. Spontaneous regression of perianal extramammary Paget's disease after partial surgical excision. Arch Dermatol. 1998;123:379–82.
47. Choi YD, Cho NH, Park YS, Cho SH, Lee G, Park K. Lymphovascular and marginal invasion as useful prognostic indicators and the role of c-erbB-2 in patients with male extramammary Paget's disease: a study of 31 patients. J Urol. 2005;174:561–5.
48. Yang WJ, Kim DS, Im YJ, et al. Extramammary Paget's disease of penis and scrotum. Urology. 2005;65:972–5.
49. O'Connor WJ, Lim KK, Zalla MJ, et al. Comparison of mohs micrographic surgery and wide excision for extramammary Paget's disease. Dermatol Surg. 2003;29:723–7.
50. Fanning J, Lambert HC, Hale TM, et al. Paget's disease of the vulva: prevalence of associated vulvar adenocarcinoma, invasive Paget's disease, and recurrence after surgical excision. Am J Obstet Gynecol. 1999;180:24–7.
51. Misas JE, Cold CJ, Hall FW. Vulvar Paget disease: fluorescein-aided visualization of margins. Obstet Gynaecol. 1991;77:156–60.
52. Lai YL, Yang WG, Tsay PK, Swei H, Chuang SS, Wen CJ. Penoscrotal extramammary Paget's disease: a review of 33 cases in a 20-year experience. Plast Reconstr Plast Reconstr Surg. 2003;112:1017–23.

53. Shieh S, Dee AS, Cheney RT, et al. Photodynamic therapy for the treatment of extramammary Paget's disease. Br J Dermatol. 2002;146:1000–5.
54. Burrows NP, Jones DH, Hudson PM, et al. Treatment of extramammary Paget's disease by radiotherapy. Br J Dermatol. 1995;132:970–2.
55. Hata M, Koike I, Wada H, Miyagi E, Kasuya T, Kaizu H, Mukai Y, Inoue T. Postoperative radiation therapy for extramammary Paget's disease. Br J Dermatol. 2015;172(4):1014–20.
56. Choi Y, Park W, Lee J, Cho EY, Moon GH. Aggressive clinical course of extramammary Paget disease after radiotherapy. Radiat Oncol J. 2014;32(2):95–8.
57. Hegarty PK, Suh J, Fisher MB, Taylor J, Nguyen TH, Ivan D, Prieto VG, Pagliaro LC, Pettaway CA. Penoscrotal extramammary Paget's disease: the University of Texas M. D. Anderson Cancer Center contemporary experience. J Urol. 2011;186(1):97–102.
58. Herrel LA, Weiss AD, Goodman M, Johnson TV, Osunkoya AO, Delman KA, Master VA. Extramammary Paget's disease in males: survival outcomes in 495 patients. Ann Surg Oncol. 2015;5:1625–30.
59. Fujisawa Y, Yoshino K, Kiyohara Y, Kadono T, Murata Y, Uhara H, Hatta N, Uchi H, Matsushita S, Takenouchi T, Hayashi T, Fujimoto M, Ohara K. The role of sentinel lymph node biopsy in the management of invasive extramammary Paget's disease: multi-center, retrospective study of 151 patients. J Dermatol Sci. 2015; pii: S0923-1811(15)00114-0.
60. Dai B, Kong YY, Chang K, Qu YY, Ye DW, Zhang SL, Zhang HL. Primary invasive carcinoma associated with penoscrotal extramammary Paget's disease: a clinicopathological analysis of 56 cases. BJU Int. 2015;115(1):153–60.

Kaposi's Sarcoma of the Penis and Scrotum

22

Kimberly A. Maciolek, E. Jason Abel, David F. Jarrard, and Tracy M. Downs

Introduction

Over 20 years ago, Yuan Chang, Patrick Moore, and their colleagues [1] made the discovery of DNA from a novel herpesvirus in biopsy specimens of human Kaposi's sarcoma (KS). That virus, now called KS-associated herpesvirus or human herpesvirus 8 (HHV-8), has since been cloned [2–4] and sequenced [2, 5], grown in culture [6], and extensively studied in vitro.

Epidemiologic studies [7, 8] provide strong evidence that infection by Kaposi's sarcoma herpesvirus (KSHV) is required for KS tumorigenesis and further links the viral genome to at least two rare lymphoproliferative disorders: primary effusion lymphoma (PEL) and multicentric Castleman disease (MCD) [9].

Kaposi's sarcoma is a systemic multifocal angiomatous tumor, characterized by multiple red to purple macular or papular skin lesions slowly evolving to nodules or plaques. Most commonly lesions first appear in the distal part of the extremities and spreading later in a more disseminated multifocal pattern. Other common and less common sites of cutaneous lesions are described in Table 22.1. Kaposi's sarcoma has a strong male predominance. External genitourinary lesions, especially on the penis, are fairly common. Therefore, the focus of this chapter is specifically on penile manifestations of Kaposi's sarcoma.

Clinically Kaposi's sarcoma is classified into four clinical variants: (1) classic that predominantly affects elderly males of Jewish, Eastern Europe, or Mediterranean origin and represents the form originally described by Moritz Kaposi; (2) endemic (African) that affects children and adults in the eastern half of equatorial Africa; (3) iatrogenic, most commonly encountered in organ transplant recipients undergoing

K.A. Maciolek, BS • E.J. Abel, MD, FACS • D.F. Jarrard, MD
T.M. Downs, MD, FACS (✉)
Department of Urology, University of Wisconsin School of Medicine and Public Health, 1685 Highland Avenue, Madison, WI 53705, USA
e-mail: kmaciolek@wisc.edu; downs@urology.wisc.edu

L. Pagliaro (ed.), *Rare Genitourinary Tumors*,
DOI 10.1007/978-3-319-30046-7_22

Table 22.1 Common and uncommon anatomical locations of Kaposi's sarcoma

Common locations	Uncommon locations
Skin	Adrenal gland
Oral mucosa	Bones and skeletal muscles
Lymph nodes (superficial and deep)	Brain and spinal cord
Lungs, endobronchial tract, and pleura	Breast
Gastrointestinal tract	Eye and ear
External genitalia	Gonads
Oropharynx	Heart, kidney, and larynx
Tonsils	Pancreas and peripheral nerves
Nasal cavity	Salivary glands (major)
Liver	Thoracic duct and thyroid gland
Spleen	Ureter and urinary bladder
Bone marrow	Wounds and blood clots

Table 22.2 Clinical variants of Kaposi's sarcoma

Variant	Risk group	Median survival	Notes
Classic	Elderly Eastern European or Mediterranean origin, Jewish (Ashkenazi) or Arabic ancestry: males > females	Years or decades	Nodular plaques on hands and feet proximally spreading to hands and feet
Endemic	African children and adults ("KS belt"), HIV+ and HIV−: males > females	Months or years	Localized disease Infection in childhood or adulthood is geographically dependent
Immunosuppression associated, transplant associated	Organ transplant recipients, especially kidney allograft recipients	Months or years	More aggressive presentation
Epidemic or AIDS associated	Persons infected with HIV with CD4 T-cell counts, especially homosexual or bisexual men	Weeks or months	Historical defining presentation of AIDS HAART cause sustained KS decline

Modified from Antman et al. [10]
KS Kaposi's sarcoma, *HIV* human immunodeficiency virus, *AIDS* acquired immune deficiency syndrome, *HAART* highly active antiretroviral therapy

immunosuppressive chemotherapy and cancer patients under chemotherapy or radiation therapy; and (4) epidemic or AIDS related (Table 22.2) [10].

Initially described in 1872 by Hungarian dermatologist Moritz Kaposi (1837–1902) [11, 12] in five male patients with aggressive "idiopathic multiple pigmented sarcoma of the skin," Kaposi's sarcoma was practically unheard of before the 1980s HIV/AIDS epidemic, comprising only 0.3 % of all cancers in men and 0.1 % in women in the United States and Europe. Afterward, the incidence of Kaposi's sarcoma increased more than a thousandfold in homosexual/bisexual men and in individuals at high risk for HIV infection peaking in 1989 in the United States, annual incidence at 9.6 per 100,000. Rates have declined to pre-HIV/AIDS levels by the use of effective combination therapy for HIV disease (i.e., highly active antiretroviral therapy, HAART) [10].

In light of recent discoveries regarding the viral pathogenesis of Kaposi's sarcoma, the four clinical variants have identical histologic features and most likely represent different manifestations of the same pathologic process [13].

Early History of Kaposi's Sarcoma

Kaposi was a leading contributor to the development of the Vienna School of Dermatology. Among his several achievements in dermatology include the following: the first description of the cutaneous and systemic manifestations of lupus erythematosus (1869/1872), idiopathic multiple pigmented sarcoma of the skin (1872) that bears his name, xeroderma pigmentosum (1882), lichen ruber moniliformis (1886), and varicelliform eruption (1887) [14].

Kaposi described a new entity observed in five men aged 40–68 years with skin lesions primarily involving the feet, which he initially named "idiopathic multiple pigmented sarcoma of the skin." The lesions appeared on the ankles and forearms and in 2–3 years progressed to the face and trunk; later they ulcerate and become gangrenous and necrotic [10]. At autopsy similar lesions were found in the trachea, esophagus, stomach, liver, and bowel. On histologic examination Kaposi noted that "they presented a picture of small cell sarcoma, with cells appearing in masses and clumps" [14].

In 1882, 10 years after Kaposi's first description, the Italian dermatologist Tommaso de Amicis (1838–1924) delineated another group of 12 patients with Kaposi's sarcoma. Except for one small child, all were Neapolitan men aged 39–44 years [10]. In 1894, Kaposi suggested replacing the term pigmented with hemorrhagic in order to make a clear distinction from "melanosarcoma", then the term for malignant melanoma [15]. Over time and after the suggestion of the dermatologist Heinrich Koebner (1838–1904), the disease instead became known as Kaposi's sarcoma [10].

Almost forgotten for more than a century, Kaposi's sarcoma came to the forefront in the 1980s after Alvin Friedman-Kien's report proving its association to HIV disease [16]. In 1994, Yuan Chang, Patrick Moore, and Ethel Cesarman, from Columbia University, linked the etiology of Kaposi's sarcoma to human herpesvirus 8 (HHV-8) [1, 17].

Boshoff and Weiss in *Kaposi Sarcoma Herpesvirus: New Perspectives* [18] summarized important events in the history of Kaposi's sarcoma and its associated virus from 1872 to 2006 (Table 22.3).

Table 22.3 Timeline: important events in the history of Kaposi's sarcoma and its associated virus

Year	Discovery
1872	Skin sarcomas described
1895	Kübner coined term Kaposi's sarcoma
1940	Kaposi's sarcoma observed in Africa
1972	Giraldo showed herpesviral particles in Kaposi's sarcoma
1981	Kaposi's sarcoma and *Pneumocystis carinii* reported in Los Angeles and New York City
1988	Gallo and colleagues show role of cytokines in Kaposi's sarcoma pathogenesis
1990	Beral and Jaffe suggest infectious cause for AIDS-Kaposi's sarcoma
1994	Molecular identification of herpesviral sequences in Kaposi's sarcoma
1995	KSHV shown to be present in most tumor cells in KS lesions
1996	Serologic surveys established link between virus and disease
1998	Viral-encoded GPCR first protein directly implicated in tumorigenesis
2001	Characterization of K3 and K5 leads way to identifying cellular homologues modulating immune responses (MIRs)
2006	Identification of KSHV fusion-entry receptor

Modified from Boshoff and Weiss [18]

Epidemiology

The Clinical Variants of Kaposi's Sarcoma

The four recognized epidemiologic-clinical forms include classic, endemic (African), iatrogenic (transplant-associated), and epidemic (AIDS-associated) Kaposi's sarcoma.

Classic Kaposi's Sarcoma

Classic KS occurs predominantly in elderly individuals of Eastern European or Mediterranean countries or those of Jewish (Ashkenazi) or Arabic ancestry. The incidence rates of classic KS in European population-based registries are also markedly variable. Low rates were reported in England, Wales, and Denmark [19]; intermediate rates were reported in Sweden, France, and Spain [20], whereas higher rates were reported in Italy, Greece, Iceland, and the Faroe Islands [21–23]. The highest incidence rates in Europe were reported in two Mediterranean Italian islands: Sardinia (24.3 per million in men and 7.7 per million in women between 1977 and 1991) [24] and Sicily (30.1 per million in men and 5.5 per million women between 1976 and 1984) [21]. Classic KS is much more common in men than in women, with a ratio as high as 15 to 1 [10]. It is an uncommon disease, and the median age at histologic diagnosis in one study of 67 men and 23 women was 64 years (range, 26–90) [25]. Classic KS clinically manifests as purple nodular plaques initially on the hands and feet that eventually extend to the arms and legs. In a small number of cases, visceral involvement occurs (10 %). Homosexual/bisexual men may be at increased risk for classic Kaposi's sarcoma, even in the absence of clinically detectable immunosuppression [10].

Endemic (African) Kaposi's Sarcoma

Before the HIV epidemic, KS was an endemic tumor in Africa with greater geographic variation in incidence than any other cancer, representing up to 9 % of all cancers in men in certain parts of sub-Saharan Africa [26]. The highest prevalence of endemic KS in Africa lies in a broad strip running from the Uganda, Sudan, and Democratic Republic of Congo border southward through Rwanda and Burundi. In the Northeastern provinces of the Democratic Republic of Congo and in Rwanda and Burundi, KS accounts for up to 17 % of adult male malignancies [27, 28]. Prevalence diminishes rapidly away from this endemic region.

The endemic form or African KS typically presents as localized disease. It can be seen in both HIV-negative and HIV-positive patients and currently accounts for 10–50 % of all cancers in adults and up to 25 % of cancers in children in certain parts of Africa. This form also affects males more than females [26].

Immunosuppression-Associated or Transplantation-Associated Kaposi's Sarcoma

Iatrogenic KS or transplant-associated KS induced by immunosuppression therapy has a protracted but aggressive course. Fortunately, in transplant recipients, KS lesions may regress after removal of immunosuppression medication. This type of KS is not only aggressive, but tends to involve the lymph nodes, mucosa, and visceral organs in about half of the patients, sometimes in the absence of skin lesions [10]. The first case of Kaposi's sarcoma associated with immunosuppressive therapy occurred in 1969, in a patient with renal transplantation. On average the median time from organ transplantation to the diagnosis of Kaposi's sarcoma is 29–31 months (range, 3–124 months) [10, 29, 30].

An epidemiologic study from the Cincinnati Transplant Tumor Registry showed that the incidence of KS in transplant patients was increased 400- to 500-fold over that seen in a control population of the same ethnic origin [31]. KS was observed mainly in kidney allograft recipients, with smaller incidence in recipients of other solid organs, mainly hearts and livers, but was rare in bone marrow (BM) allograft recipients. Another study from the Collaborative Transplantation Research Group of the Ile de France reported a higher incidence of KS in liver (1.24 %) than in kidney (0.45 %) and heart (0.41 %) transplant recipients, but confirmed the rarity of KS occurrence in BM transplant patients [31]. The incidence of posttransplant KS varies in different ethnic groups, being higher in those which are at increased risk for classic KS, and originates from endemic areas for HHV-8 infection [10]. Consistent with this, despite similar immunosuppression regimens, KS was more frequent in transplant patients from Southern (2.98 %) compared with Northern Italy (1.6 %) reflecting the distribution of HHV-8 seroprevalence rates in the same Italian regions [10]. It has been proposed that posttransplant KS is primarily due to HHV-8 reactivation in endemic areas with high HHV-8 seroprevalence and to primary infection in non-endemic areas [32–34]. HHV-8 transmission is less common from the donor allograft but has been reported from the kidney allograft in two recipients, following transplantation, suggesting that the kidney might be a site for latent virus infection and a possible source of transmission [34].

The lack of a gold standard in the serologic assays for anti-KSHV/HHV-8 antibodies represents a major obstacle to implementation of screening programs of organ donors/recipients in transplantation centers. The rapid immunostaining for latency-associated nuclear antigens (LANA) in the renal biopsies at the time of transplantation could be an additional useful tool to assess KSHV/HHV-8 status of potential organ donors.

Epidemic Kaposi's Sarcoma

In 1981, a disseminated and fulminant form of Kaposi's sarcoma was described in homosexual or bisexual men and was first reported as part of an epidemic now known as AIDS [35]. The immune dysfunction and deregulation of the immune system predispose patients to the development of a wide range of opportunistic infections and unusual neoplasm such as Kaposi's sarcoma.

In HIV-infected persons, KS is an AIDS-defining illness. This form of epidemic KS usually, but not exclusively, arises in HIV-positive patients with low CD4 T-cell counts. Epidemic KS is a more aggressive disease that typically manifests with disseminated lesions and visceral involvement. This may be attributed to the fact that HIV infection augments human herpesvirus 8 (HHV-8) replication [36].

The proportion of AIDS patients with Kaposi's sarcoma has declined dramatically since the outbreak of the disease was identified in 1981 [37].

Roughly 48 % of patients diagnosed with AIDS presented with Kaposi's sarcoma at diagnosis in 1981; by August 1987, this proportion had declined to less than 20 %. The introduction of highly active antiretroviral therapy (HAART) in 1996 has led to a sustained decline in the incidence of Kaposi's sarcoma among patients with AIDS [38–40]. Recent reports indicate that the incidence of KS has decreased from 30/1,000 patient-years in the pre-HAART era to 0.003/1,000 patient-years in the HAART era [39]. While incidence rates have dramatically declined, KS remains the most common AIDS-associated cancer in the United States [10]. The clinician should be reminded that a less aggressive presentation in patients already receiving highly active antiretroviral therapy (HAART) can occur. This exacerbation, known as a KS flare, can occur after therapy (i.e., corticosteroids, rituximab) or subsequent to immune reconstitution inflammatory syndrome that may occur when initiating HAART in HIV-infected persons [41]. In the era of potent antiretroviral therapy (ARV), malignancies, such as Kaposi's sarcoma, that were found to have high incidence in HIV-infected individuals, as mentioned previously, have decreased in developed nations, but still poses a major problem in developing and resource-limited countries where HIV-1 incidence is high and ARV is still not yet widely available [42].

Kaposi's Sarcoma Belt: Seroprevalence in Sub-Saharan Africa

HHV-8 is a geographically restricted HHV [43]. On the basis of reported incidences, the world can be divided into three zones: (1) high incidence (>50 %) zones of Africa and parts of the Amazon basin; (2) intermediate incidence (5–20 %) zones in

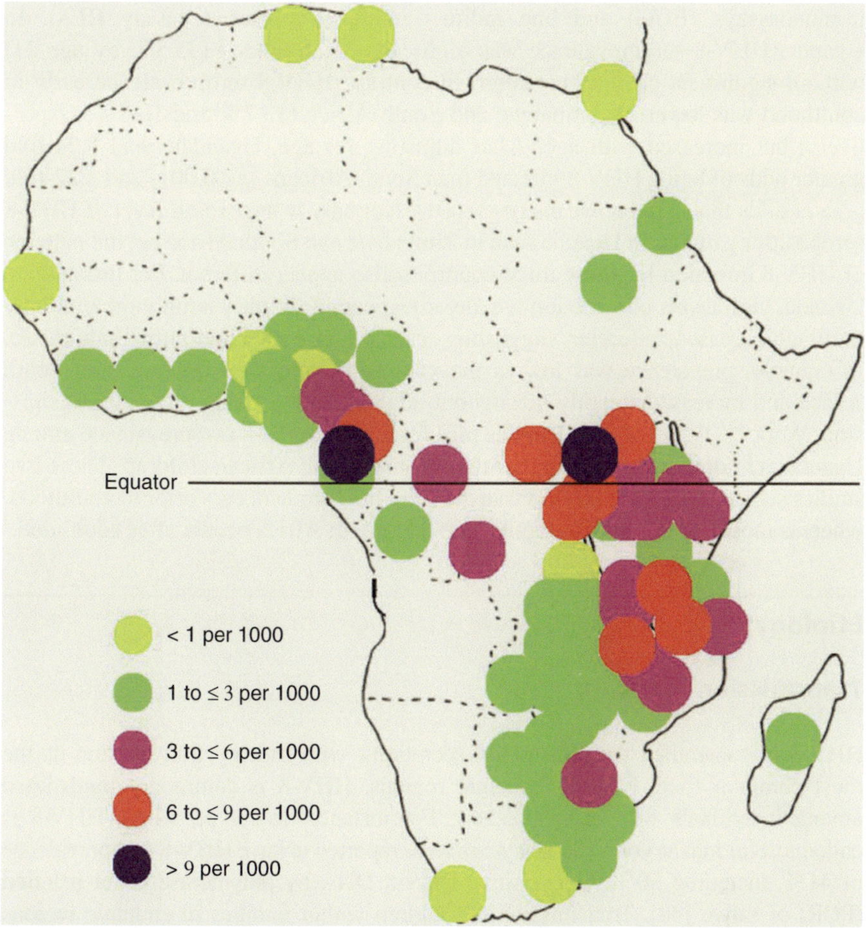

Fig. 22.1 Cumulative incidence from birth to age 64 years of endemic (non-HIV-related) Kaposi's sarcoma among men in Africa. Estimates are from Cook-Mozaffari et al. [26] (Graphic from Dollard et al. [45])

Mediterranean countries, Middle-Eastern countries, and the Caribbean; and (3) low incidence (<5 %) zones of North America, Northern Europe, and Asia [44].

Even prior to the HIV epidemic, the incidence of Kaposi's sarcoma in equatorial Africa was among the highest in the world. In portions of Uganda, Tanzania, and what is now known as the Democratic Republic of Congo, the lifetime incidence of KS approached 16 per 1,000 [26], thus earning the region the name (Fig. 22.1).

Due to challenges with accurate case reporting of KS, Dollard et al. analyzed regional differences in HHV-8 seroprevalence in three African countries with different pre-AIDS epidemic incidences of KS: Uganda with high KS incidence versus Zimbabwe and South Africa with lower KS incidence [45]. A total of 2,375 study participants were examined for antibodies to KSHV with two enzyme immunoassays (EIAs) and one indirect immunofluorescence assay (IFA). In Uganda, HHV-8 seroprevalence was high early in adulthood (35.5 % by age 21) without significant change thereafter. In contrast, HHV-8 seroprevalence early in adulthood was lower in Zimbabwe and South Africa (13.7 % and 10.8 %, respectively) but increased with age. After adjusting for age, Ugandans had 3.24-fold greater odds of being HHV-8 infected than South Africans ($p < 0.001$) and 2.22-fold greater odds than Zimbabweans ($p < 0.001$). Not only is the overall level of HHV-8 seropositivity higher in Uganda than in Zimbabwe and South Africa but the patterns of HHV-8 infection for these three countries also appear different. For instance, in Uganda, high levels of infection are already apparent by early adulthood with only minimal increases thereafter, suggesting scant primary infection during adulthood. In contrast, prevalence was low in the youngest adults in Zimbabwe and South Africa and increased steadily throughout adulthood suggesting ongoing transmission. Work by Butler and colleagues [46] found that HHV-8 seroprevalence among Ugandan children was much higher than among South African children. These two studies suggest that most HHV-8 transmission in Uganda occurs prior to adulthood, whereas most transmission in Zimbabwe and South Africa occurs after adulthood.

Etiology

Transmission of HHV-8

HHV-8 is transmitted through bodily secretions, with salivary transmission as the most common route [47]. In endemic regions, HHV-8 is commonly transmitted among individuals with close contacts. For instance, in Egypt, where HHV-8 is endemic, children as young as 1–4 years were reported to have HHV-8 seroprevalence of 41 %, including 30 % with positive HHV-8 DNA by polymerase chain reaction (PCR) of saliva [48]. Transmission to children within families in endemic regions such as the Mediterranean and subequatorial Africa is not likely to be sexually transmitted, further supporting a salivary and close contact mode of transmission [49, 50].

HHV-8 can also be acquired through sexual intercourse [33,51]. Immunocompromised patient populations have higher rates of HHV-8 seroprevalence compared with healthy individuals [52], with rates from 13.7 to 44.9 % depending on geography [43]. Some reports describe higher seroprevalence among homosexual and bisexual men [43]. Sexual transmission predominates with low prevalence of HHV-8, typically in developed countries. There was a linear relationship between HHV-8 seropositivity and the number of male sexual partners especially with receptive anal intercourse and history of sexually transmitted diseases [10, 47]. Multiple studies have reported that HHV-8 has been detected in seminal mononuclear cells and sperm in 90 % HIV+ endemic KS male's semen samples compared to 33 % of control group HIV+ [53–55]. Furthermore, multiple studies have shown 100 % HHV-8 detection in prostate gland of HIV-positive men [56]. Intermittent replication of HHV-8 occurs in the prostate allowing subsequent shedding of the virus in semen [56, 57]. There is debate regarding the rates of prevalence of HHV-8 in the prostate gland of HIV-negative men [57, 58].

Pathologic changes in the skin due to friction from intercourse could allow the endothelial cells of the skin and eventually microvasculature to become susceptible to HHV-8 and other infectious agents. All herpesviruses can establish latent infection within specific tissues, which are characteristic for each virus. The penis represents 3 % of all primary cases of AIDS-related KS. In HIV-seronegative individuals, primary penile KS is less common and reported in a few published case reports. Additionally, the penis can represent a secondary site of infection (secondary penile KS) as part of the systemic disease [59] in which up to 20 % of individuals will have genital involvement. Micali et al. reviewed the non-HIV cases with penile KS in 2003 and could collect only 12 documented cases of primary penile non-HIV KS in the English literature [60]. Micali and colleagues noted that most cases of primary penile KS reported since 1985, especially in young or middle-aged patients, are strongly associated with immunosuppression due to HIV infection. Penile KS in HIV-negative patients usually occurs in the elderly [60].

HHV-8 as a Sexually Transmitted Disease (STD): Does the Glove Fit?

Epidemiologic data showing much higher KS rates in gay men than IVDU with HIV led Beral and Jaffee to hypothesize that KS was a sexually transmitted disease caused by a pathogen distinct from HIV-1 [61]. However, what is still unclear is the mode of acquisition of HHV-8 – which mucosal sites in the genital tract harbor HHV-8 and whether any intervention in sexual practice reduces acquisition or transmission [62].

The specific sexual activity or activities that appear to result in acquisition are at present unclear [63]. Traditionally, such studies are directed by evaluation of mucosal shedding patterns of the transmissible agent. Studies of mucosal and genital secretion shedding of HHV-8 have not defined a consistent genitourinary source of HHV-8 in either men or women for transmission of HHV-8. Early reports of high prevalence in semen were influenced by contamination in the PCR reaction [58, 64]. Detection of HHV-8 in genitourinary secretions, whether they be semen, urethral swabs, or prostatic secretions, is inconsistent [65]. Among 26 studies reporting on HHV-8 DNA detection in semen, HHV-8 DNA was detected in about 9 % of samples (59 of 681). Even among persons with KS, HHV-8 DNA has been found in only 16 % of semen samples and invariably in low copy number. Prostatic biopsy samples have also shown relatively infrequent evidence of HHV-8 DNA (12 %). Urethral and anorectal secretions have given even lower rates of positivity [66]. Kival and colleagues tested rectal mucosal biopsies from 200 HHV-8- and HIV-1-seropositive men who have sex with men (MSM) who practiced anal receptive intercourse; none had HHV-8 DNA detected by solution- or tissue-based PCR (unpublished data; refer to this paper) [65]. Thus, available data indicate that shedding of HHV-8 DNA in the male genitourinary tract does occur, but it is uncommon, even among men with KS. Thus, the link between sexual activity and HHV-8 is at present one that is based upon sexual history data, has largely been defined among MSM, and is not well corroborated by virological studies.

The Role of KSHV in Kaposi's Sarcoma

Widespread occurrence of KS in AIDS patients in the 1980s leads investigators to initially suspect that HIV might be the etiologic cause. Two findings put this idea to rest: (1) HIV proviral DNA was not present in the tumor; and (2) not all HIV-positive individuals were equally at risk of KS. KS risk was much greater in homosexual men with AIDS than in any other AIDS risk group [61]. Despite the finding that individuals with parenteral and sexual transmission of HIV both became equally immunodeficient, the cases linked to sexual transmission of HIV had higher risk of KS. This finding suggested that, in addition to HIV infection, a second agent, linked to sexual activity, must be involved, eventually leading to the discovery of KSHV by Chang and Moore [1].

The discovery of the KSHV genome allowed rapid development of both PCR tests for viral DNA and serologic tests for antiviral antibodies. This important advancement made possible population-based research studies that delineated the key facts of KSHV epidemiology – all of which supported a central role for KSHV infection in KS development [36].

The major pillars of this association can be summarized as follows: (a) all KS lesions whether HIV positive or HIV negative harbor KSHV DNA [67–69]; (b) in KS tumors, KSHV infection specifically localizes to the spindle cells, the cell type whose proliferation is thought to drive KS histogenesis [68]; (c) in any given locale, KSHV seroprevalence is high (30–60 %) in AIDS risk groups in which KS is frequent and low (2–4 %) in groups in which AIDS is rare [70, 71]; (d) globally, KSHV prevalence mirrors the distribution of classical KS, high [72] (15–60 %) in regions where classical KS is common (Southern Mediterranean and Africa) and low (1–5 %) in regions where classical KS is rare (e.g., the United States) [7, 71]; and (e) KSHV infection precedes KS development [73] and prospectively predicts elevated KS risk [74]. Taken together, these facts strongly imply that KSHV is the agent predicted by KS epidemiology and is necessary for KS development – KS is never observed in the absence of KSHV. It is also important to remember that while KSHV is necessary for KS development, it requires additional events to trigger KS.

Pathogenesis

KSHV Virology

All forms of KS are associated with human herpesvirus type 8 infection (HHV-8), also known as KS-associated herpesvirus (KSHV). HHV-8 or KSHV is a DNA virus that belongs to the gammaherpesvirus subfamily. Several viral homologues exist in nonhuman primates, but HHV-8 is the only known member of the genus *Rhadinovirus* (RDV) that infects humans. *Rhadinovirus*, a term of Greek origin that means "fragile" or "slender," characterizes the appearance of the virus under electron microscopy [75].

Classification of Herpesviruses

More than 100 herpesviruses have been discovered, of which all are double-stranded DNA viruses that can establish latent infections in their respective vertebrate hosts; however, only eight regularly infect humans. The *Herpesviridae* family is subdivided into three subfamilies: the *Alpha-, Beta-, or Gammaherpesvirinae* [75].

The *Gammaherpesvirinae* have a host range that is found within organisms that are part of the family or order of the natural host. In vitro replication of the viruses occurs in lymphoblastoid cells, but some lytic infections occur in epithelial and fibroblasts for some viral species in this subfamily. Gammaherpesviruses are specific for either B or T cells with latent virus found in lymphoid tissues. Only two human gammaherpesviruses are specific for either B or T cells with latent virus found in lymphoid tissues. Only two human gammaherpesviruses are known, human herpesvirus 4, referred to as Epstein-Barr virus (EBV), and human herpesvirus 8, referred to as HHV-8 or Kaposi's sarcoma-associated herpesvirus (KSHV) [75]. HHV-8 is the only *Rhadinovirus* (RDV) discovered in humans, and several human host cells are permissive for HHV-8 infection: B cells of the body cavity-based lymphoma (BCBL) or pleural effusion lymphoma (PEL) [76] and the spindle cells characteristic of Kaposi's sarcoma (KS) [77].

HHV-8 Immune Responses and Infectivity

Following primary infection, HHV-8 establishes lifelong latency in cells of lymphoid origin. The natural reservoirs of HHV-8 are CD19+ B cells [78]. HHV-8 also infects endothelium-derived spindle cells, macrophages, and epithelial cells [75].

HHV-8 may exist in latent and lytic state. It exists "by default" in the latent state, where it is maintained as episomes attached to the chromosome [36]. Because most viral genes are not expressed during latency, there is no cytotoxicity in this subclinical state.

The primary B cells infected with KSHV do not become immortalized nor transformed, in contrast to Epstein-Barr virus (EBV) where in its latency phase infected B cells do become immortalized. One cell type that does show phenotypic changes when infected by KSHV is the primary endothelial cell. When these cells are exposed to KSHV, morphologic changes occur producing an elongated morphology strongly reminiscent of that of the spindle cell [79, 80].

The best characterized latent proteins are latency-associated nuclear antigen (LANA), viral cyclin, viral FLICE-inhibitory protein, and kaposins A, B, and C [75]. LANA expression is necessary for persistent infection, although it also has a potential role in tumorigenesis [81]. LANA's principal role in viral replication is to promote replication of the latent viral episome – a property mediated by its ability to bind specifically to sequences within the terminal repeats of the viral genome [82–87]. LANA likely makes additional and more direct biochemical contributions to tumorigenesis, since it has also been shown to bind and (partially) inhibit the cellular tumor suppressor genes p53 [88] and Rb [89].

The finding that KSHV encodes a functional cyclin D homologue (termed v-cyclin) [90] in latency provoked great interest, given the known roles of the family of proteins in the regulation of the cell cycle and the fact that v-cyclin-dependent kinase 6 (cdk6) is more refractory to the inhibitory effects of cdk inhibitors such as p27 [91–93]. The role of the adjacent v-FLIP gene, which encodes a homologue of known cellular FLIPs, is much better understood. Cellular FLIPs are known to inhibit Fas-mediated caspase activation, promoting resistance to Fas-mediated apoptosis [94]. Kaposin A is a tiny (60 amino acid) transmembrane protein whose overexpression in fibroblasts can lead to their transformation in vitro suggesting that the molecule can stimulate signaling pathways linked to growth deregulation [95]. Kaposin B is a second latent gene product that promotes the proinflammatory microenvironment so characteristic of KS lesions.

From latency, HHV-8 can be "induced" to upregulate protein expression and transition to the lytic state. The signal that promotes reactivation is not well understood.

Using peripheral blood mononuclear cells (PBMCs) from KS patients and grown in culture, Monini et al. showed that reactivation of HHV-8 required at least the inflammatory cytokine (IC) INF-γ [96]. They also proposed that a likely scenario of KS pathogenesis is the recruitment of circulating monocytes into peripheral skin tissues, where upon exposure to inflammatory cytokines, their latent HHV-8 genomes enter into the lytic phase. The monocytes then rupture and free virus is available to infect local tissues.

In the human host, the principal site of lytic virus replication is the oropharynx, most likely in B cells of tonsillar or other pharyngeal lymphoid tissue; tough growth in pharyngeal epithelium is another possibility [97]. Careful clinical studies have shown that shedding of KSHV virions, reflecting periodic bouts of lytic reactivation, is intermittent and generally asymptomatic [66, 98]. This biology underlies much of the epidemiology of KSHV, which is presumed to be driven by mucosal exposure to salivary virus, both in sexual transmission among adults [74] and in horizontal spread of virus among prepubertal children in the endemic zones of Africa and the Mediterranean basin [7].

Neutralizing Antibodies (nAb) and KSHV Disease Progression

Neutralizing antibodies (nAb) are an important component of the humoral immune response and have been implicated in controlling the progression of herpesvirus-associated disease [99]. Kumar et al. studied a cohort of patients in Zambia, located in the "KS belt," and noted that the overall prevalence of neutralizing antibodies (nAb) in KS patients was 66.7 % (24 out of 36) and 6.5 % (15 out of 231) in asymptomatic individuals (p-value <0.001) [100]. A positive correlation between the KSHV antibody titer and neutralizing antibody titer was present in the KS patients (correlation coefficient 0.33) and asymptomatic patients (correlation coefficient 0.40). KS patients had both higher KSHV antibody titers and higher neutralizing antibody titers than asymptomatic control patients.

This finding is different from Kimball et al. who found lower neutralizing antibody titers in a US cohort of KS patients [101]. These differences could be attributable to different study populations that have vastly different KSHV prevalence in the general population. It is likely that neutralizing antibody titer increases over the course of KSHV infection and this increase is driven by higher levels of antigenic stimulation. It is possible that neutralizing antibodies have very different roles during primary KSHV infection than later in the disease process seen in patients' with persistent long-term infection. For instance, in chronically infected patients, neutralizing antibodies may be elevated and have a limited role only in controlling the spread of the virus. However, during primary infection, neutralizing antibodies may be lower but still able to prevent KSHV infection if they are present at the time of exposure as would be the case if elicited by a vaccine prior to primary infection.

Pathobiology of Kaposi's Sarcoma

Kaposi's sarcoma (KS) is an unconventional neoplasm that differs from more common tumors in many respects [102]. It is unfortunate that the term sarcoma was applied to the disease by Kübner in the nineteenth century [103]. The name implies a similarity of this entity to traditional mesenchymal tumors, but in fact the differences between KS and classical cancers outnumber their similarities [102]. Unlike most cancers, which are histologically monotonous clonal outgrowths of a single cell type, KS lesions display a remarkable diversity of cell types whose proportions vary with the stage of the disease [104–107].

Patch lesions are the earliest recognizable foci of KS; these are not masses, but flat lesions in the dermis that display prominent numbers of inflammatory cells (T and B cells, monocytes) and abundant neovascularity (Fig. 22.2). These features are equally as characteristic of granulation tissue as of cancer. At this initial stage, angiogenesis is so pronounced that gross lesions appear red to the naked eye. A key difference in KS and classical cancers is that neovascularity in KS begins prior to the establishment of a mass, in contrast to classical tumors, in which angiogenesis only begins after proliferation results in outgrowing the antecedent vascular supply (leading to upregulation of proangiogenesis genes termed the "angiogenic switch") [108]. Patch lesions do in fact contain the elongated, spindle-shaped cells that will come to dominate the lesion at its later stages, but these so-called spindle cells are only one of many elements at this stage.

Over time, dermal KS progresses to the *plaque stage* – whereby the lesion is more indurated, often becoming edematous, and characteristically is intensely red or even violaceous in color (Fig. 22.3). Next, as the spindle cell proliferation continues, the lesions progress to the *nodular stage*, characterized by visible masses dominated histologically by spindle cells but also accompanied by inflammatory cells and the continued elaboration of slit-like neovascular spaces (Fig. 22.4a–c). These new vessels, one of the histologic hallmarks of KS, are prone to leakage of fluid and extravasation of red blood cells (RBCs). It is this extravasation of blood that gives the lesions their bruise-like purplish appearance.

Spindle cells are recognized as the driver of KS pathogenesis and the principle target of KSHV infection in the lesion [68, 109]. While spindle cells are often referred to as the "malignant" cells of KS, this designation is not precisely correct. In fact, spindle cells have few properties in common with malignantly transformed cells: (1) they lack clonality, even in well-developed lesions; (2) they are typically

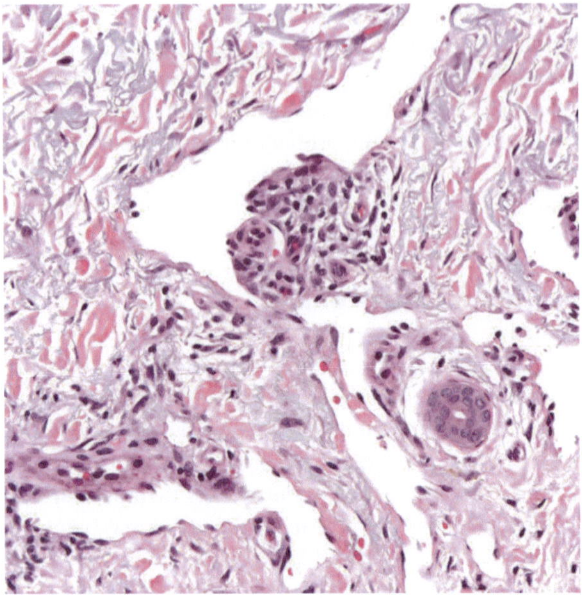

Fig. 22.2 Characteristic promontory sign (new vessels growing into vascular space) of KS lesion in patch stage (H&E stain) (Graphic from Grayson et al. [107])

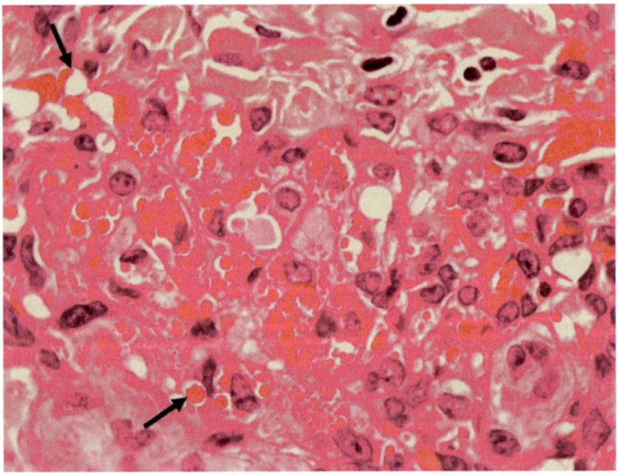

Fig. 22.3 KS lesion in plaque stage. H&E staining reveals intra- and extracellular eosinophilic hyaline globules. *Arrows* indicate autolumination of extravasated effete erythrocytes in paranuclear vacuoles (Graphic from Grayson et al. [107])

diploid, a sharp contrast to classical cancers, which are usually strikingly aneuploidy; and (3) when put into culture, most spindle cells fail to display a malignant phenotype: a reduced dependence on extracellular growth factors. Spindle cells on the contrary display the opposite phenotype, an exaggerated dependence on growth

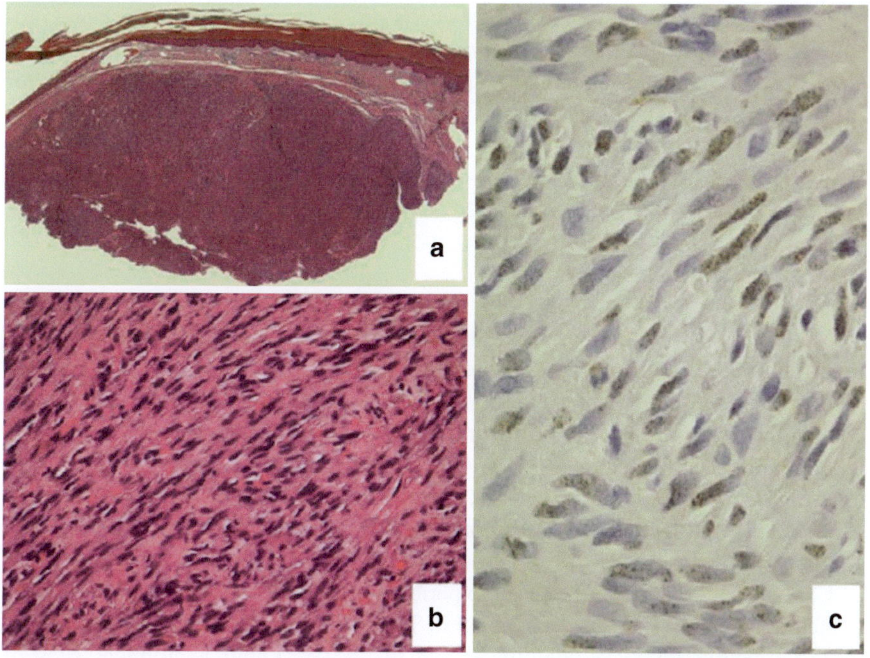

Fig. 22.4 KS lesion in nodular stage. (**a**) Expansion of the dermis by solid tumor as seen on H&E stain. (**b**) Slit-like vascular channels surrounded by monomorphic spindle cell fascicles. (**c**) Cell nuclei are immunoreactive to HHV-8 with LNA-1 immunohistochemical stain (Graphic from Grayson et al. [107])

factors, and cannot grow in culture without being incubated in a medium laden with cytokines and growth factors [110–112].

Everything we know about the clinical behavior of KS also supports the distinction from traditional malignancy. In classical KS, the lesions progress very slowly, such that many patients do not require therapy. On the other hand, when these lesions do progress, most progression is local, with widespread dissemination being very uncommon. Epidemic or AIDS-associated KS can be widespread, involving large areas of the body surface; life-threatening complications can arise from its propensity for visceral involvement, especially of the lungs (respiratory failure) or the gastrointestinal tract (GI bleed). To underscore the nonmalignant phenotype, multifocal lesions in epidemic or AIDS-associated KS do not spread from a primary lesion, but instead appear to be from separate independent occurrences (multicentricity) [113]. Molecular analysis of KSHV genomes from KS lesions has demonstrated that different lesions from the same patient often harbor genomes of differing terminal structure, suggesting they arose from independent infection events [114].

KS is a disease, in which three parallel processes, proliferation (spindle cells), inflammation, and angiogenesis, are simultaneously at work from the inception (patch lesion) and remain continuously necessary for the lesion to progress. Our current paradigm for KS highlights that no single process is autonomous; instead, all three processes are at work – spindle cells producing proinflammatory and proangiogenic factors leading to recruitment of inflammatory cells and neovascular elements that in turn provide the necessary growth factors and other substances for spindle cell survival and proliferation [111, 115, 116].

Clinical Findings in Kaposi's Sarcoma

General Manifestations

The course of Kaposi's sarcoma (KS) ranges from indolent, with only skin manifestations, to fulminant with extensive visceral involvement [117]. KS occurs most frequently in mucocutaneous sites, typically the skin of the lower extremities, face, trunk, genitalia, and oropharyngeal mucosa (see Table 22.1). Kaposi's sarcoma affects all ages, but lymph node involvement is more frequent in children and adolescents. The disease predominantly affects men [118], and the lower limbs are reported to be the predominant site affected in Africans [118–121].

Chalya et al. reported the 10-year experience of Kaposi's sarcoma in 248 patients treated at a single tertiary care hospital in Tanzania [122]. The lower limb was the most frequently involved anatomical site in 28.9 %. Other anatomical sites of involvement included the following: the trunk (21.7 %), oropharynx (14 %), ocular (12.4 %), upper limb (11.6 %), lymph node (6.7 %), viscera (3.1 %), genitalia (1 %), and face (0.5 %).

Lesions present as palpable and non-pruritic macules, papules, nodules, or plaques. Sizes range in diameter from few millimeters to few centimeters. Lesions are discrete or confluent, typically in a symmetrical linear distribution along tension skin lines. Colors range from pink to brown to violet. Lymphedema is found in dependent areas of the lower extremities or face due to lesions causing secondary obstruction of lymphatic vessels [38].

Occasionally visceral disease precedes cutaneous disease. Lesions along the gastrointestinal (GI) tract are typically associated with an advanced HIV infection. Patients with GI involvement report symptoms of pain, GI bleeding, nausea, vomiting, or intestinal obstruction. Pulmonary lesions can be incidental findings on imaging or cause exudative and/or hemorrhagic pleural effusion [38].

The duration of symptoms of Kaposi's sarcoma ranges from 1 to 14 months with a median of 6 months (IQR = 4–8 months) [122]. Symptoms of KS were present in 212/248 patients (85.5 %). The most common symptoms were swelling of the extremities (58.5 %), pain (46.2 %), and cosmetic disabilities (25.5 %). Fourteen percent (14 %) of patients had no symptoms of KS, and the diagnosis was made during routine clinical evaluation of other diseases. In an endemic (African) cohort [122] of HIV patients, KS was the AIDS-defining disease in 67.2 % of patients, while in the remaining 32.8 %, KS was diagnosed between 1 and 15 months after the initial diagnosis of AIDS.

Genitourinary Manifestations

Genitourinary manifestations of Kaposi's sarcoma are nearly identical to that of other cutaneous sites and common to all four Kaposi's sarcoma clinical variants. The most common site of genitourinary manifestations of Kaposi's sarcoma involves the skin of the penis. Involvement of other genitourinary sites is exceedingly rare.

Urinary Tract

KS of the urinary system has only been rarely reported, despite the fact that HHV-8 is shed in the urine from infected patients [123]. There have been three accounts of KS of the urinary bladder [124–126]. Interestingly, all three patients were renal transplant recipients. In one patient KS involved a transplanted kidney, ureter, and urinary bladder [125]. Infrequently, urethral meatal lesions may cause outlet obstruction and urinary retention [127, 128].

Kaposi's Sarcoma: Penis and Scrotum

It is worth mentioning that Kaposi's sarcoma is distinctively different from malignant and benign mesenchymal tumors, which represent 5 % of tumors involving the penis. These mesenchymal neoplasias are classified as superficial or deep-seated if they derive from the structures forming the spongy body and the cavernous bodies [129].

One of the earliest reports of Kaposi's involving the scrotum was published by Dorffel in 1932 [130]. Hopkins and Hudson, in 1953, published a review of the literature on KS and two cases of patients with penile and scrotal KS lesions [131]. Linker et al. presented four cases with the initial lesion on the glans penis and 13 cases with secondary involvement of the external genitalia in 1975 [132].

Table 22.4 summarizes the well-documented cases ($N=29$) of primary penile KS in HIV-negative subjects (age range, 34–80; mean age, 53 years), and Table 22.5 summarizes an additional nine cases of primary penile KS, in immunocompetent aged patients (age range, 55–77; mean age, 67 years) not tested for HIV infection. Cases of primary penile KS reported before the introduction of HIV testing are difficult to classify.

Kaposi's sarcoma lesions commonly present with a single nontender hyperpigmented nodules ranging from reddish or bluish purple to black or bruise-like in color. Typically the glans penis (most common site), coronal sulcus, or foreskin is involved. The shaft of the penis is rarely involved [144, 152, 156, 166]. Single primary lesions range from 5 to 20 mm in diameter (Figs. 22.5 and 22.6). The presence of multiple primary penile lesions has been well described in the literature [135, 139, 141, 142, 164, 167]. Lesions are typically soft and spongy initially and solidify over time. Verrucous or wartlike lesions are also possible (Fig. 22.7a) [134, 161, 169]. Kaposi's sarcoma is not typically associated with enlarged lymph nodes.

A wide variety of KS lesions have been reported in the literature. One report described a KS lesion in the same dermatome after herpes zoster flare suggesting

Table 22.4 Cases of primary genitourinary Kaposi's sarcoma in HIV-seronegative patients in English literature

Ref. #	Age (years)	Clinical features	Treatment	Course and follow-up
Marquart [133]	44	Single red-brown nodule (Ø 5 mm) on the glans	Local excision + IFN-α	New lesions on the toe, the thigh, and the knee at 2 years
Zambolin [134]	47	Single brown pedunculate lesion on prepuce	Circumcision	No recurrence at 10 months
Lands [135]	54	Multiple blue-purple to brown macules, papules (Ø 2–6 mm) on the glans	Radiation therapy	No recurrence at 3.5 years
	50	Maroon linear growth (Ø 8 mm) on the glans	Radiation therapy	No recurrence at 1.5 years
Myslovaty [136]	70	Single purplish, slightly raised nodule (Ø 5 mm) on the glans	Local excision	NS
Guy [137]	69	Single smooth reddish-violet nodule on the glans (Ø 15 mm)	Local excision	No recurrence at 6 months
Grunwald [138]	75	Single, nontender, purplish papule (Ø 5 mm) on the glans	Local excision	Onset of new lower extremity lesions at 2 years
Ruszczack [139]	78	Multiple violaceous, crusted nodules (Ø 5–10 mm) on the glans, coronal sulcus, and foreskin; massive edema of distal shaft	Radiation therapy	No recurrence at 2 years
Koyuncuoglu [140]	52	Single painless nodule on the glans	Local excision	No recurrence at 2 years
Chun [141]	54	Multiple, dark-brownish plaques on the glans and shaft	CO2 laser therapy	Onset of 3 new lesions on shaft at 1 year
Schwartz [142]	45	Lymphedema then 2.5 years later two verrucous lesions on the glans and on the ventral shaft (Ø 30 mm)	Local excision + radiation therapy	Persistence of slight edema at 1 year
	43	Two reddish and smooth papules (Ø 4 mm) on the glans and coronal sulcus	Local excision	New lesion on the dorsum of the left hand at 5 months
Chitale [143]	38	Painless 10×5 mm cystic purplish lump on the glans near external urethral meatus	Excision	NS
Pacifico [144]	39	Solitary reddish-brown papule on the glans penis, 3 papules on glans 2 months later	Excision	No recurrence at 6 months
Micali [60]	45	Single asymptomatic reddish macule on coronal sulcus, excised. Additional macule on prepuce	Local excision	No recurrence at 3 years
Morelli [145]	53	Isolated reddish, elevated lesion (Ø 7 mm) on glans	Excision	NS

Serrano [146]	75	Brown-blue purpuric nodules on the scrotum, red-purple macules (Ø 3–10 mm) on the legs and thighs	Chemotherapy	No recurrence at 1.5 years
Ekmekci [147]	52	Seven nontender, smooth-surfaced, purplish papules (Ø 2 mm) on the dorsal glans penis	Radiation	No recurrence at 6 months
Gonen [148]	55	Two reddish papules on the coronal sulcus (Ø 5 mm) and glans (Ø 2 mm)	Excision	No recurrence at 1 year
Zargari [149]	71	Purplish macular lesions over glans, mildly edematous penis	Radiotherapy	No recurrence at 6 months
Curatolo [150]	80	Isolated reddish-brown painful nodule (Ø 20 mm) on the glans penis and numerous purplish papules (Ø 5–8 mm) on the coronal sulcus	Failed surgical excision → electrochemotherapy	No recurrence at 14 months
Mukai [151]	64	Violet lesion on the urethral meatus with altered urinary stream, excision. Additional lesions	Excision → radiotherapy	No recurrence at 1 month
Kim [152]	68	Painless dark-reddish ulcerated nodule on the penile skin	NS	No recurrence at 2 years
Seleit [153]	34	Bluish firm nodule (Ø 1 cm) on the glans penis	NS	No recurrence at 6 months
Cecchi [154]	52	Nodular translucent, dome-shaped, reddish nodule (Ø 0.8 cm) on the glans penis	Excision	No recurrence at 2 years
Emadi [155]	58	Multiple red, violaceous papules coalescing to an impetiginized plaque with yellow-brown scale crust on glans penis and sulcus corona. Generalized dermatophytosis (T-cell lymphoma/Sézary syndrome)	Chemotherapy and IM IFN-α	Deceased 1 year later
Kamari [156]	47	Isolated pruritic violet papules (Ø 5 mm) around coronal sulcus, extended over 3 months with multiple lesions in coronal area	Radiation	NS
Kampantais [157]	50	Two isolated bluish nodules (Ø 5 mm) on prepuce	Excision	No recurrence at 6 months
Ozmen [158]	71	Three black nodular lesions on the scrotum (Ø 5 mm)	Surgical excision	NS

Modified from Micali et al. [60]
Ø diameter, *NS* Not stated

Table 22.5 Cases of primary genitourinary Kaposi's sarcoma in patients with nonspecified HIV serology in English literature

Ref. #	Age (years)	Clinical features	Treatment	Course and follow-up
Girgis [159]	72	Pedunculated, verrucous, and ulcerated lesion on ventral glans (Ø 1 mm) that is rapidly progressing in size over 2 months	Excision	NS
Vyas [160]	74	Posterior ulcer with circumscribed small hard area with edema of the penis and scrotum	Orchiectomy	No recurrence at 1 year
Conger [161]	55	Single painless bluish wartlike lesion on the frenulum	Local excision	No recurrence at 5 years
	67	Single purplish nodule (Ø 10 mm) on the glans near the frenulum	Local excision	Onset of new lesion on the toe at 1 year
Maiche [162]	70	Single nodule (Ø 5 mm) on the glans; local swelling	Local excision	Local recurrence after 1.5 years; no recurrence at 3 years
Jaimowich [163]	74	Single painless, firm, smooth, and purple nodule (Ø 5 mm) on the glans	Not performed	Spontaneous regression of primary lesion, onset of a new lesion on the back, both legs and conjunctiva at 1 year
Casado [164]	77	Six red smooth papulonodules (Ø 3–7 mm) on the glans and inner foreskin	Not performed	Spontaneous regression of the primary lesions at 1 year; no recurrences after 1.5 years
Berkmen [165]	55	Single purplish ulcerated nodule on the glans	Local excision	NS
	60	Single purplish ulcerated nodule on the glans	Local excision + chemotherapy	NS

Modified from Micali et al. [60]
Ø diameter, *NS* not stated

role of local immunosuppression [170]. Outflow obstruction and urinary retention can result from urethral meatal lesions (Fig. 22.7b) [171]. Lesions can progress to ulceration; this occurrence is uncommon, but has been described with severe disease and lymphatic involvement with severe deformity of the penis and surrounding pelvic structures [142, 165, 166]. Penile gangrene is rare and also associated with severe immunosuppression and advanced disease [172]. In cases of severe disease, lesions on the scrotum and surrounding groin skin have been reported [172]. Table 22.6 summarizes well-documented cases of primary penile KS in HIV-seropositive patients with unique presentations.

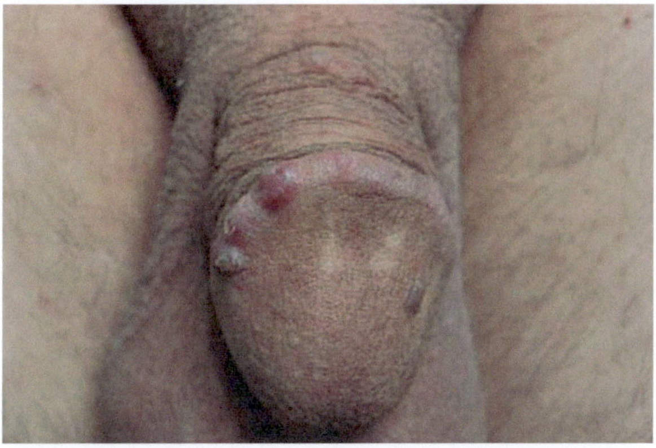

Fig. 22.5 Common penile presentation of KS. Five smooth, nontender, 2-mm diameter purplish papules on the dorsal aspect of the glans penis with no surrounding lymphadenopathy (Graphic from Ekmekci et al. [147])

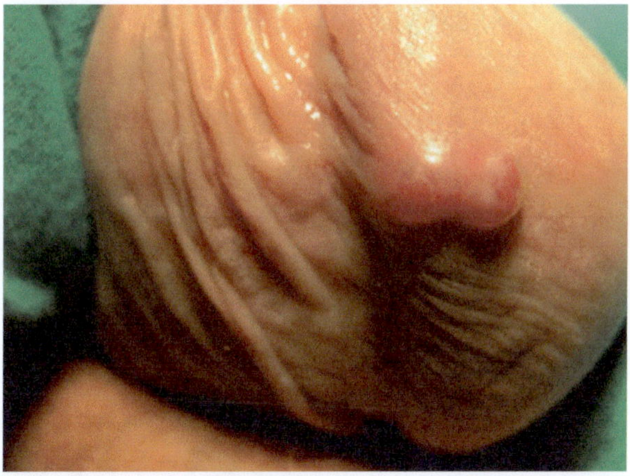

Fig. 22.6 Common penile presentation of KS. Single raised translucent reddish 8-mm nodule located on the glans penis near the coronal sulcus with no surrounding lymphadenopathy (Graphic from Cecchi et al. [154])

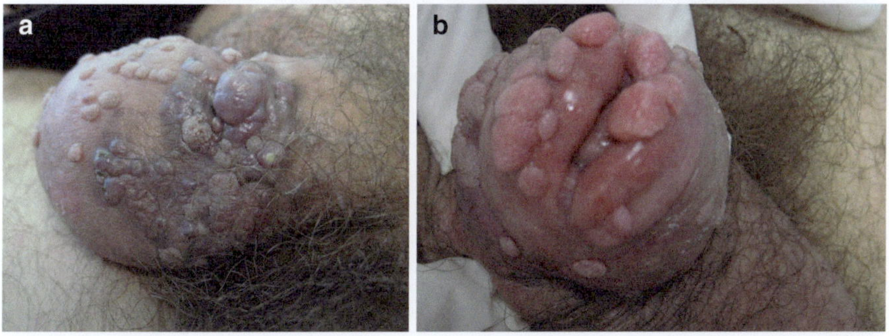

Fig. 22.7 More severe presentation of KS. (**a**) Multiple pigmented confluent violaceous nodules ranging from 5 to 10 mm in diameter circumferentially over the corona. (**b**) Multiple nonpigmented verrucous papules from 2 to 5 mm in diameter on the foreskin and glans penis (Graphics from Pinto-Almeida et al. [168])

Table 22.6 Cases of advanced primary genitourinary Kaposi's sarcoma in HIV-seropositive patients in English literature

Ref. #	Classification	Age (years)	Clinical features	Treatment	Course and follow-up
Hayes [173]	HIV+	50	Multiple firm bluish-red verrucous nodular lesions covering dorsal surface of coronal sulcus, 2 nodules on the glans with edema of the distal penis, progress to ulceration	Refused partial amputation, radiotherapy	Recurrence at 9 months, partial amputation performed and patient refused further follow-up
Swierzewski [171]	HIV+	36	Purplish lesion involving the entire glans penis and meatus causing tight meatal stricture and outflow obstruction	Simple urethral serial dilation	Deceased 6 months later
Klein [172]	HIV+	47	Massive KS lesions of the penis, scrotum, and lower extremities	Radiotherapy + chemotherapy	Acute urinary retention → deceased
	HIV+	34	Painful bleeding lesions on the penis, scrotum, and groin	Chemotherapy	Acute urinary retention → deceased
Pinto-Almeida [168]	HIV+	47	Multiple exuberant nontender violaceous confluent nodules (Ø 5–10 mm) over the entire corona circumference with multiple verrucous papules (Ø 2–5 mm) over the foreskin and glans	HAART for 20 months	No recurrence after 1 year
Lebari [174]	HIV+	40	2 skin colored lesions on prepuce	NS	NS

Modified from Micali et al. [60]
Ø diameter, *NS* not stated

Additional diagnosis to consider in the differential diagnosis based on the physical examination includes pyogenic granuloma, condyloma acuminata, glomus tumor, and molluscum contagiosum.

Squamous Cell Cancer of the Penis Versus Penile Kaposi's Sarcoma

Woldrich et al. identified 2,870 cases of penile cancer from 1988 to 2004 in the California Cancer Registry (CCR). Squamous cell carcinoma accounted for 87 % of all penile cancer ($n=2507$), and penile Kaposi's sarcoma (PKS) was the second most common cancer, accounting for 4.6 % ($n=132$) of cases of penile cancer. Patients diagnosed with PKS were significantly younger at diagnosis (mean age 43.7 years versus 62.6 years, $p<0.001$) [175].

Squamous cell carcinoma of the penis almost always presents with a skin abnormality or a palpable lesion on the penis of a male patient with an average age of 50 years or older. In a series of 243 men with newly diagnosed squamous cell cancer of the penis, the most common signs were a painless lump (25 %) or ulcer (13 %) [176]. Inguinal adenopathy is present in 30–60 % at diagnosis, and malignant infiltration of the lymph node has been demonstrated in approximately half of these cases (range 47–85 %), while adenopathy in the remainder likely represents an inflammatory reaction [176].

In penile Kaposi's sarcoma (PKS), the penile KS lesions have the classic hyperpigmented nodule appearance and typically involve the glans penis while sparing the shaft of the penis [144, 152 156, 166]. Squamous cell carcinoma of the penis can equally involve the glans penis along with the shaft of the penis. Unlike squamous cell carcinoma, PKS is not typically associated with enlarged lymph nodes.

To establish the diagnosis of squamous cell carcinoma, a biopsy is usually performed (incisional, excisional) or fine-needle aspiration. For PKS, excisional biopsy of a single lesion can aid in establishing the diagnosis; there is no role for FNA, needle biopsy, or incisional biopsy for PKS.

Treatment options for patients with squamous cell carcinoma of the penis include surgery, radiation therapy, and chemotherapy (systemic and topical). Surgical treatment options for squamous cell carcinoma of the penis range from circumcision, Mohs microscopic-guided surgery, laser surgery, partial penectomy, and total penectomy.

Likewise for PKS, several treatment options are available ranging from local excision, topical, chemotherapy, and HAART. To date there have been no reports of penectomy nor microscopically controlled surgery (Mohs surgery) being used to treat patients with PKS. Lastly, inguinal lymph node dissection (ILND) has a role in managing local and regional disease in squamous cell carcinoma of the penis, but there is no role for ILND in PKS given the fact that PKS is not typically associated with enlarged lymph nodes.

Diagnosis

High clinical suspicion of Kaposi's sarcoma is often attributed to clinical history and appearance of skin lesions. Definitive diagnosis is made by excluding bacillary angiomatosis with biopsy; this is especially important for lesions with systemic symptoms or rapid progression [38]. Complete clinical workup for suspected Kaposi's sarcoma lesions includes clinical evaluation, histology, laboratory assessment, and imaging. In cases of suspected penile KS, excisional biopsy should be the rule and needle biopsy avoided.

Histology

Kaposi's sarcoma is a low-grade vascular neoplasm derived from mesenchymal multipotent cells. Lesions are characterized by activation of endothelial cells and immune dysregulation including CD8+ Tcell activation, Th1 cytokines production, and angiogenesis [156]. Kaposi's sarcoma progresses through the following three stages: *patch stage to plaque stage to nodular stage*.

The earliest and most histologically variable phase of cutaneous KS is the *patch stage* (Fig. 22.2). Commonly the dermis appears hypercellular like mild inflammation. Close examination reveals abnormal outward proliferation of endothelial cells lining small blood vessels (promontory sign). This growth extends outward from native vessels to penetrate between adjacent collagen bundles. This process creates "stellate" and "ectatic" blood vessels that are open to surrounding tissue [107]. Tiny blood vessels lack basement membrane causing microhemorrhages and deposition of hemosiderin in tissue causing visual discoloration of the skin [38]. Erythrocytes in the vascular space are characteristic of the patch stage. Extravasation of red blood cells could contribute to hyperpigmented ecchymotic appearance of lesion upon gross inspection. Mild infiltration of inflammatory cells – lymphocytes, plasma cells, and hemosiderin-laden macrophages – is seen surrounding native vessels [107]. A broad differential diagnosis remains at this stage.

The intermediate *plaque stage* is characterized by more diffuse dermal vascular infiltrate with many erythrocytes (Fig. 22.3). Some infiltrations progress into adjacent subcutaneous adipose tissue. Inflammation around vascular channels continues. Spindles are more readily seen and are arranged in fascicles that appear sievelike on cross section. Few mitotic figures and little cellular atypia are seen. Hyaline globules likely from extravasated effete erythrocytes are present intra- and extracellularly. Autolumination occurs when an erythrocyte enclosed in clear paranuclear vacuole is seen inside the cytoplasm of a spindled epithelial cell. Differential diagnosis is more limited, including tufted angioma, targetoid hemosierotic hemangioma, microvenular hemangioma, and acroangiodermatitis ("pseudo-Kaposi's sarcoma") [107]. Less than 10 % of cells in ectatic vessels contain HHV-8 [67].

Nodular stage histology is more readily identifiable as Kaposi's sarcoma. Nodule is formed by circumscribed dermal expansion due to variable sized fascicles. Fascicles are composed of proliferated monomorphic neoplastic spindle-shaped cells. Intra- and extracellular hyaline globules, likely composed of old erythrocytes, are prominent [53, 148]. Hyaline globules are eosinophilic and periodic acid shift (PAS) positive. Tumor cells are flanked by mixed inflammatory reactions and hemosiderin-laden macrophages [148] (Fig. 22.4a–c).

Positive immunohistochemical staining of endothelial nuclei for HHV-8-latent nuclear antigen (LNA-1) confirms the diagnosis [53]. Using in situ polymerase chain reaction and immunohistochemistry, HHV-8 DNA can be detected in greater than 90 % of the spindle cells and microvascular endothelial cells in all forms of KS [53, 67]. Normal endothelial cells will not stain for HHV-8. HHV-8 colocalizes with vascular endothelial growth factor receptor 2 (VEGFR-3). VEGFR-3 serves as a marker of lymphatic and precursor endothelium [67]. Less specific CD31 or CD34 vascular markers are useful but do not delineate lesional and non-lesional endothelial cells well [53, 152].

Differential diagnosis includes bacillary angiomatosis, other vascular tumors, fibrohistiocytic tumors, resolving dermal fasciitis, spindle cell melanoma, and other spindle cell mesenchymal neoplasms [107]. Warthin-Starry staining of tissue is expected to be negative to rule out bacillary angiomatosis [178]. A small ulcerated lesion could be mistaken for a pyogenic granuloma, and therefore excisional biopsies are preferred over superficial shave biopsies [53].

Other less common forms of KS are seen. *Anaplastic KS* is the only variant associated with aggressive behavior. It is extremely rare and characterized by increased cellular pleomorphism and increased propensity for deep invasion or even metastasis. It has not been reported following iatrogenic immunosuppression KS variant. KS from lymphatic origins shows intimate association of abnormal lymphatics and can occur after chronic lymphedema. Furthermore, reason or outcomes associated with progressive histology differentiation are unknown. Certain variants might have prognostic relevance, but further studies into the role of HHV-8 and host immune response may provide some insight [107].

Laboratory Assessment

Laboratory assessment is especially important to assess immune status, classify KS, and further investigate systemic symptoms. Possible workup includes complete blood count with differential, electrolyte panel, erythrocyte sedimentation rate, liver function tests, and kidney function tests. HIV-I and HIV-II enzyme-linked immunosorbent assays should be performed twice at a 6-month interval. In the absence of positive HIV testing, lymphocyte subset analysis including CD4+/CD8+ ratio and assessment of other causes of immunocompromised diseases should be considered. Assessment for other sexually transmitted diseases should also be performed including chlamydia and gonorrhea screening as well as Venereal Disease Research Laboratory test for syphilis. HHV-8 IgG antibody titers should be performed [178].

Imaging

Imaging is not required for diagnosis of cutaneous lesions but can be useful for evaluation of systemic symptoms or exclusion of visceral disease. Patients with confirmed KS lesions must undergo bronchoscopy as well as upper and lower gastrointestinal endoscopy for prognostic value (see Stage and Prognosis section). The appearance of lesions on computed tomography (CT) is commonly nonspecific [178]. Restrepo and Ocazionez reported that a distinctive feature of KS lymphadenopathy (pelvic and retroperitoneal) is its rich vascularity, which manifests as increased density on contrast-enhanced CT (80 % sensitivity and 79 % positive predictive value) [179].

Additional studies have described using chest x-ray, abdominal ultrasounds, and esophagogastroduodenoscopy for further evaluation. One report used magnetic resonance imaging (MRI) to evaluate KS. KS has a nonspecific appearance of a well-circumscribed contrast-enhancing mass on MRI. However, MRI provides contrast and multiplane imaging to demonstrate anatomic detail of tumor limits and absence of deep invasion to determine degree of excision required [137].

FDG-PET/CT has been shown to be effective in detecting clinically occult KS lesions that are difficult to diagnose with traditional imaging techniques in more advanced stages of KS [180, 181]. Since visceral involvement predicts survival in patients with AIDS-associated KS [182], thus, accurate staging and identification of more sites with FDG-PET/CT can be useful in the management of patients with advanced disease.

Stage and Prognosis

The AIDS Clinical Trial Group (ACTG) proposed a staging method for epidemic KS (associated with seropositive HIV status) that incorporates tumor load, immune status, and systemic involvement (Table 22.7). Each criterion was shown to be independently associated with patient survival; worsening of the immune system, especially below a CD4 count of 150 cells/mm^3, was the most important individual predictor of survival. Of note, ACTG studies were performed prior to ready availability of HAART [38].

Table 22.7 ACTG classification of Kaposi's sarcoma for HIV-seropositive patients

	Low risk (0)	High risk (1)
	Any of the following findings:	Any of the following findings:
Tumor (T)	Confined to the skin and/or lymph nodes and/or minimum oral disease[a]	Edema or ulceration associated with tumor
		Extensive oral disease
		Gastrointestinal disease
		Visceral disease other than lymph node
Pulmonary involvement (p)	Absence of pulmonary lesions	Presence of pulmonary lesions
Immune system (I)	Pre-HAART era: CD4 cells $\geq 200\ \mu L^{-1}$	Pre-HAART era: CD4 cells $< 200\ \mu L^{-1}$
Systemic disease (S)	Absence of history of opportunistic infections or canker sores	History of opportunistic infections or canker sores
	Absence of symptoms B	Presence of symptoms B
	Performance status	Performances <70
	(PS) $\geq$70	Another HIV-related disease (neurological, lymphoma)

Adapted from AIDS Clinical Trials Oncology Committee (ACTG) [18, 38]
Symptoms B = unexplained fever, night sweats, >10 % weight loss, or persistent diarrhea lasting >2 weeks
PS = Karnofsky scale
[a]Non-nodular disease confined to the palate

HAART era studies suggest elimination of the immune system (I) category to only use extent of tumor (T) and systemic disease (S) to predict survival. High risk of death is considered T1S1; low risk is considered T0S0, T1S1, and T0S1. The presence (p1) or absence (p0) of pulmonary involvement was the most prognostic indicator of tumor burden. Survival analysis with scoring involving pulmonary disease and systemic disease only provided the best distribution of risk. Hazard ratios progress toward death: Tp0S0 (HR=1), Tp0S1 (HR=2.68), Tp1S0 (HR=4.98), and Tp1S1 (HR=7.65) [183]. Pulmonary presentations had worse prognosis than systemic disease [38, 183].

No universal staging or classification method has been defined for classic KS. Mortality in individuals with classic KS is rarely from KS itself. Hiatt et al. reported outcomes of patients in the United States with classic Kaposi's sarcoma from 1980 to 2000. A single lesion was reported in 77 % of classic Kaposi's sarcoma patients. Follow-up at mean of 4.8 years (range: <1–19 years) showed that 24 % of patients died of second malignancy ($n=26$), 22 % died of other medical conditions ($n=24$), 2 % died of treatment-related complications ($n=2$), and 2 % patients died of widespread disease ($n=2$). Thirty-five percent are alive with no evidence of disease ($n=38$) and 15 % with persistent disease ($n=16$) [184].

Treatment

Treatment goals include relief of symptoms, prevention of disease progression, and reduction in tumor size to alleviate subsequent edema, organ dysfunction, and psychological stress (Fig. 22.8).

Highly Active Antiretroviral Therapy (HAART)

Highly active antiretroviral therapy (HAART) is a first-line treatment for HIV and associated epidemic Kaposi's sarcoma regardless of CD4 count. HAART is a combination of nucleoside analogue reverse transcriptase inhibitors and protease inhibitors or non-nucleoside reverse transcriptase inhibitors. HAART has significantly increased survival associated with HIV. There are no randomized controlled trials comparing treatment of KS with and without HAART.

Increasing use of HAART correlates with dramatically decreased incidence and progression of KS in the HIV-seropositive population [185]. One cohort study found that the relative risk of development of Kaposi's sarcoma during the HAART era (1997 and 1998) to pre-HAART era (1992–1994) was 0.08 (95 % CI, 0.03–0.22) [186]. A different study showed that pre-HAART era (1990–1996, $n=366$) and HAART era (1997–2002, $n=40$) patients had similar mean counts of CD4 and HIV RNA, but HAART era was associated with significantly decreased overall risk of death (HR, 0.24) [187]. Furthermore, HAART has been shown to cause partial or complete disappearance of spindle-shaped cells manifesting as a parallel disappearance of KS lesions [38, 188].

Initiation of HAART can acutely exacerbate KS lesions. Immune reconstitution inflammatory syndrome (IRIS) occurs when regeneration of the immune

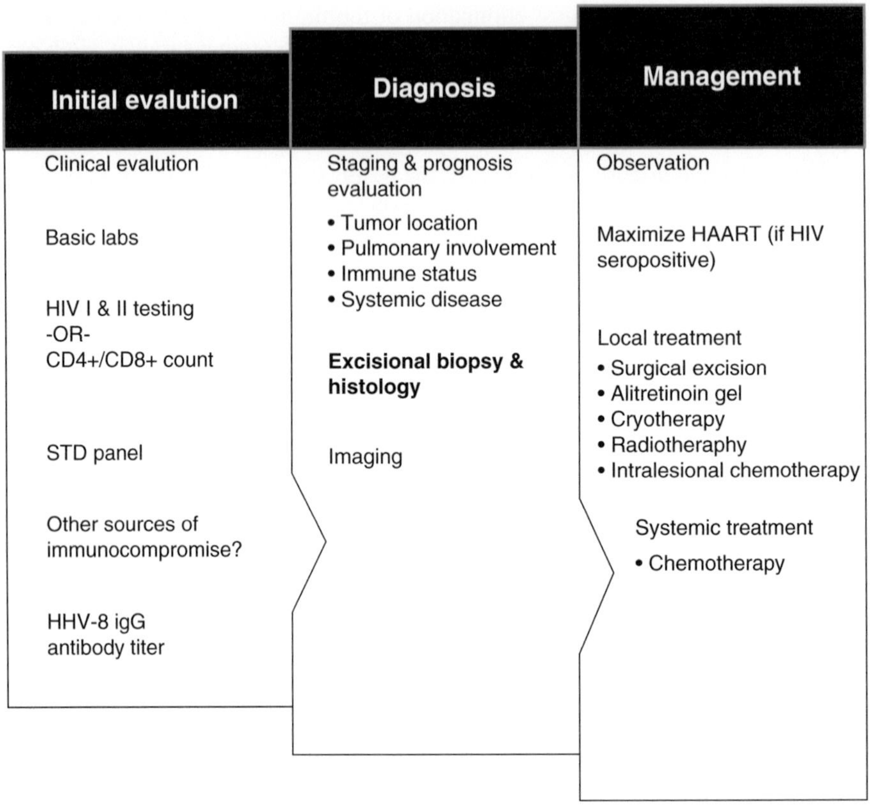

Fig. 22.8 Algorithm for management of penile KS

system causes an exuberant immune attack on opportunistic infections and cancers. This is associated with an increase in CD4 cells and a decrease in HIV viral load. One study reported KS progression with initiation of HAART was reported in 7 % of treatment-naive patients [38]. Progression occurs at an average of 5 weeks after initiation of HAART [38]. Upregulation of steroid receptor expression was hypothesized as a similar exacerbation occurs with corticosteroid treatment [38].

Effects of HAART on KS are not completely clear. HIV suppression with subsequent immune reconstitution is the obvious answer and the best predictor of response. HIV suppression results in inhibition of HHV-8 replication as well as decrease of HIV-associated Tat protein and subsequent decrease in its angiogenic and anti-apoptotic effects. HAART may also have a direct anti-angiogenic effect on KS [185]. Immune reconstitution increases the ability to attack HHV-8 [168, 185]. However, not all patients respond to HAART alone. KS has been reported in the presence of undetectable HIV levels [174]. Further studies are needed to understand the molecular pathways and also unlock new insights into novel-targeted therapies.

Antiviral Agents

HHV-8 viremia is correlated with increased risk of KS lesion presentation. However, the use of antiviral agents has not shown clear therapeutic benefit. Studies have shown conflicting HHV-8 sensitivities to acyclovir, ganciclovir, foscarnet, and cidofovir. Moreover, these medications have little effect on the latent form of the virus and therefore are unlikely that they are effective against established lesions. These drugs have significant systemic side effects persuading against long-term prophylaxis [38].

Local Treatments

Local treatments are ideal for small localized cutaneous KS lesions. Single lesions can be adequately treated with excisional biopsy. In cases of suspected penile KS, excisional biopsy should be the rule and needle biopsy avoided. One study reported 56 % (29 out of 52 patients) showed no recurrence for a median of 15 months (range: 1–162 months). Common excision methods include surgical excision, electrodesiccation and curettage, and cryotherapy. Local radiotherapy of cutaneous and oral cavity lesions has achieved excellent results with 20 Gy or higher doses [38]. One study reported radiation doses ranging from 10 to 30 Gy according to tumor response, and toxicity resulted in complete response in 69.4 % (34 out of 49) of HIV-seropositive patients [189]. Radiotherapy is less effective for treatment of visceral lesions, especially pulmonary or gastrointestinal lesions. Topical imiquimod 5 % cream (Aldara) was shown to treat a localized genital KS lesion in an HIV-seronegative man [190]. One study showed that conservative palliative treatment including serial urethral dilation with or without radiation was well tolerated and has been effective for resolution of hesitancy and improvement of urinary stream for rare presentation of KS lesion causing urethral obstruction [191].

Cytotoxic Agents

Systemic chemotherapy should be initiated in patients with severe disease, such as:

All types of KS

- Pulmonary involvement
- Symptomatic visceral lesions
- Lymphedema secondary to Kaposi's sarcoma
- Rapidly progressive skin disease

AIDS-related KS

- S1T1 status
- Progression of clinical disease after introduction of HAART (immune reconstitution inflammatory syndrome) by Kaposi's sarcoma
- New lesions with regular use of HAART, regardless of disease stage

Additionally, systemic chemotherapy should be considered if there is delay to start HAART, there is failure of response to HAART or local therapy, or there are cosmetically disfiguring lesions [38].

Immunotherapy

Before the availability of HAART and liposomal anthracyclines, the use of biological response modifier interferon-α was approved for the treatment of Kaposi's sarcoma. The objective response rate with interferon-α was 40 % in patients with epidemic Kaposi's sarcoma [192, 193]. Response rates in patients differed significantly based on extent of disease, prior or coexistent opportunistic infections, previous treatment with chemotherapy, CD4 lymphocyte counts <200 cells/mm^3, the presence of circulating acid-labile interferon-α, and increased β2-microglobulin.

Response rates to interferon-α often require continuous treatment for 6 months or more, and the average time to response may take a minimum of 4 months. Interferon-α is contraindicated in progressive or visceral disease. Toxicity of high doses of interferon-α (i.e., fever, chills, neutropenia, and depression) is common. Patients with low CD4 cell counts are poor responders to immunotherapy. Currently, interferon-α is seldom used because it is less effective in patients with AIDS and has a high toxicity profile (Ref. [28]). Interleukin-12 has also shown promise with a response rate of 71 % (95 % CI, 48–89 %) in the treatment of Kaposi's sarcoma in a phase I study involving 24 patients [194].

Conclusion

Penile KS is a virus-induced neoplasm affecting primarily men who are HIV positive, have other forms of immunosuppression, or are of Mediterranean or African origin. The proportion of PKS tumors has declined in recent years, reflecting improvements in HIV treatment. Excisional biopsy and histology including intralesional HHV-8 testing are done to establish the diagnosis.

References

1. Chang Y, et al. Identification of herpesvirus-like DNA sequences in AIDS-associated Kaposi's sarcoma. Science. 1994;266:1865–9.
2. Russo J, et al. Nucleotide sequence of the Kaposi sarcoma-associated herpesvirus (HHV8). Proc Natl Acad Sci. 1996;93:14862–7.
3. Zhong W, et al. Restricted expression of Kaposi sarcoma-associated herpesvirus (human herpesvirus 8) genes in Kaposi sarcoma. Proc Natl Acad Sci. 1996;93:6641–6.
4. Nicholas J, et al. Kaposi's sarcoma associated human herpesvirus-8 encodes homologues of macrophage inflammatory protein-1 and interleukin-6. Nat Med. 1997;3(3):287–92.
5. Neipel F, Albrecht J-C, Fleckenstein B. Cell-homologous genes in the Kaposi's sarcoma-associated rhadinovirus human herpesvirus 8: determinants of its pathogenicity? J Virol. 1997;71(6):4187–92.
6. Renne R, et al. Lytic growth of Kaposi's sarcoma-associated herpesvirus (human herpesvirus 8) in culture. Nat Med. 1996;2(3):342–6.
7. Schultz T. Epidemiology of Kaposi's sarcoma-associated herpesvirus/human herpesvirus 8. Adv Cancer Res. 1999;76:121–60.
8. Cohen A, et al. Kaposi's sarcoma-associated herpesvirus: clinical, diagnostic, and epidemiological aspects. Crit Rev Clin Lab Sci. 2005;42(2):101–53.
9. Mainati M, et al. Human herpesvirus 8 (HHV-8/KSHV) and hematologic malignancies. Rev Clin Exp Hematol. 2003;7(4):375–405.
10. Antman K, Chang Y. Kaposi's sarcoma. N Engl J Med. 2000;342:1027–38.

11. Ellis H. Moritz (Maurice) Kaposi: Kaposi's sarcoma. J Perioper Pract. 2013;23(9):208.
12. Oriel J. Mortiz Kaposi (1837–1902). Int J STD AIDS. 1997;8(11):715–7.
13. Chang Y, Moore P. Twenty years of KSHV. Viruses. 2014;6(11):4258–64.
14. Holubar K, Fatovic-Ferencic S. 1902–2002: a hundred years later. Moritz Kaposi 1837–1902: a historical reappraisal. Wien Klin Wochenschr. 2001;113:885–93.
15. Sanders C. Kaposi's sarcoma in retrospect. Genitourin Med. 1997;73(6):571–4.
16. Friedman-Kien A, et al. Disseminated Kaposi's sarcoma syndrome in young homosexual men. J Am Acad Dermatol. 1981;5:468–71.
17. Moore P, Chang Y. Detection of herpesvirus-like DNA sequences in Kaposi's sarcoma in patients with and without HIV infection. N Engl J Med. 1995;332:1181–5.
18. Boshoff C, Weiss R. In: Boshoff C, Weiss R, editors. Kaposi sarcoma herpesvirus: new perspectives, vol. 312. Heidelberg: Springer Science; 2006. 42.
19. Grulich A, Veral V, Swerdlow A. Kaposi's sarcoma in England and Wales before the AIDS epidemic. Br J Cancer. 1992;66(6):1135–7.
20. Dictor M, Attewell R. Epidemiology of Kaposi's sarcoma in Sweden prior to the acquired immunodeficiency syndrome. Int J Cancer. 1988;42:346–51.
21. Geddes M, et al. Kaposi's sarcoma in Italy before and after the AIDS epidemic. Br J Cancer. 1994;69(2):333–6.
22. Touloumi G, et al. The epidemiologic profile of Kaposi's sarcoma in Greece prior to and during the AIDS era. Int J Cancer. 1997;70:538–41.
23. Hjalgrim H, et al. High incidence of classical Kaposi's sarcoma in Iceland and the Faroe Islands. Br J Cancer. 1998;77(7):1190–3.
24. Cottoni F, De Marco M, Montesu A. Classical Kaposi's sarcoma in north-east Sardinia: an overview from 1977 to 1991. Br J Cancer. 1996;73(9):1132–3.
25. DiGiovanna J, Bijan S. Retrospective study of 90 cases with particular emphasis on the familial occurrence, ethnic background and prevalence of other diseases. Am J Med. 1981;71:779–83.
26. Cook-Mozaffari P, et al. The geographical distribution of Kaposi's sarcoma and of lymphomas in Africa before the AIDS epidemic. Br J Cancer. 1998;78:1521–8.
27. Taylor J, et al. Kaposi's sarcoma in Uganda: geographic and ethnic distribution. Br J Cancer. 1972;26(6):483–97.
28. Ziegler J. Endemic Kaposi's sarcoma in Africa and local volcanic soils. Lancet. 1993;342(8883):1348–51.
29. Montagnino G, et al. Clinical features and course of Kaposi's sarcoma in kidney transplant patients: report of 13 cases. Am J Nephrol. 1994;14:121–6.
30. Parola L, et al. Kaposi's sarcoma in renal-transplant recipients: experience at the Catholic University in Rome, 1988–1996. Dermatology. 1997;194:229–33.
31. Penn I. Kaposi's sarcoma in transplant recipients. Transplantation. 1997;64(5):669–73.
32. Luppi M, et al. HHV-8 infection in the transplantation setting: a concern only for solid organ transplant patients? Leuk Lymphoma. 2002;43(3):517–22.
33. Luppi M, et al. Bone marrow failure associated with human herpesvirus 8 infection after transplantation. N Engl J Med. 2000;343(19):1378–85.
34. Sarid R, et al. Detection of human herpesvirus-8 DNA in kidney allografts prior to the development of Kaposi's sarcoma. Clin Infect Dis. 2001;32(10):1502–5.
35. Centers for Disease Control (CDC) (1981) Kaposi's sarcoma and pneumocystis pneumonia among homosexual men – New York City and California. MMWR Morb Mortal Wkly Rep 30(25):305–8
36. Ganem D. KSHV and the pathogenesis of Kaposi sarcoma: listening to human biology and medicine. J Clin Invest. 2010;120(4):939–49.
37. Selik R, Starcher E, Curran J. Opportunistic diseases reported in AIDS patients: frequencies, associations, and trends. AIDS. 1987;1(3):175–82.
38. Arruda E, et al. Consensus of the Brazilian society of infectious diseases and Brazilian society of clinical oncology on the management and treatment of Kaposi's sarcoma. Braz J Infect Dis. 2014;18(3):315–26.

39. Portsmouth S, et al. A comparison of regimens based on non-nucleoside reverse transcriptase inhibitors or protease inhibitors in preventing Kaposi's sarcoma. AIDS. 2003;17(11): F17–22.
40. Lodi S, et al. Kaposi sarcoma incidence and survival among HIV-infected homosexual men after HIV seroconversion. J NCI. 2010;102:784–92.
41. Sharma S, Soneja M. HIV and immune reconstitution inflammatory syndrome (IRIS). Indian J Med Res. 2011;134(6):866–77.
42. Wood C, Harrington Jr W. AIDS and associated malignancies. Cell Res. 2005;15(11–12):947–52.
43. Cannon G. Out of the box. Public Health Nutr. 2003;6(5):427–9.
44. Moore PS, Chang Y. Molecular virology of Kaposi's sarcoma-associated herpesvirus. Philos Trans R Soc Lond B Biol Sci. 2001;356(1408):499–516.
45. Dollard S, et al. Substantial regional differences in human herpesvirus 8 seroprevalence in sub-Saharan Africa: insights on the origin of the "Kaposi's sarcoma Belt". Int J Cancer. 2010;127:2395–401.
46. Butler L, et al. Kaposi sarcoma associated herpesvirus (KSHV) seroprevalence in population based samples of African children: evidence for at least 2 patterns of KSHV transmission. J Infect Dis. 2009;200:430–8.
47. Pica F, Volpi A. Transmission of human herpesvirus 8: an update. Curr Opin Infect Dis. 2007;20(2):152–6.
48. Al-Otaibi LM, et al. Extensive oral shedding of human herpesvirus 8 in a renal allograft recipient. Oral Microbiol Immunol. 2009;24(2):109–15.
49. Bourboulia D, et al. Serologic evidence for mother-to-child transmission of Kaposi sarcoma-associated herpesvirus infection. JAMA. 1998;280(1):31–2.
50. Andreoni M, et al. High seroprevalence of antibodies to human herpesvirus-8 in Egyptian children: evidence of nonsexual transmission. J Natl Cancer Inst. 1999;91(5):465–9.
51. Regamey N, et al. Transmission of human herpesvirus 8 infection from renal-transplant donors to recipients. N Engl J Med. 1998;339(19):1358–63.
52. Ariza-Heredia EJ, Razonable RR. Human herpes virus 8 in solid organ transplantation. Transplantation. 2011;92(8):837–44.
53. Bobroski S, Bagasra A, Patel D, Saikumari P, Memoli M, Abbey MV, Wood C, Sosa C, Bagasra O. Localization of human herpesvirus type 8 (HHV-8) in the Kaposi's sarcoma tissues and the semen of specimens of HIV-1 infected and uninfected individuals by utilizing in situ polymerase chain reaction. J Reprod Immunol. 1998;41:149–60.
54. Lin JC LS, Mar EC, Pellett PE, Stamney F, Stewart J, Spira TJ. Is Kaposi's sarcoma-associated herpesvirus detectable in semen of HIV-infected homosexual men? Lancet. 1995;346:160–2.
55. Viviano E, Vitale F, Ajello F, Perna AM, Villafrate MR, Bonura F, Arico M, Mazzola G, Romano N. Human herpesvirus type 8 DNA sequences in biological samples of HIV-positive and negative individuals in Sicily. AIDS. 1997;11:607–12.
56. Diamond C, Brodie S, Krieger JN, Huang ML, Koelle DM, Diem K, Muthui D, Corey L. Human herpesvirus 8 in the prostate glands of men with Kaposi's sarcoma. J Virol. 1998;72(7):6223–7.
57. Corbellino M, Galli M, Parravicini C. Absence of HHV-8 in prostate and semen. N Engl J Med. 1996;335:1237–9.
58. Monini P, de Lellis L, Fabris M, Rigolin F, Cassai E. Kaposi's sarcoma-associated herpesvirus DNA sequences in prostate tissue and human semen. N Engl J Med. 1996;334(18):1168–72.
59. Lowe F, Lattimer D. Kaposi's sarcoma of the penis in patients with acquired immunodeficiency syndrome. J Urol. 1989;142:1475–7.
60. Micali G, et al. Primary classic Kaposi's sarcoma of the penis: report of a case and review. J Eur Acad Dermatol Venereol. 2003;17:320–3.
61. Beral V, et al. Kaposi's sarcoma among persons with AIDS: a sexually transmitted infection? Lancet. 1990;335(8682):123–8.

62. Grulich A, et al. Kaposi's sarcoma-associated herpesvirus: a sexually transmissible infection? J AIDS Hum Retrovirol. 1999;20:387–93.
63. Beral V, et al. Risk of Kaposi's sarcoma and sexual practices associated with faecal contact in homosexual or bisexual men with AIDS. Lancet. 1992;339:632–5.
64. Gupta P, et al. Detection of Kaposi's sarcoma herpesvirus DNA in semen of homosexual men with Kaposi's sarcoma. AIDS. 1996;10:1596–8.
65. Corey L, et al. HHV-8 infection: a model for reactivation and transmission. Rev Med Virol. 2002;12:47–63.
66. Pauk J, Huang M, Brodie SJ, Wald A, Koelle DM, Schacker T, Celum C, Selke S, Corey L. Mucosal shedding of human herpesvirus 8 in men. N Engl J Med. 2000;343(19):1369–77.
67. Dupin N, et al. Herpesvirus-like DNA sequences in patients with Mediterranean Kaposi's sarcoma. Lancet. 1995;345(8952):1043–4.
68. Boshoff C, et al. Kaposi's sarcoma-associated herpesvirus in HIV negative Kaposi's sarcoma. Lancet. 1995;345(8956):1043–4.
69. Collandre H, et al. Kaposi's sarcoma and new herpesvirus. Lancet. 1995;345(8956):1043.
70. Kedes D, et al. The seroepidemiology of human herpesvirus 8 (Kaposi's sarcoma-associated herpesvirus): distribution of infection in KS risk groups and evidence for sexual transmission. Nat Med. 1996;2(8):918–24.
71. Gao SJ, et al. KSHV antibodies among Americans, Italians and Ugandans with and without Kaposi's sarcoma. Nat Med. 1996;2(8):925–8.
72. Simpson G, et al. Prevalence of Kaposi's sarcoma associated herpesvirus infection measured by antibodies to recombinant capsid protein and latent immunofluorescence antigen. Lancet. 1996;348(9035):1133–8.
73. Moore P, et al. Kaposi's sarcoma-associated heepwacieua indwxrion peioe ro onawr od Kaposi's sarcoma. AIDS. 1996;10(2):175–80.
74. Martin J, et al. Sexual transmission and the natural history of human herpesvirus 8 infection. N Engl J Med. 1998;338(14):948–54.
75. Edelman D. Human herpesvirus 8 – a novel human pathogen. Virol J. 2005;2:78.
76. Cesarman E, et al. Kaposi's sarcoma-associated herpesvirus-like DNA sequences in AIDS-related body cavity-based lymphomas. N Engl J Med. 1995;332:1186–91.
77. Sturzl M, et al. Expression of HHV-8 latency-associated T0.7 RNA in spindle cells and endothelial cells of AIDS-associated, classical and African Kaposi's sarcoma. Int J Cancer. 1997;72(1):68–71.
78. Coleman C, Nealy M, Tibbetts S. Immature and transitional B cells are latency reservoirs for a gammaherpesvirus. J Virol. 2010;84(24):13045–52.
79. Ciufo D, et al. Spindle cell conversion by Kaposi's sarcoma associated herpesvirus: formation of colonies and plaques with mixed lytic and latent gene expression in infected primary dermal microvascular endothelial cell cultures. J Virol. 2001;75(12):5614–26.
80. Grossman C, et al. Activation of NF-kb by the latent v-FLIP gene of KSHV is required for the spindle shape of virus-infected endothelial cells and contributes to their pro-inflammatory phenotype. J Virol. 2006;80(14):7179–85.
81. Wen K, Damania B. Kaposi sarcoma-associated herpesvirus (KSHV): molecular biology and oncogenesis. Cancer Lett. 2010;289(2):140–50.
82. Ballestas M, Chatis P, Kaye K. Efficient persistence of extrachromosomal KSHV DNA mediated by latency-associated nuclear antigen. Science. 1999;284(5414):641–4.
83. Ballestas M, Kaye K. Kaposi's sarcoma-associated herpesvirus latency-associated nuclear antigen 1 mediates episome persistence through cis-acting terminal repeat (TR) sequence and specifically binds TR DNA. J Virol. 2001;75(7):3250–8.
84. Cotter M, Robertson E. The latency-associated nuclear antigen tethers the Kaposi's sarcoma-associated herpesvirus genome to host chromosomes in body cavity-based lymphoma cells. Virol J. 1999;264(2):254–64.
85. Cotter M, Subramanian C, Robertson E. The Kaposi's sarcoma-associated herpesvirus latency-associated nuclear antigen binds to specific sequences at the left end of the viral genome through its carboxy-terminus. Virol J. 2001;291(2):241–59.

86. Garber A, et al. DNA binding and modulation of gene expression by the latency-associated nuclear antigen of Kaposi's sarcoma-associated herpesvirus. J Virol. 2001;75(17):7882–92.
87. Garber A, Hu J. Latency-associated nuclear antigen (LANA) cooperatively binds to two sites within the terminal repeat, and both sites contribute to the ability of LANA to suppress transcription and to facilitate DNA replication. J Biol Chem Renne R. 2002;277(30):27401–11.
88. Friborg JJ, et al. p53 inhibition by the LANA protein of KSHV protects against cell death. Nature. 1999;402(6764):889–94.
89. Radkov S, Kellam P, Boshoff C. The latent nuclear antigen of Kaposi sarcoma-associated herpesvirus targets the retinoblastoma-E2F pathway and with the oncogene Hras transforms primary rat cells. Nat Med. 2000;6(10):1121–7.
90. Chang Y, et al. Cyclin encoded by KS herpesvirus. Nature. 1996;82(6590):410.
91. Swanton C, et al. Herpes viral cyclin/Cdk6 complexes evade inhibition by CDK inhibitor proteins. Nature. 1997;390:184–7.
92. Ellis M, et al. Degradation of p27(Kip) cdk inhibitor triggered by Kaposi's sarcoma virus cyclin-cdk6 complex. EMBO J. 1999;18(3):644–53.
93. Mann D, et al. Modulation of p27(Kip1) levels by the cyclin encoded by Kaposi's sarcoma-associated herpesvirus. EMBO J. 1999;18(3):654–63.
94. Thome M, et al. Viral FLICE-inhibitory proteins (FLIPs) prevent apoptosis induced by death receptors. Nature. 1997;386(6624):517–21.
95. Muralidhar S, et al. Identification of kaposin (open reading frame K12) as a human herpesvirus 8 (Kaposi's sarcoma associated herpesvirus) transforming gene. J Virol. 1998;72(6): 4980–8.
96. Monini P, et al. Reactivation and persistence of human herpesvirus-8 infection in B cells and monocytes by TH-1 cytokines. Blood. 1999;93(12):4044–58.
97. Duus K, et al. Wild-type Kaposi's sarcoma-associated herpesvirus isolated from the oropharynx of immune-competent individuals has tropism for cultured oral epithelial cells. J Virol. 2004;78(8):4074–84.
98. Casper C, et al. Frequent and asymptomatic oropharyngeal shedding of human herpesvirus 8 among immunocompetent men. J Infect Dis. 2007;195(1):30–6.
99. XU J, et al. The Epstein-Barr virus (EBV) envelope glycoprotein gp350/220 specific antibody reactivities in the sera of patients with different EBV-associated diseases. Int J Cancer (Pred Oncol). 1998;79:481–6.
100. Kumar P, et al. Higher levels of neutralizing antibodies against KSHV in KS patients compared to asymptomatic individuals from Zambia. PLoS One. 2013;8(8):e71254.
101. Kimball L, et al. Reduced levels of neutralizing antibodies to Kaposi sarcoma-associated herpesvirus in persons with a history of Kaposi sarcoma. J Infect Dis. 2004;189:2016–22.
102. Ganem D. KSHV and Kaposi's sarcoma: the end of the beginning? Cell. 1997;91:157–60.
103. Kaposi M. Idiopathisches multiples pigmentsarkom her haut. Arch Dermatol Shypillol. 1872;4:265–73.
104. Regezi J, et al. Oral Kaposi's sarcoma: a 10-year retrospective histopathologic study. J Oral Pathol Med. 1993;22(7):292–7.
105. Regezi J, et al. Human immunodeficiency virus-associated oral Kaposi's sarcoma. A heterogeneous cell population dominated by spindle-shaped endothelial cells. Am J Pathol. 1993;143(1):240–9.
106. Herndier B, Ganem D. The biology of Kaposi's sarcoma. Cancer Treat Res. 2001;104:89–126.
107. Grayson W, Pantanowitz L. Histological variants of cutaneous Kaposi sarcoma. Diagn Pathol. 2008;3:31.
108. Hanahan D, Folkman J. Patterns and emerging mechanisms of the angiogenic switch during tumorigenesis. Cell. 1996;86(3):353–64.
109. Staskus K, et al. Kaposi's sarcoma-associated herpesvirus gene expression in endothelial (spindle) tumor cells. J Virol. 1997;71(1):715–9.
110. Ensoli B, Sturzl M. Kaposi's sarcoma: a result of the interplay among inflammatory cytokines, angiogenic factors and viral agents. Cytokine Growth Factor Rev. 1998;9(1):63–83.

111. Ensoli B, et al. Biology of Kaposi's sarcoma. Eur J Cancer. 2001;37(10):1251–69.
112. Ensoli B, et al. AIDS-Kaposi's sarcoma-derived cells express cytokines with autocrine and paracrine growth effects. Science. 1989;243(4888):223–6.
113. Brooks J. Kaposi's sarcoma: a reversible hyperplasia. Lancet. 1986;2(8519):1309–11.
114. Duprez R, et al. Evidence for a multiclonal origin of multicentric advanced lesions of Kaposi sarcoma. J Natl Cancer Inst. 2007;99(14):1086–94.
115. Kirshner J, et al. The expression of the ORF 74 (G protein coupled receptor) gene of Kaposi's sarcoma-associated herpesvirus: implications for KS pathogenesis. J Virol. 1999;73(7):6006–14.
116. Cesarman E, Mesri E, Gershengorn M. Viral G protein-coupled receptor and Kaposi's sarcoma: a model of paracrine neoplasia? J Exp Med. 2000;191(3):417–22.
117. Krown S. Therapy of AIDS-associated Kaposi's sarcoma: targeting pathogenetic mechanisms. Hematol Oncol Clin N Am. 2003;17:763–83.
118. Mandong B, et al. Histopathological study of Kaposi's sarcoma in JOS: a 16-year review. Ann Afr Med. 2004;3(4):174–6.
119. Wabinga H, et al. Trends in cancer incidence in Kyadondo County, Uganda, 1960–1997. Br J Cancer. 2000;82(9):1585–92.
120. Bassett M, et al. Cancer in the African population of Harare, Zimbabwe, 1990–1992. Int J Cancer. 1995;63(1):29–36.
121. Ahmed A, Muktar H, Bugaje M. Epidemiological and clinical features of AIDS-Associated Kaposi's Sarcoma in Northern Nigeria. Arch Int Surg. 2013;3(1):29–34.
122. Chalya P, et al. Kaposi's sarcoma: a 10-year experience with 248 patients at a single tertiary care hospital in Tanzania. BMC Res Notes. 2015;8:1–10.
123. Santos-Fortuna E, Caterino-de-Araujo A. Confirming shedding of human herpesvirus 8 in urine from infected patients in Brazil. J Clin Microbiol. 2005;43(2):1008.
124. Biermann C, Gasser T, Rutishauser G. Kaposi's sarcoma of the urinary bladder after kidney transplantation. Helv Chir Acta. 1992;59(3):503–5.
125. Rha S, et al. Kaposi sarcoma involving a transplanted kidney, ureter and urinary bladder: ultrasound and CT findings. Br J Radiol. 2000;73:1221–3.
126. Yangm C, et al. Acute graft dysfunction due to Kaposi sarcoma involving the bladder in a renal transplant recipient. Nephrol Dial Transplant. 2001;16:625–7.
127. Lebovitch S, Mydlo J. HIV-AIDS: urologic considerations. Urol Clin North Am. 2008;35:59–68.
128. John H, Pestalozzi D, Hauri D. Kaposi sarcoma of the glans penis with meatal obstruction. Case Report and literature review (article in German). Swiss Surg. 1996;3:134–6.
129. Antunes A, et al. Deep-seated sarcoma of the penis. Int Braz J Urol. 2005;31(3):245–50.
130. Dorffel J. Arch Dermatol Syph. 1932;26:608.
131. Hopkins J, Hudson P. Kaposi's sarcoma: penile and scrotal lesions. Br J Urol. 1953;25(3):233–6.
132. Linker D, Lieberman P, Grabstald H. Kaposi's sarcoma of the genitourinary tract. Urology. 1975;5:684–7.
133. Marquart KH, Oehlschlaegel G, Engst R. Disseminated Kaposi's sarcoma that is not associated with acquired immunodeficiency syndrome in a bisexual man. Arch Pathol Lab Med. 1986;110:346–7.
134. Zambolin T, Simeone C, Baronchelli C, Cunico SC. Kaposi's sarcoma of the penis. Br J Urol. 1989;63:645–6.
135. Lands RH, Ange D, Hartman DL. Radiation therapy for classic Kaposi's sarcoma presenting only on the glans penis. J Urol. 1992;147:468–70.
136. Myslovaty B, Kyzer S, Koren R, Chaimoff C. Kaposi sarcoma limited to the glans penis. Plast Reconstr Surg. 1993;92:764.
137. Guy M, Singer D, Barzilai N, Eisenkraft S. Primary classic Kaposi's sarcoma of glans penis-appearance on magnetic resonance imaging. Br J Urol. 1994;74:521–2.
138. Grunwald MH, Amichai B, Halevy S. Purplish penile papule as a presenting sign of Kaposi's sarcoma. Br J Urol. 1994;74:517.

139. Ruszczack Z, Stadler R, Schwartz RA. Kaposi's sarcoma limited to the penis treated with cobalt-60 radiotherapy. J Med. 1996;27:211–20.
140. Koyuncuoglu M, Yalcin N, Ozkan S, Kirkali Z. Primary Kaposi's sarcoma of the glans penis. Br J Urol. 1996;77:614–5.
141. Chun Y, Chang SN, Park WH. A case of classical Kaposi's sarcoma of the penis showing a good response to high energy pulsed carbon dioxide laser therapy. J Dermatol. 1999;26:240–3.
142. Schwartz RA, Cohen J, Watson RA, et al. Penile Kaposi's sarcoma preceded by chronic penile lymphoedema. Br J Dermatol. 2000;142:153–6.
143. Chitale SV, Peat D, Meaden JD, Johnson HB, Burgess NA. Kaposi's sarcoma of the glans penis in an HIV negative patient. Int Urol Nephrol. 2002;34:251–3.
144. Pacifico A, Piccolo D, Fargnoli MC, Peris K. Kaposi's sarcoma of the glans penis in an immunocompetent patient. Eur J Dermatol. 2003;13:582–3.
145. Morelli L, Pusiol T, Piscioli F, Höfler H, Weirich G, Werner M, Cabras AD. Herpesvirus 8-associated penile Kaposi's sarcoma in an HIV-negative patient: first report of a solitary lesion. Am J Dermatopathol. 2003;25(1):28–31.
146. Serrano C, Sánchez G, del Mar Serrano M, Linares J, Dulanto C, Naranjo R. Violaceous nodules and plaques on the scrotum and thigh. Actas Dermosifiliogr. 2005;96(2):127–9. [Spanish].
147. Ekmekci TR, Kendirci M, Kizilkay O, Koslu A. Sildenafil citrate-aided radiotherapy for the treatment of Kaposi's sarcoma of the penis. J Eur Acad Dermatol Venereol. 2005;19(5):603–4.
148. Gonen M, Cenker A, Kiyici H, Kalkan M. Penile Kaposi's sarcomas in a circumcised and HIV-seronegative patient. Int J Urol. 2006;13:318–20.
149. Zargari O. Exclusive penile Kaposi's sarcoma: report of an HIV-negative man successfully treated with radiotherapy. J Eur Acad Dermatol Venereol. 2006;20(3):318–20.
150. Curatolo P, Mancini M, Ruggiero A, Clerico R, Di Marco P, Calvieri S. Successful treatment of penile Kaposi's sarcoma with electrochemotherapy. Dermatol Surg. 2008;34:839–43.
151. Mukai MM, Chaves T, Caldas L, Fillus Neto J, Santamaria JR. Sarcoma de Kaposi primário do pênis. An Bras Dermatol. 2009;84(5):524–6.
152. Kim KH, Choi J, Ryu KH, Kang IH, Leng YH, Lee JW, Lee JW, Kim YJ, Lee JK. Primary classic Kaposi's sarcoma of the penis in an HIV-negative patient. Korean J Urol. 2010;51(11):803–6.
153. Seleit I, Attia A, Maraee A, Samaka R, Bakry O, Eid E. Isolated Kaposi sarcoma in two HIV negative patients. J Dermatol Case Rep. 2011;5(2):24–6.
154. Cecchi R, Troiano M, Ghilardi M, Bartoli L. Kaposi sarcoma of the penis in an HIV-negative patient. J Cutan Med Surg. 2011;15(2):118–20.
155. Emadi SN, Babamahmoodi F, Poursaleh Z, Sayad-Noori SS, Soroush MR, Maleki AR, Izadi M, Khodaei-Ardakan MR, Emadi SE. Sézary syndrome, Kaposi sarcoma and generalized dermatophytosis 15 years after sulfur mustard gas exposure. J Dermatol Case Rep. 2012;6(3):86–9.
156. Kamari H, Bagher-Tabrizi, Yaghoobi M. Primary Kaposi sarcoma of penis in HIV negative patient. Iran J Cancer Prev. 2012;5(4):225–7.
157. Kampantais S, Gourvas V, Ioannidis S. Penile Kaposi's sarcoma in a HIV negative HHV-8 positive man. Hippokratia. 2013;17(1):96.
158. Ozmen H, Baba D, Kacagan C, Kayikci A, Cam K. Case report: HIV negative isolated scrotal Kaposi's sarcoma. Int J Surg Case Rep. 2014;5(12):1086–7.
159. Girgis AS, Bergman H, Rosenthal H, Solomon L. Unusual penile malignancies in circumcised Jewish men. J Urol. 1973;110:696–702.
160. Vyas S, Manabe T, Herman JR, Newman HR. Kaposi's sarcoma of the scrotum. Urology. 1976;8(1):82–5.
161. Conger K, Sporer A. Kaposi sarcoma limited to glans penis. Urology. 1985;26:173–5.
162. Maiche AG, Holsti P, Grohn P, Wasenius P. Kaposi's sarcoma of penis. Br J Urol. 1986; 58:557.

163. Jaimowich L, Calb I, Kaminsky A. Kaposi's sarcoma of the conjunctiva. J Am Acad Dermatol. 1986;14:589–92.
164. Casado M, Jimenez F, Borbujo J, Almagro M. Spontaneous healing of Kaposi's angiosarcoma of the penis. J Urol. 1988;139:1313–4.
165. Berkmen F, Celebioğlu A. Adult genitourinary sarcomas: a report of seventeen cases and review of the literature. J Exp Clin Cancer Res. 1997;16:45–8.
166. Kagu MB, Nggada HA, Garandawa HI, Askira BH, Durosinmi MA. AIDS-associated Kaposi's sarcoma in Northeastern Nigeria. Singapore Med J. 2006;47(12):1069–74.
167. Zargar-Shoshtari K, et al. Establishing criteria for bilateral pelvic lymph node dissection in the management of penile cancer: lessons learned from an International Multicenter Collaboration. J Urol. 2015;194:696–701.
168. Pinto-Almeida T, Torres T, Rosmaninho A, Sanches M, Alves R, Caetano M, Selores M. Letter: penile Kaposi sarcoma: a case of complete resolution with highly active antiretroviral therapy alone. Dermatol Online J. 2011;17(6):12.
169. Asuquo ME, Ogunkeyede A, Bassey EE, Ebughe G. Kaposi sarcoma: changing trend in Calabar, southeastern Nigeria. Ann Afr Med. 2008;7(3):98–101.
170. Ruocco E, Valenzano F, Brunetti G, Schwartz RA, Ruocco V. Monolesional Kaposi sarcoma at the site of slow healing herpes zoster in an HIV+ patient: immunocompromised district in an immunocompromised patient. Am J Dermatopathol. 2013;35(8):e139–24.
171. Swierzewski III SJ, Wan J, Boffini A, Faerber GJ. The management of meatal obstruction due to Kaposi's sarcoma of the glans penis. J Urol. 1993;150(1):193–5.
172. Klein LT, Lowe F. Penile gangrene associated with extensive Kaposi's sarcoma in patients with acquired immunodeficiency syndrome. Urology. 1995;46(3):425–8.
173. Hayes CW, Clark RM, Politano VA. Kaposi's sarcoma of the penis. J Urol. 1971;105:525–7.
174. Lebari D, Gohil J, Patnaik L, Wasef W. Isolated penile Kaposi's sarcoma in an HIV-positive patient stable on treatment for three years. Int J STD AIDS. 2014;25(8):607–10.
175. Woldrich J, et al. Penile Kaposi sarcoma in the state of California. Can Urol Assoc J. 2012;19(2):6178–82.
176. Ritchie A, Foster P, Fowler S. Penile cancer in the UK: clinical presentation and outcomes in 1998/99. BJU Int. 2004;94(9):1248–52.
177. Heyns C, Mendoza-Valdes A, Pompeo A. Diagnosis and staging of penile cancer. Urology. 2010;76(2 Suppl 1):S15–23.
178. Kavak A, Akman R, Alper M, Buyukbabani N. Penile Kaposi's sarcoma in a human immunodeficiency virus-seronegative patient. Br J Dermatol. 2001;144(1):207–8.
179. Restrepo CS, Ocazionez D. Kaposi's sarcoma: imaging overview. Semin Ultrasound CT MR. 2011;32(5):456–69.
180. Caponetti G, et al. Kaposi sarcoma of the musculoskeletal system. Cancer. 2007;109: 1040–52.
181. Restrepo CS, et al. Imaging findings in musculoskeletal system: a review of 66 patients. Radiographics. 2004;24:1029–49.
182. Restrepo CS, Martínez S, Lemo JA MD, Carrillo JA, Lemos DF, Ojeda P, Koshy P. Imaging manifestations of Kaposi sarcoma. RadioGraphics. 2006;26:1169–85.
183. Nasti G, et al. Impact of highly active antiretroviral therapy on the presenting features and outcome of patients with acquired immunodeficiency syndrome-related Kaposi sarcoma. Cancer. 2003;98:2440–6.
184. Hiatt K, et al. Classic Kaposi sarcoma in the United States and over the last two decades: a clinicopathologic and molecular study of 438 non-HIV-related Kaposi sarcoma patients with comparison to HIV-related Kaposi Sarcoma. Mod Pathol. 2008;21(5):572–82.
185. Stebbing J, Portsmouth S, Gazzard B. How does HAART lead to the resolution of Kaposi's sarcoma? Antimicrob Chemother. 2003;51:1095–8.
186. Ledergerber B, Telenti A, Egger M. Risk of HIV-related Kaposi's sarcoma and non-Hodgkin's lymphoma with potent antiretroviral therapy: prospective cohort study. Swiss HIV Cohort Study. BMJ. 1999;319:23–4.

187. Gallafent JH, Buskin S, De Turk PB, Aboulafia DM. Profile of patients with Kaposi's sarcoma in the era of highly active antiretroviral therapy. J Clin Oncol. 2005;23:1253–60.
188. Cheung T. AIDS-related cancer in the era of highly active antiretroviral therapy (HAART): a model of the interplay of the immune system, virus, and cancer. "On the offensive – the Trojan Horse is being destroyed" – part A: Kaposi's sarcoma. Cancer Invest. 2004;22(5):774–86.
189. Le Bourgeois JP, Frikha H, Piedbois P, Le Pechoux C, Martin L, Haddad E. Radiotherapy in the management of epidemic Kaposi's sarcoma of the oral cavity, the eyelid, and the genitals. Radiother Oncol. 1994;30(3):263–6.
190. Fairley J, et al. Topical imiquimod 5% as a treatment for localized genital Kaposi's sarcoma in an HIV-negative man: a case report. Int J STD AIDS. 2012;23(12):907–8.
191. Milan-Rodriguez F, Montilleó-González M, Rosales-Bordes A, Segarra-Tomas J, Salvador-Bayarri J. Kaposi's sarcoma of the urethral meatus: management by urethral dilation. Br J Urol. 1995;75(4):559.
192. Real F, Oettgen H, Krown S. Kaposi's sarcoma and the acquired immunodeficiency syndrome: treatment with high and low doses of recombinant leukocyte A interferon. J Clin Oncol. 1986;4:544–51.
193. Groopman J, Gottlieb M, Goodman J. Recombinant alpha-2-interferon therapy for Kaposi's sarcoma associated with the acquired immunodeficiency syndrome. Ann Intern Med. 1984;100:671–6.
194. Little R, Pluda J, Wyvill K. Activity of subcutaneous interleukin-12 in AIDS-related Kaposi sarcoma. Blood. 2006;107:4650–7.

Rare Tumors of the Vulva

23

Mila Pontremoli Salcedo, Marcela G. del Carmen, and Kathleen M. Schmeler

Introduction

Vulvar cancer is the fourth most common gynecologic cancer in the United States and comprises 5 % of cancers of the female genital tract. There are an estimated 5,000 new vulvar cancer cases and 1,100 related deaths each year in the United States [29]. The most common type of vulvar malignancy is squamous cell carcinoma, which comprises over 90 % of cases and includes two subtypes: (1) keratinizing/differentiated/simplex type and (2) classic/warty/Bowenoid type. The keratinizing/differentiated/simplex type occurs in older women and is associated with vulvar dystrophies such as lichen sclerosis, and it is not associated with human papillomavirus (HPV) infection. In contrast, the classic/warty/Bowenoid type occurs in younger women and is associated with HPV infection. Both of these types of squamous cell carcinoma of the vulva are preceded by a preinvasive phase known as vulvar intraepithelial neoplasia (VIN). Other less common types of vulvar cancer include melanoma (5–10 %), basal cell carcinoma (2 %), sarcoma (1–2 %), Bartholin's gland carcinoma (<1 %), verrucous carcinoma (<1 %), and Paget's disease of the vulva (<1 %), all of which will be reviewed in this chapter.

M.P. Salcedo
The Department of Obstetrics and Gynecology, Federal University of Health Sciences Porto Alegre (UFCSPA)/Irmandade Santa Casa de Misericordia de Porto Alegre, Porto Alegre, Brazil

M.G. del Carmen, MD
Division of Gynecologic Oncology, Vincent Obstetrics and Gynecology, Massachusetts General Hospital, Harvard Medical School, Boston, MA, USA

K.M. Schmeler, MD (✉)
Department of Gynecologic Oncology and Reproductive Medicine, The University of Texas MD Anderson Cancer Center, 1515 Holcombe Blvd., Houston, TX 77030, USA
e-mail: kschmele@mdanderson.org

L. Pagliaro (ed.), *Rare Genitourinary Tumors*,
DOI 10.1007/978-3-319-30046-7_23

Vulvar Melanoma

Melanoma is the second most common histologic type following squamous cell carcinoma and accounts for 5–10 % of vulvar malignancies [8, 33]. It occurs primarily in postmenopausal Caucasian women. The median age at diagnosis is 68 years, which is much higher than cutaneous melanomas at other sites where the age at diagnosis is often less than 45 years [31, 32]. Patients with vulvar melanoma usually present with a pigmented lesion, but amelanotic lesions are also possible. In general, vulvar melanoma is very aggressive and prognosis is poor. Risk factors for melanoma of the vulva include chronic inflammatory disease, viral infections, chemical irritants, as well as genetic factors [36].

The most common symptoms for vulvar melanomas are a vulvar mass, pain, bleeding, and/or pruritus [35]. However, many patients are asymptomatic and the lesion is noted on routine gynecologic exam (Fig. 23.1). The most common sites are the periclitoral area and the labia majora. In addition, approximately 20 % of women have multifocal disease at diagnosis [26]. The recommended evaluation includes a complete physical exam and imaging to assess for metastatic disease. Stage at diagnosis is the most important prognostic factor with 5-year survival rates of approximately 70 % for stage I disease, 50 % for stage II, 48 % for stage III, and 24 % for stage IV [11].

The primary treatment for vulvar melanoma is surgical resection. For localized disease, a wide radical excision of the vulva with sentinel inguinal lymph node biopsy is performed. A complete inguinofemoral lymphadenectomy is required for patients with positive sentinel lymph nodes. More radical surgery with pelvic exenteration has also been described but is associated with significant morbidity. Neoadjuvant and adjuvant radiotherapy, chemotherapy, and/or biologic agents such as interferon may benefit a select group of patients, although the response rates are limited and most patients with vulvar melanoma ultimately develop distant metastatic disease regardless of the primary therapy. However, further research is ongoing to develop novel targeted therapies for vulvar melanoma, particularly in the area of immunotherapy, which has been shown to improve survival in patients with

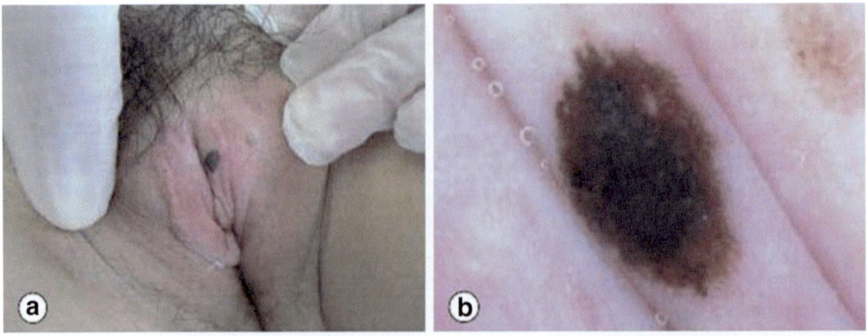

Fig. 23.1 (a) Invasive vulvar melanoma. (b) Higher-pwer view of invasive vulvar melanoma

melanoma at other sites. It is suggested that all patients undergo molecular testing of their tumors including evaluation for c-KIT and BRAF V600E mutations. Furthermore, patients with this rare disease should be strongly encouraged to participate in clinical trials [18].

Basal Cell Carcinoma

Basal cell carcinomas (BCCs) represent approximately 2 % of all vulvar cancers [13]. They are tumors derived from the nonkeratinized cells, which originate from the basal cell layer of the epidermis. BCC primarily affects postmenopausal Caucasian women. Risk factors include exposure to ultraviolet light, chronic arsenic exposure, radiation therapy, long-term immunosuppressive therapy, as well as some genetic factors and the basal cell nevus syndrome. BCCs may be locally invasive but they rarely metastasize. The recommended treatment is complete excision with negative histological margins. The prognosis for BCC is excellent, but long-term close follow-up is recommended due to the substantial risk (10–20 %) of local recurrence [1, 24].

Sarcoma

Sarcomas of the vulva are neoplasms with mesenchymal origin that arise from the soft tissues and viscera. They comprise 1–2 % of all vulvar cancers and include leiomyosarcomas, rhabdomyosarcomas, liposarcomas, angiosarcomas, neurofibrosarcomas, epithelioid sarcomas, and undifferentiated/unclassified soft tissue sarcomas [30]. Sarcomas of the vulva are characterized by rapid growth, high metastatic potential, frequent recurrences, aggressive behavior, and a high mortality rate [9]. Most patients present with a vulvar mass, bleeding, or pain. The recommended evaluation includes a comprehensive physical and pelvic examination with measurement of the size of the primary tumor, palpation of regional lymph nodes, and assessment of direct tumor extension to adjacent structures. Imaging studies should also be performed to rule out metastatic disease given the aggressive nature of these tumors.

The most common histologic type of vulvar sarcoma is leiomyosarcoma [2, 28]. It can be difficult to distinguish leiomyosarcomas from benign leiomyomas pathologically. On gross inspection, both lesion types have a whorled-sectioned surface characteristic of benign smooth muscle tumors. However, if necrotic or hemorrhagic foci are present, careful evaluation is needed as these findings are characteristic of leiomyosarcoma [21]. A less common type of vulvar sarcoma is epithelioid sarcoma. This histologic type of vulvar cancer tends to occur in young to middle-aged women, and the tumor is often multinodular. Most patients are asymptomatic and unfortunately are diagnosed at advanced stages with a poor prognosis [15, 27]. A very rare form of vulvar carcinoma is rhabdomyosarcoma (RMS). In comparison to other vulvar sarcomas, RMS has a favorable outcome.

Surgery is the primary treatment modality for all vulvar sarcomas and usually includes local excision with possible inguinal lymph node dissection. Given the rarity of vulvar sarcomas, there are limited data regarding adjuvant therapy with radiation therapy and/or chemotherapy, with the exception of RMS, which is chemosensitive [2].

Bartholin's Gland Carcinoma

Primary Bartholin's gland carcinoma (BGC) accounts for less than 1 % of all vulvar carcinomas. Criteria for the diagnosis of BGC were originally described by Honan in 1897 and subsequently revised by Chamlian and Taylor to include the following: (1) The tumor involving the area of Bartholin's gland is histologically compatible with the origin from Bartholin's gland, (2) areas of apparent transition from normal elements to neoplastic ones are found in histologic study, and (3) there is no evidence of primary tumor elsewhere [7]. Presentation of primary BGC is usually late as lesions are deep within the vulva and often misdiagnosed as a Bartholin's gland abscess or cyst. BGC is usually a slow-growing tumor with a marked propensity for perineural and local invasion. Approximately 50 % of BGCs are of squamous histology and are thought to originate in Bartholin's duct, and the remaining 50 % include adenocarcinoma and adenoid cystic carcinoma, which mimics the behavior of salivary gland carcinoma of the same histology [10, 19, 22].

The largest published series of patients with BGC is by Copeland and colleagues who retrospectively evaluated 30 years of clinical experience involving 36 patients diagnosed with BGC from 1954 to 1983 at MD Anderson Cancer Center [10]. They noted that 47 % of patients had nodal involvement at diagnosis. In addition, 25 % of patients developed recurrent disease and the 5-year overall survival rate was 84 %. In a similar study, Cardosi and colleagues reported a 15-year experience of 12 patients with primary BGC [6]. Seven of 12 patients (58.3 %) had stage III/IV disease at presentation, and the majority of patients received adjuvant radiation and/or chemotherapy. The authors reported an overall survival rate of 67 %. A more recent study by Bhalwal et al. compared 33 patients with BGC to 396 patients with non-BGC vulvar carcinoma [3]. Twenty-nine of the 33 patients (87.9 %) had squamous cell histology and 4 (12.1 %) had adenocarcinoma. When compared with non-BGC-related vulvar carcinoma, patients with primary BGC had a younger age at diagnosis (median 57 vs. 63 years, $p=0.045$), had higher rate of stage III/IV disease (60.6 % vs. 35.8 %, $p=0.008$), and were more likely to receive radiation therapy. However, there were no significant differences between the two groups with regard to histologic subtype, lymphovascular space involvement, perineural invasion, positive margins, recurrence-free survival, or overall survival.

The management of BGC is similar to the more common squamous cell carcinoma of the vulva. For localized disease, radical vulvectomy with sentinel lymph node biopsy and/or groin lymphadenectomy is performed. Postoperative radiotherapy is given to patients with positive margins, positive lymph nodes, or other high-risk features. For locally advanced disease, radiotherapy with weekly cisplatin (chemoradiation) is preferred over radical surgery. Patients with metastatic disease have a very poor prognosis and are treated with palliative chemotherapy and/or supportive care.

Verrucous Carcinoma

Verrucous carcinoma of the vulva is a rare variant of squamous cell carcinoma of the vulva that occurs primarily in elderly women. It is characterized by a well-differentiated squamous cell carcinoma morphology with minimal nuclear atypia [20]. The lesions typically have a large cauliflower-like appearance. They grow slowly and rarely metastasize to lymph nodes, but may be locally destructive [8, 16]. Local excision is usually adequate treatment but suspicious lymph nodes should be biopsied or excised. Radiation therapy has not been shown to provide any survival benefit for verrucous carcinoma [5].

Paget's Disease of the Vulva

Paget's disease of the vulva is a rare vulvar neoplasm most commonly seen in postmenopausal women. Mammary Paget's disease involving the nipple and areola was first described in 1874 by Sir James Paget [23]. The first case of extramammary Paget's disease was subsequently described in 1889 affecting the scrotum and penis [12]. This was followed by the first description of Paget's disease of the vulva in 1901 [14]. The mean age at diagnosis of Paget's disease of the vulva has been reported to range between 50 and 80 years, and it is most common in Caucasian women [4, 17, 25, 34]. It usually presents as a pink eczematous lesion with white islands of hyperkeratosis accompanied by pruritus (Fig. 23.2). Pathologically it resembles mammary Paget's of the nipple and areola.

Paget's disease of the vulva is often limited to the epidermis and mucosa without invasion. The optimal management of Paget's disease of the vulva remains unclear.

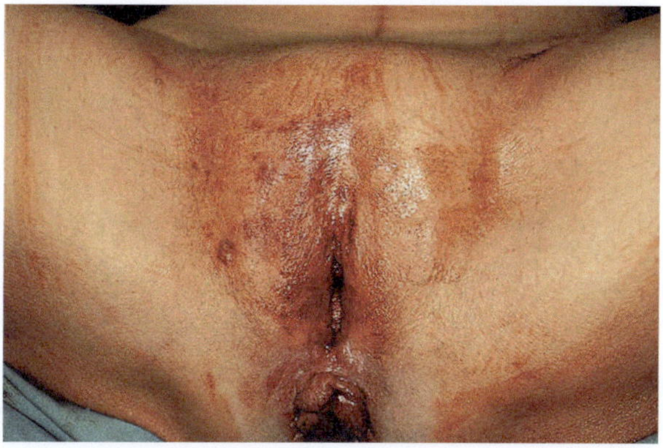

Fig. 23.2 Paget's disease of the vulva

Surgical excision is usually the primary therapy; however, 30–60 % of patients develop recurrent disease. Furthermore, the lesions often extend past clinically apparent borders resulting in positive margins, and surgical excision is limited by the anatomy of the vulva. In addition, the disease is often multifocal. Many patients require multiple excisions resulting in significant morbidity. Alternative treatment strategies with topical agents such as imiquimod are being investigated. It also appears that the risk of invasive disease is low and more conservative approaches are being considered. Interestingly, patients with Paget's disease of the vulva have a high incidence of a second synchronous or metachronous neoplasm including colorectal adenocarcinoma, cervical adenocarcinoma, carcinoma of the transitional epithelium from the renal pelvis to the urethra, and/or breast carcinoma [25]. Routine screening with colonoscopy, Pap/HPV test, and mammogram is therefore recommended.

References

1. Benedet JL, Miller DM, Ehlen TG, Bertrand MA. Basal cell carcinoma of the vulva: clinical features and treatment results in 28 patients. Obstet Gynecol. 1997;90(5):765.
2. Bhattacharyya T, Patel FD, Srinivasan R, Rai B, Saha P, Nijhawan R. Rhabdomyosarcoma of vulva in a young lady: a rare case report with review of literature. J Cancer Res Ther. 2015;11(3):650. doi:10.4103/0973-1482.138116.
3. Bhalwal AB, Nick AM, dos Reis R, Chen CL, Munsell MF, Ramalingam P, et al. Carcinoma of the Bartholin Gland: A Review of 33 Cases. Int J Gynecol Cancer 2016. [Epub ahead of print].
4. Black D, Tornos C, Soslow RA, Awtrey CS, Barakat RR, Chi DS, et al. The outcomes of patients with positive margins after excision for intraepithelial Paget's disease of the vulva. Gynecol Oncol. 2007;104(3):547–50.
5. Boujoual M, Hachi H, Rimani M, El Khannoussi B, Bougtab A. Verrucous carcinoma of the vulva: report of four cases. Pan Afr Med J. 2014;17:303.
6. Cardosi RJ, Speights A, Fiorcia JV, Grendys EC, Hakam S, Hoffman MS. Bartholin's gland carcinoma: a 15 year experience. Gynecol Oncol. 2001;82:247–51.
7. Chamlian DL, Taylor HB. Primary carcinoma of Bartholin's gland. A report of 24 patients. Obstet Gynecol. 1972;39(4):489–94.
8. Chokoeva AA, Tchernev G, Castelli E, Orlando E, Verma SB, Grebe M, et al. Vulvar cancer: a review for dermatologists. Wien Med Wochenschr. 2015;165(7–8):164–77. doi:10.1007/s10354-015-0354-9.
9. Chokoeva AA, Tchernev G, Cardoso JC, Patterson JW, Dechev I, Valkanov S, et al. Vulvar sarcomas: short guideline for histopathological recognition and clinical management. Part 1. Int J Immunopathol Pharmacol. 2015;28(2):168–77. doi:10.1177/0394632015576029.
10. Copeland LJ, Sneige N, Gershenson DM, McGuffee VB, Abdul Karim F, Rutledga FN. Bartholin gland carcinoma. Obstet Gynecol. 1986;67:794–801.
11. Creasman WT, Phillips JL, MEnck HR. A survey of hospital management practices for vulvar melanoma. J Am Coll Surg. 1999;188(6):670.
12. Crocker HR. Paget's disease, affecting the scrotum and penis. Trans Pathol Soc Lond. 1889; 40:187–91.
13. De Giorgi V, Salvini C, Massi D, Raspollini MR, Carli P. Vulvar basal cell carcinoma: retrospective study and review of the literature. Gynecol Oncol. 2005;97(1):192.
14. Dubreuilh W. Paget's disease of the vulva. Br J Dermatol. 1901;13:403–13.
15. Guillou L, Wadden C, Coindre JM, Krausz T, Fletcher CD. "Proximal-type" epithelioid sarcoma, a distinctive aggressive neoplasm showing rhabdoid features. Clinicopathologic, immunohistochemical, and ultrastructural study of a series. Am J Surg Pathol. 1997;21:130–46.

16. Iavazzo C, Fotiou S, Salakos N, Bakalianou K, Kondi-Pafiti A. HPV-related verrucous carcinoma of the vulva. A case report and literature review. Eur J Gynaecol Oncol. 2011;32(6): 680–1.
17. Kay JM, Southwood WF. Paget's disease of the vulva associated with an unusual bladder tumour. Br J Cancer. 1964;18:233–7.
18. Leitao MM Jr. Management of vulvar and vaginal melanomas: current and future strategies. Am Soc Clin Oncol Educ Book. 2014;e277–81. doi: 10.14694/EdBook_AM.2014.34.e277.
19. Leuchter RC, Hacker NF, Voet RL, Berek JS, Townsend DE, Lagasse LD. Primary carcinoma of the Bartholin gland: a report of 14 cases and review of the literature. Obstet Gynecol. 1982;60:361–8.
20. Nascimento AF, Granter SR, Cviko A, Yuan L, Hecht JL, Crum CP. Vulvar acanthosis with altered differentiation: a precursor to verrucous carcinoma? Am J Surg Pathol. 2004;28(5): 638–43.
21. Nielsen GP, Rosenberg AK, Koerner FC, et al. Smooth-muscle tumors of the vulva: a clinicopathological study of 25 cases and review of the literature. Am J Surg Pathol. 1996;20: 779–93.
22. Ouldamer L, Chraibi Z, Arbion F, Barillot I, Body G. Bartholin's gland carcinoma: epidemiology and therapeutic management. Surg Oncol. 2013;22:117–22.
23. Paget J. On disease of the mammary areola preceding cancer of the mammary gland. Bartholomew's Hosp Rep. 1874;10:87.
24. Piura B, Rabinovich A, Dgani R. Basal cell carcinoma of the vulva. J Surg Oncol. 1999;70(3): 172.
25. Preti M, Micheletti L, Ghiringhello B, Privitera S, Condello V, Chieppa P, et al. Vulvar Paget's disease. Clinico-pathologic review of the literature. Minerva Ginecol. 2000;52(5):203–11.
26. Ragnarsson-Olding BK, Kanter-Lewensohn LR, Lagerlöf B, Nilsson BR, Ringborg UK. Malignant melanoma of the vulva in a nationwide, 25-year study of 219 Swedish females: clinical observations and histopathologic features. Cancer. 1999;86(7):1273–84.
27. Rodrigues AI, Lopes HI, Lima O, Marta S. Proximal-type epithelioid sarcoma-unusual presentation: unilateral vulvar mass. BMJ Case Rep. 2015. pii: bcr2014208488. doi:10.1136/bcr-2014-208488.
28. Salehin D, Haugk C, William M, Hemmerlein B, Thill M, Diedrich K, et al. Leiomyosarcoma of the vulva. Eur J Gynaecol Oncol. 2012;33(3):306–8.
29. Siegel RL, Miller KD, Jemal A. Cancer statistics 2015. CA Cancer J Clin. 2015;65:5–29.
30. Sleijfer S, Seynaeve C, Verweij J. Gynaecological sarcomas. Curr Opin Oncol. 2007;19: 492–6.
31. Stang A, Streller B, Eisinger B, Jöckel KH. Population-based incidence rates of malignant melanoma of the vulva in Germany. Gynecol Oncol. 2005;96(1):216.
32. Suwandinata FS, Bohle RM, Omwandho CA, Tinneberg HR, Gruessner SE. Management of vulvar melanoma and review of the literature. Eur J Gynaecol Oncol. 2007;28(3):220–4.
33. Sugiyama VE, Chan JK, Shin JY, Berek JS, Osann K, Kapp DS. Vulvar melanoma: a multivariate analysis of 644 patients. Obstet Gynecol. 2007;110(2):296.
34. Tebes S, Cardosi R, Hoffman M. Paget's disease of the vulva. Am J Obstet Gynecol. 2002;187(2):281–3.
35. Verschraegen CF, Benjapibal M, Supakarapongkul W, Levy LB, Ross M, Atkinson EN, et al. Vulvar melanoma at the M. D. Anderson Cancer Center: 25 years later. Int J Gynecol Cancer. 2001;11(5):359–64.
36. Wechter ME, Gruber SB, Haefner HK, Lowe L, Schwartz JL, Reynolds KR, Johnston CM, Johnson TM. Vulvar melanoma: a report of 20 cases and review of the literature. J Am Acad Dermatol. 2004;50(4):554.

16. Iavazzo C, Fotiou S, Salakos N, Bakalianou K, Kondi-Pafiti A. HPV-related verrucous carcinoma of the vulva. A case report and literature review. Eur J Gynaecol Oncol. 2011;32(6): 680–1.
17. Kay JM, Southwood WF. Paget's disease of the vulva associated with an unusual bladder tumour. Br J Cancer. 1964;18:233–7.
18. Leitao MM Jr. Management of vulvar and vaginal melanomas: current and future strategies. Am Soc Clin Oncol Educ Book. 2014;e277–81. doi: 10.14694/EdBook_AM.2014.34.e277.
19. Leuchter RC, Hacker NF, Voet RL, Berek JS, Townsend DE, Lagasse LD. Primary carcinoma of the Bartholin gland: a report of 14 cases and review of the literature. Obstet Gynecol. 1982;60:361–8.
20. Nascimento AF, Granter SR, Cviko A, Yuan L, Hecht JL, Crum CP. Vulvar acanthosis with altered differentiation: a precursor to verrucous carcinoma? Am J Surg Pathol. 2004;28(5): 638–43.
21. Nielsen GP, Rosenberg AK, Koerner FC, et al. Smooth-muscle tumors of the vulva: a clinicopathological study of 25 cases and review of the literature. Am J Surg Pathol. 1996;20: 779–93.
22. Ouldamer L, Chraibi Z, Arbion F, Barillot I, Body G. Bartholin's gland carcinoma: epidemiology and therapeutic management. Surg Oncol. 2013;22:117–22.
23. Paget J. On disease of the mammary areola preceding cancer of the mammary gland. Bartholomew's Hosp Rep. 1874;10:87.
24. Piura B, Rabinovich A, Dgani R. Basal cell carcinoma of the vulva. J Surg Oncol. 1999;70(3): 172.
25. Preti M, Micheletti L, Ghiringhello B, Privitera S, Condello V, Chieppa P, et al. Vulvar Paget's disease. Clinico-pathologic review of the literature. Minerva Ginecol. 2000;52(5):203–11.
26. Ragnarsson-Olding BK, Kanter-Lewensohn LR, Lagerlöf B, Nilsson BR, Ringborg UK. Malignant melanoma of the vulva in a nationwide, 25-year study of 219 Swedish females: clinical observations and histopathologic features. Cancer. 1999;86(7):1273–84.
27. Rodrigues AI, Lopes HI, Lima O, Marta S. Proximal-type epithelioid sarcoma-unusual presentation: unilateral vulvar mass. BMJ Case Rep. 2015. pii: bcr2014208488. doi:10.1136/bcr-2014-208488.
28. Salehin D, Haugk C, William M, Hemmerlein B, Thill M, Diedrich K, et al. Leiomyosarcoma of the vulva. Eur J Gynaecol Oncol. 2012;33(3):306–8.
29. Siegel RL, Miller KD, Jemal A. Cancer statistics 2015. CA Cancer J Clin. 2015;65:5–29.
30. Sleijfer S, Seynaeve C, Verweij J. Gynaecological sarcomas. Curr Opin Oncol. 2007;19: 492–6.
31. Stang A, Streller B, Eisinger B, Jöckel KH. Population-based incidence rates of malignant melanoma of the vulva in Germany. Gynecol Oncol. 2005;96(1):216.
32. Suwandinata FS, Bohle RM, Omwandho CA, Tinneberg HR, Gruessner SE. Management of vulvar melanoma and review of the literature. Eur J Gynaecol Oncol. 2007;28(3):220–4.
33. Sugiyama VE, Chan JK, Shin JY, Berek JS, Osann K, Kapp DS. Vulvar melanoma: a multivariate analysis of 644 patients. Obstet Gynecol. 2007;110(2):296.
34. Tebes S, Cardosi R, Hoffman M. Paget's disease of the vulva. Am J Obstet Gynecol. 2002;187(2):281–3.
35. Verschraegen CF, Benjapibal M, Supakarapongkul W, Levy LB, Ross M, Atkinson EN, et al. Vulvar melanoma at the M. D. Anderson Cancer Center: 25 years later. Int J Gynecol Cancer. 2001;11(5):359–64.
36. Wechter ME, Gruber SB, Haefner HK, Lowe L, Schwartz JL, Reynolds KR, Johnston CM, Johnson TM. Vulvar melanoma: a report of 20 cases and review of the literature. J Am Acad Dermatol. 2004;50(4):554.

MIX
Papier aus verantwortungsvollen Quellen
Paper from responsible sources
FSC® C105338

If you have any concerns about our products, you can contact us on
ProductSafety@springernature.com

In case Publisher is established outside the EU, the EU authorized representative is:
Springer Nature Customer Service Center GmbH
Europaplatz 3, 69115 Heidelberg, Germany

Printed by Libri Plureos GmbH
in Hamburg, Germany